INSTITUTE FOR RESEARCH INTO MENTAL RETARDATION

Study Group No. 3

THE BRAIN IN UNCLASSIFIED MENTAL RETARDATION

IRMR STUDY GROUPS

1. Infantile Autism: Concepts, Characteristics and Treatment
2. Cellular Organelles and Membranes in Mental Retardation
3. The Brain in Unclassified Mental Retardation
4. Mental Retardation and Behavioural Research
5. Psychological Assessment of the Mentally Handicapped

The Brain in Unclassified Mental Retardation

STUDY GROUP NO. 3

Study Group held at the Ciba Foundation, London under the auspices of the Institute for Research into Mental Retardation

EDITED BY

PROFESSOR J. B. CAVANAGH, MD, MRCP

The Director, MRC Research Group
in Applied Neurobiology

Churchill Livingstone
Edinburgh and London 1972

First Published 1972

International Standard Book Number
0 443 00916 3

Any correspondence relating to this volume should be directed to the publishers at 104 Gloucester Place, London W1H 4AE.

Printed in Great Britain by
The Whitefriars Press Ltd., London and Tonbridge

Preface

The contents of this volume are a distillation of a discussion about one of the most neglected, and yet socially and economically one of the more important problems that face psychiatry, paediatrics, pathology and biochemistry today. As with geriatrics, mental retardation is one of those subjects that the public will not face, and in consequence the public purse will not provide for, at least not much beyond the means of daily subsistence. Yet mental retardation is in more than any other subject one which must be closely examined in a clear light if adequate means of treatment of the present problem is to be sought, and the prevention of future harm is to be attained. Prevention is the only just solution, but because this crosses into the territories of ethics, morals and social philosophy these are not fields through which the scientist and enquirer would care to travel for long. His place is to unravel the causes and point to the remedy. Unless the conditions are defined, the causes cannot be determined, and it is this definition of the clinical and pathological entities that might conceivably come to make up Unclassified Mental Retardation that is the subject of this symposium.

In truth, it cannot be said that this exercise was in one sense rewarding. It is clear from this discussion that many, if not most, of these conditions are unfortunate accidents, or often a concatenation of small accidents, that eventually have come to distort the structure and diminish the function of the most delicate of mechanisms, brain function. Some of these small accidents, indeed probably many of them, are no doubt preventable; some certainly arise from ignorance, others neglect, perhaps others too from well-meaning, but misguided, actions. But it is also clear from this discussion that there is much in the substratum of mental retardation that is not understood at all, and it is this perhaps more than anything that this symposium has emphasised: this, and also the urgent necessity for bringing the problem into the open for further discussion and action.

J. B. CAVANAGH, MD, MRCP
Editor and Adviser to the Study Group

Acknowledgements

We acknowledge the co-operation and financial assistance of the Ciba Foundation for the Promotion of International Co-operation in Medical and Chemical Research and the Wellcome Trust. Without their help this Study Group would not have been realised.

For their most generous advice and time, we thank Dr. Crome, Dr. Kirman and Dr. Stern of the Queen Mary's Hospital for Children, Carshalton.

We also thank Professor Cavanagh and his staff at the M.R.C. Research Group in Applied Neurobiology for their assistance in producing papers and the Proceedings.

Foreword

B. H. KIRMAN (Chairman)

I would like first on your behalf and that of the Institute of Research into Mental Retardation to thank the CIBA Foundation for these premises and for their hospitality. I do think that it is very valuable to have the many disciplines that are represented here. I was first attracted to the subject of mental handicap when I was a young man because everybody said nobody knows anything about it, and I think that this is something that has attracted many of us. Perhaps it is still the situation despite the great accumulation of knowledge recently. I think we all know that the problem of unclassified mental retardation is a big challenge because it still makes up the majority of cases, and I think we all know that in the past people have gone ahead more or less in blinkers with their own approach and the limitation of the work in this field has been the assumption that their approach has been the only valid one. In consequence they have made assumptions which have been in the main quite unjustified, so that a good deal of the work has to be destructive or critical in order to clear the ground for a multidisciplinary approach. We are very fortunate in having so many authorities present who can produce a synthesis of existing knowledge. Clearly the value of the meeting is the cross fertilisation and the effect of it will be manifest perhaps years afterwards. In many instances we have gone for consideration of aetiology and prevention each in our way, but in these unclassified cases we have not always looked at the multifactorial aspect. I think that the paranatal mortality survey and similar work in the United States have underlined the importance of looking at multiple factors in aetiology. If we can get together using the sophisticated techniques in a carefully measured way that are available, then clearly there are enormous areas where very little attention has so far been paid to this important subject.

It is a subject which attracts scientific enquiry and curiosity. But it is also of fundamental importance for the future of mankind, because it is an aspect of enquiry which questions the function of the human brain and of human endeavour, and could throw a clear light on a whole area of human function and society.

Contents

		Page
Preface		v
Acknowledgements		vi
Foreword		vii
THE DEVELOPING BRAIN AND CONTROL MECHANISMS		
D. H. M. Woollam	Vascularisation of the developing brain	3
M. Prestige	On numbers and neurones	13
A. Giroud	Sensitivity of the developing nervous system	23
J. Dobbing	General discussion	41
BIOCHEMICAL ASPECTS OF THE DEVELOPING BRAIN		
J. S. Wigglesworth	The effects of pre-natal growth inhibition on brain composition	49
R. Balázs	Hormonal aspects of brain development	61
J. E. Cremer	Changes in enzyme activity and the developing brain	77
A. N. Davison	General discussion	91
MUTAGENIC AGENTS AND THEIR EFFECTS ON THE DEVELOPING BRAIN		
I. Zlotnik	Virus infection and brain development	103
P. Kleihues	Alkylating agents and their effects on the adult mammalian brain	117

W. Wechsler Teratogenic and oncogenic effects of ethylnitrosourea on the developing nervous system of rats 133

P. N. Magee General discussion 145

AETIOLOGY AND EPIDEMIOLOGY OF UNCLASSIFIED MENTAL RETARDATION

C. M. Drillien Perinatal factors affecting mental development of low birthweight infants 155

A. T. Rundle Somatic growth in severe mental retardation 173

B. H. Kirman Psychiatric aspects of unclassified mental retardation 187

K. S. Holt General discussion 205

PSYCHOLOGICAL, ELECTROPHYSIOLOGICAL AND BIOCHEMICAL ASPECTS OF UNCLASSIFIED MENTAL RETARDATION

B. E. Clayton Clinical biochemistry and unclassified mental retardation 213

R. Harris EEG aspects of unclassified mental retardation 225

N. O'Connor Brain injury and mental subnormality 243

J. Stern General discussion 261

MORPHOLOGICAL ASPECTS OF UNCLASSIFIED MENTAL RETARDATION

K. M. Laurence Defects in CSF pathways and unclassified mental retardation 269

L. Crome Non-specific developmental abnormalities and unclassified mental retardation 283

K. Jellinger Neuropathological features of unclassified mental retardation 293

P. E. Sylvester	General discussion	313
B. H. Kirman	Chairman's summary	317
List of Participants		321
Index		324

1

The Developing Brain and Control Mechanisms

Vascularisation of the Developing Brain

D. H. M. WOOLLAM

Introduction

To a considerable extent the title of this paper ensures that it must be an essay in teleology, except when a direct description is given of what is actually observable under the microscope. The problems of teleology constantly bedevil the study of structure and function in the adult as well as in the embryo and foetus. One single aspect of the situation must be clarified at once. It is perfectly permissible to suggest from the structure and distribution of the cerebral vessels that their role is in maintaining the embryonic and foetal brain, but the statement must always be seen as merely a suggestion and not as a truth. It may be that even when two structures such as capillaries taken from different organs have identical electron microscopic appearances that, physiologically, their functions and behaviour are entirely different. It is my contention that whenever an anatomist or histologist fails constantly to stress the teleological element inevitably present in his statements, he is in peril and extremely likely to lead his non-structurally orientated colleagues into waters where they will sink without trace. It is my endeavour in this short paper to make it clear when I am dealing with fact and when I am speculating on the significance of those facts.

The Functional Aspects of Cerebral Vascular Architectonics

I base my concept of the *raison d'être* and function of both embryonic and adult vascular architecture in the brain on a very pertinent statement made by Feeney and Watterson (1946), namely that 'there exists a very close relationship between the metabolic requirements of the nervous tissue and the final distribution of intraneural vessels in the adult, a relationship which functions in such a way as to provide the nervous system with a blood supply just adequate for its minimal needs'. If this supposition represents the truth of the matter a number of problems in embryonic and foetal neuro-embryology and neuropathology are clarified. For example the description of cell death as a perfectly normal feature of the development of the nervous system (Glucksmann, 1951; Boyd, 1955) is explicable on a vascular basis, if it is assumed that so important is the evolutionary significance of having as many neurons as possible that neurons develop beyond the capacity of the vascular supply, and some must die off each day. Similarly one can explain why it should be that an adult is alleged to lose 60,000 or more nerve cells every day. Again if this concept of the interrelationship between blood supply and nervous tissue is correct, it is easy to support the view of Craigie (1955) that anoxia is the main factor responsible for vascularisation of the embryonic nervous system.

The Importance of Anoxia in Cerebral Vascularisation

If anoxia is indeed the main factor responsible for vascularisation of the nervous system, this does not put the nervous system in a peculiar position isolated from all other tissues. As Hamilton, Boyd and Mossman (1962) have pointed out, at the 7-somite stage (that is the beginning of the fourth week of gestation), when the chorionic sac is about 1 cm in diameter, the distance of the embryonic body from the nearest maternal blood in the early placental blood lacunae is probably not more than 3 mm. They regard this distance, however, as being too great to allow adequate nutrition by direct diffusion, and suggest that, at this stage, the circulation of blood is required to overcome the deficiencies of nutrition by simple diffusion, and it is at this stage that the circulation of blood does in fact commence. Indeed, even earlier there is evidence of the importance of blood supply to the central nervous system since, after the earliest vasculature has appeared in the walls of the yolk sac and gut, the neural tube is the first place to which they spread, reaching it in the 14-somite stage (24th day of gestation) before the tube has had the opportunity to close and immediately after the establishment of a circulation of any kind.

The Development of the Cerebral Blood Vessels

The blood vessels which reach the brain surround it in a plexiform manner, so that by the 8 mm stage (about the 35th day of gestation) the surface of the brain and spinal cord is covered by a network of what are often termed 'capillaries'. This nomenclature, although justified if one judges the question solely by diameter, is somewhat misleading since some of these vessels are destined to disappear completely and others to receive media and adventitia and thus be converted into the major tributaries of the arteries and veins supplying the brain and spinal cord. One thing is certain, namely, that for a considerable period before birth as well as after birth there will be no capillaries on the surface of the brain and spinal cord, only arteries and veins.

Very shortly after the network of blood vessels appears on the surface of the brain and spinal cord, vascular twigs appear which penetrate the central nervous system to supply the tissue which is becoming progressively further removed from the surface and thus from its sources of nutriment by diffusion. We know virtually nothing of the factors which control this important event. It is all too easy to attribute it to genetic causes or local haemodynamic effects, neither of which explain how or why it occurs.

Intra-cerebral Capillaries

It is as vessels of capillary size that the twigs from the surface vessels enter the brain. By the 13 mm stage (early part of sixth week of gestation) the capillary bed is at its peak of development and is evenly spread between the white and grey matter. From then onwards to adult life the story is of the development of an overwhelming superiority in the capillary supply of the grey matter with a corresponding decline in that of the white matter. The supply to the grey and white matter is not however constant but varies from site to site. Nevertheless, in capillary density the poorest supply to the grey matter is half as great again as the richest supply to the white matter. In various areas of the grey matter there is considerable difference in the density of the capillary bed. On the whole the sensory nuclei have a much more extensive supply than the motor nuclei. This phenomenon appears to be correlated directly with the number of synapses at a neuron. The trigeminal ganglion, for example, with no synapses, has a relatively poor blood supply (Dunning and Wolff, 1937), whilst the main sensory nuclei in the spinal cord have a much richer supply than the ventral horn. Somewhat strangely, in view of the fact that nerve cells must of necessity receive their nutriment virtually entirely at the cell body, there is a marked range of difference in the blood supply to the white matter, albeit at a much lower level than that to the grey matter. The pyramidal tract, for example, receives about twice the supply of the fasciculus cuneatus (Woollam and Millen, 1958).

Whether it is in fact the number of synapses (Scharrer, 1944), the oxidase content (Campbell, 1938), or the density of mitochondria in the neurons (Scharrer, 1945) which provides the closest correlation between the anatomical features of the neurons and the density of the capillary network surrounding them, it seems reasonable to conclude that it is activity, and, in particular, metabolic activity which is the prime factor in determining the vascularity of individual areas of the nervous system. A further pointer to this comes from comparative anatomical studies. In mammals the blood supply to the central nervous system is much more abundant than in lower forms; in the rat the white matter of the medial longitudinal bundle is as well supplied as the richest area of grey matter in the turtle (Craigie, 1955).

The Influence of the Position of Intracerebral Blood Vessels in Relation to Nerve Cells

In lower forms there are several examples in which the pattern of vascular distribution determines quite clearly the arrangement of nervous tissue, a good example being the optic lobe of the squid. In mammals this type of relationship is not unknown as for example in the nucleus supraopticus accessorius of the hypothalamus (Scharrer, 1944).

The Relationship Between the Metabolic Requirements of Certain Special Areas in the Central Nervous System and the Capillary Network

Cells, such as secreting nerve cells, which are thought to have exceptionally high metabolic requirements may be surrounded by veritable capillary baskets (Scharrer and Scharrer, 1940). In some cases, as, for example, occasionally in human pyramidal cells (Scharrer, 1937), capillaries may be endocellular. It must be acknowledged that the authority with probably the widest experience of cerebral vascular anatomy (Craigie, 1955), whilst not denying the possibility that endocellular capillaries occur, indicates that he personally has never encountered them. It is indeed extremely difficult to distinguish a truly endocellular situation of a capillary from that degree of close proximity to the neuron which may make the capillary appear to be endocellular in histological section.

The Anatomical and Physiological Significance of the Vascular Supply to the Brain in Embryonic and Foetal Life

In the last few weeks of pregnancy it would seem that the whole object of the foetal circulation is to see that the most richly oxygenated blood which comes from the placenta via the umbilical vein and ductus venosus into the right atrium passes through the foramen ovale into the left atrium and is thus distributed by means of the internal carotid and vertebral arteries to the brain and spinal cord. Similarly once the nervous system has removed the oxygen all the blood returns to the right atrium via the superior vena cava, that from the spinal cord reaching the superior vena cava through the azygos system of veins. This deoxygenated blood passes into the right ventricle being directed thence rather than through the foramen ovale by the intervenous tubercle, and since the lungs do not require blood passes largely via the ductus arteriosus to the aorta immediately below the point at which the left subclavian artery (the parent of one vertebral artery) arises. From here the blood travels back to the placenta for reoxygenation via the umbilical arteries.

At an earlier stage of development the arteries of the pharyngeal arches pass between the cartilages of the arches and thus connect the ventral and dorsal aortae. They are in fact the only connections between the heart and the vessels which supply the brain and spinal cord. Any interruption to them would result in the destruction of a large part of the nervous system and possibly all. It can be argued (Woollam and Millen, 1962) that the function of the pharyngeal arches and in particular of their cartilages is to protect the arteries of the arches from compression. In many ways it seems preferable to use this teleological argument to account for the passage of the embryo through the stage at which the pharyngeal arches are present rather than to adopt the concept that it is obliged to follow this pathway of development because its forebears were fishes and had to have gills in the neck region. I make no apology in this regard for following the attitude of the great embryologist, Streeter, who is recorded as saying in a conversation with the then Professor of Anatomy at Harvard:

'You know, Wislocki, many people think that the stages of placental and embryonic development lead up to the final stage when suddenly the placenta and foetus are ready to function, but I have never agreed with them. I grew up in a small town as the son of a merchant and I am reminded when I observe the growth and differentiation of the embryo of a sign which appeared now and then in my father's store which read: "Open for business during alterations." I think that each successive stage in embryonic differentiation must be regarded as a functional stage, albeit the functions may be quite different from those which the tissues and organs will ultimately assume when development is completed.'

'Business as usual during alterations' seems to sum up the whole story of the development of the blood supply to the central nervous system.

Mental Defect and Cerebral Vascularisation

Although a wide range of new techniques now exist for studying cerebral vascularisation, including the injection of acrylic resins, neoprene, colloidal carbon and various pigments (Woollam and Millen, 1955), as well as a variety of staining methods which have been made available in the past 30 years, very few attempts have been made to correlate accurately blood supply and mental defect. Only rarely are the brains of those mental defectives who come to post-mortem examination considered in detail from the point of view of blood supply. A few scattered and possibly important observations exist. For example, Eayrs (1954) showed that in cretinism the capillary bed is less dense than normal. It may be that his observation ought to be interpreted as meaning that in cretinism more extracellular fluid is present than usual. Nevertheless, both situations come to the same thing as far as the brain is concerned, it is liable to suffer a relative anoxia.

Taking the problem away from the vascular side to the significance of the shape and size of the brain in mental retardation, I offer for consideration the size and shape of the massa intermedia in the brain (Fig. 1), which comes from a case of unclassified mental retardation aged 39. The massa intermedia is considerably larger than any I have seen in the many thousands of brains I have examined in the past 20 years. Curiously it resembles very closely the massa intermedia of many lower forms of life and is particularly comparable to that of the ox brain and thus recalls Galen's description of the third ventricle which we now know was taken from the ox brain and transferred to the human as if there could not possibly be any difference between the brains of the two species. I give this description in Singer's (1956) translation.

'There is a large duct below in the base of the third ventricle which receives the waste products from the anterior ventricle by the holes (that is the interventricular foramina) above and there is another duct from the tissues above also. Those ignorant of this ventricle are naturally unaware of the duct extending backward whereby the conarium is supported, and, if it is bared of the surrounding veins and broken off at the base, a hole is seen there higher up.'

I make this digression in order to summarise what I want to say about the significance of cerebral vascularisation in relation to mental defect. Here is a simple but apparently rare abnormality, a grossly large massa intermedia. Normally neurologists assign no particular function to the massa intermedia which is frequently absent in brains taken from normal individuals. Neither of course do neurologists assign any

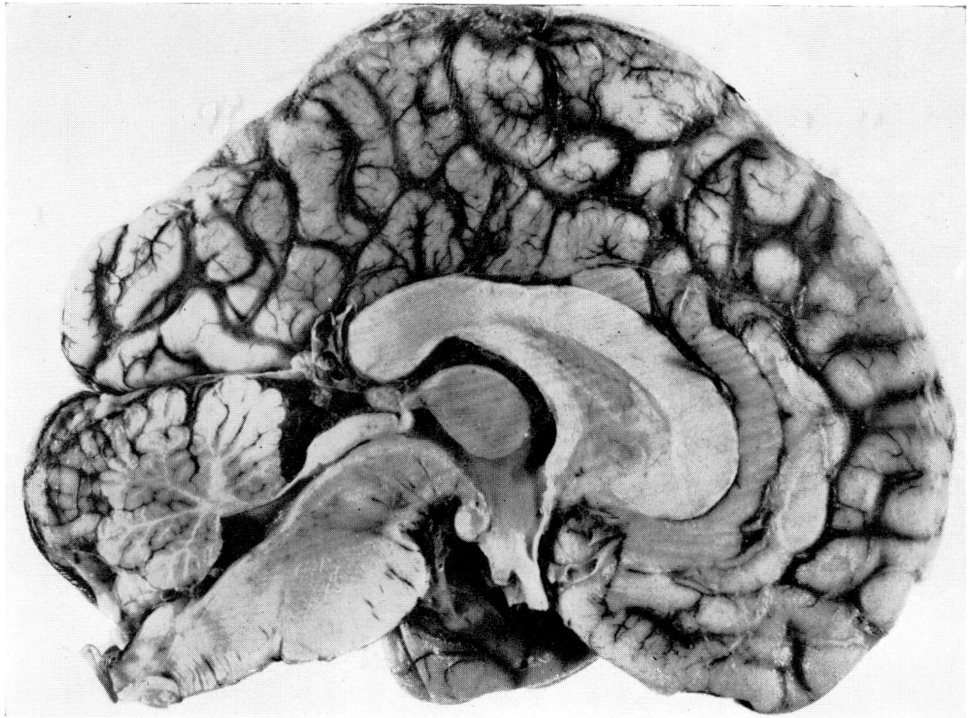

Fig. 1. Sagittal section through third ventricle of brain from case of unclassified mental retardation. Aged 39. Note extremely large massa intermedia.

[To face p. 8

particular significance to abnormal features in the anatomy of the ventricular system, with the sole exception of hydrocephalus. Yet there can be little doubt that the large massa intermedia seen in this case must have been accompanied by gross alterations from normal in the architecture of blood vessels in the neighbourhood of the thalamus. This seems to me a point of the very greatest importance to determine, namely which is first in determining neural development, the cerebral cortex or its vascular supply. Does one determine the form of the other or do they develop *pari passu?* If we see something unusual in the vascular or other architecture of the brain of a mental defective, have we any right to say that this anomaly was responsible for the occurrence of the defect? I take an anatomist's view and, just as at the present time I would say that autosomal trisomy was associated with Down's syndrome but would not go so far as to say it caused it, I would not be inclined to give any abnormality of cerebral vascular arrangement priority as a cause of mental deficiency. The organism must be studied as a whole. It is not sufficient to draw conclusions sometimes from this system and sometimes from the other. It is my contention that the study of cerebral vascular distribution in mental defect is well overdue for close examination, and an essential precursor to this will be the attempt to obtain very much more information than we have at present about the distribution of cerebral blood vessels in the normal individual.

REFERENCES

Boyd, J. D. (1955). In Waelsch, H. (Ed.). 'Biochemistry of the Developing Nervous System', p. 17. New York: Academic Press.

Campbell, A. C. P. (1938). *Res. Publ. Ass. nerv. ment. Dis.* **18**, 69.

Craigie, E. H. (1955). In Waelsch, H. (Ed.) 'Biochemistry of the Developing Nervous System', p. 28. New York: Academic Press.

Dunning, H. S. and Wolff, H. G. (1937). *J. Comp. Neurol.* **67**, 433.

Eayrs, J. T. (1954). *J. Anat., Lond.* **88**, 164.

Feeney, J. F. and Watterson, R. L. (1946). *J. Morph.* **78**, 231.

Glucksmann, A. (1951). *Biol. Rev.* **26**, 59.

Hamilton, W. J., Boyd, J. D. and Mossman, H. W. (1962). 'Human Embryology', p. 159. Cambridge: Heffer.

Scharrer, E. (1937). *Z. ges. Neur. Psychiat.* **158**, 93.

Scharrer, E. (1944). *Quart. Rev. Biol.* **19**, 308.

Scharrer, E. (1945). *J. comp. Neurol.* **83**, 237.

Scharrer, E. and Scharrer, B. (1940). *Res. Publ. Ass.. nerv. ment. Dis.* **20**, 170.

Singer, C. (1956). 'Galen on Anatomical Procedures'. London: Oxford University Press.

Woollam, D. H. M. and Millen, J. W. (1955). *J. Anat., Lond.* **89**, 193.

Woollam, D. H. M. and Millen, J. W. (1958). *Proc. roy. Soc. Med.* **51**, 540.

Woollam, D. H. M. and Millen, J. W. (1962). *Clin. Physiol.* **4**, 1.

DISCUSSION

Laurence: Dr. Woollam mentioned the matter of the massa intermedia in its relation to blood supply and the formation of mental defect. It is an almost invariable accompaniment of spina bifida cystica and Arnold-Chiari malformation and relatively few of these children have basic mental defect. The massa intermedia in these cases is sometimes so large as to obliterate the third ventricle and cause the two thalamic bodies to be almost completely fused. Secondly, the question of chromosome trisomy and abnormality. For some years I have studied trisomy 13 and arhinencephaly finding that very few of the latter condition are associated with trisomy 13/15. By contrast 13/15 is invariably associated with arhinencephaly. The relationship between that chromosome abnormality and the somatic malformations is far from constant.

Crome: I would like to hear Professor Woollam's comment on the role of C.S.F. in the development of the brain. Some years ago Professor Klosowskii, I think, in Moscow said that in the beginning the C.S.F. in the embryo is very different in composition from later, containing more chloride, glucose and glycogen, and the nutrition of the growing brain is at first by diffusion from the ventricles. Later this becomes inadequate, and a slow switch-over to the vascular system occurs on the surface of the brain. This switch-over at the surface is one of the factors in the migration of the neuroblasts. This theory seems to be complementary to Woollam's views.

Woollam: In answer to Dr. Laurence, all I wished to say was that mongolism was associated with a chromosome abnormality, but this did not necessarily cause it, and a third factor may be responsible. In answer to Crome's point. The C.S.F. is rather a negative substance and its appearance in the spinal cord comes from a breakthrough from the ventricular system, as suggested by Weed.

Balázs: You said that the blood supply may develop as a function of the particular brain region, but how would you define the functional activity of a brain region, and what factors would be involved in inducing the blood supply?

Woollam: From the morphological standpoint the more synapses there are the greater the blood supply, but why one species higher in the animal kingdom has a greater blood supply than another cannot be explained by morphology alone.

Balázs: In germinative sites not much oxygen is needed so there is a mutual interplay between certain stages of development and the necessity for a rich vascularisation, and this interplay changes very much during development. Can you give a lead to this?

Woollam: I'm afraid I can't.

Richter: Is anything known about the chemical signals that tell the developing blood vessels whether they should sprout capillaries or develop into arterioles? Is anoxia a sufficient signal?

Woollam: No, so far as I know.

Crome: There are exceptions and paradoxes in neuropathology known, such as in Leigh's encephalomyelopathy where there is a devastation of neurones associated with increased vascularisation.

Kirman: Does the supposed relatively simple relationship leading to retrolental fibroplasia illustrate this question, where the overgrowth of capillaries is stimulated by the anoxia?

Richter: There must be more than one signal since the endothelium has to decide whether to sprout into capillaries or form arterioles and veins.

Dobbing: The closest analogy is that of inflammation in which chemical stimuli lead to vascular proliferation.

Zlotnik: I wanted to ask Dr. Woollam about the loss of 60,000 neurones. There has never been any proof of this. At this rate statistically speaking by the age of 30 a man would probably have no neurones left!

Woollam: I don't know the reason. It constantly appears in the text-books.

Dobbing: There can be no sort of evidence, can there? It is inconceivable that anyone has counted them. On the DNA estimation there might even be more DNA with age from gliosis.

Prestige: The evidence comes from measurements of the surface area of the cortex and the numbers of neurones per unit area, and this shows a considerable decline from age 20, but the double measurement has to be done, so that the inaccuracy is substantial, but the general change is too great to be thrown over. There are also some individual counts of Purkinje cells which definitely go down, but there are some regions such as the ventrocochlear nucleus which do not go down. Also, data on rats show that the motor neurones do not go down.

Crome: Without any doubt the weight of the brain begins to diminish in middle-age and becomes appreciatively smaller. Furthermore with the microscope there is an increase in the glial cell population. Without any doubt the neuronal population begins to vanish at accelerated rates.

Dobbing: Concentration of the neurones due to shrinkage of the tissue without loss of cells must also of course be taken into account.

Prestige: I suspect that the main reason for reduction in brain weight is not loss of neurones but shrinkage of white matter.

Crome: What's your evidence?

Prestige: The pictures!

Zlotnik: There must also be loss of fluid in old age.

Wigglesworth: I would support Dr. Woollam in his plea for more study of brain vascularity. During the third trimester, many babies I see die of intraventricular haemorrhage, and while we have lots of theories of the cause of this, we do need a lot more study of the developmental changes in the vascular system. This is one of the major causes of death in the premature baby in the immediate neonatal period, and seems to be closely related to some anatomical change.

On Numbers and Neurones

MARTIN PRESTIGE

On the Total Number of Neurones

'Men are bigger and better than rats', concluded C. Judson Herrick (1926) at the end of his classic book on the cerebral cortex. But it is probable that in this he was allowing himself a modicum of prejudice, and so before discussing the control of cell number in a specific population of nerve cells, I shall briefly consider what the relation may be between the total number of neurones within a nervous system and its potentialities. While we no longer accept Lashley's law of mass action, we do intuitively recognise that nervous systems do better with a larger number of elements, but there is at the moment no answer to the question of how we may best construct one, given *n* nerve cells. This is partly because we are still searching for a formal definition of what the C.N.S. does, partly because we would not then have the theoretical insight to be able to design the best engineering solution and partly because we are still largely unaware of the limitations that cell biology and evolution impose. What is clear is that any system cannot possibly process all the information that is available to it, and that therefore classification must be accompanied by rejection. That the nervous system does classify is implicit in the structure of the neurone. It is therefore important that this process is appropriate, evaluated both in terms of the life of the organism and the survival of the species. We do not though understand what is appopriate ('reinforcing') nor how the decision is taken.

Furthermore, since we believe that complex pattern-recognising units are built up serially from simpler ones, it follows that their construction is more demanding in terms of neural numbers. Thus the *n* neurones available for classification must at least be shared between the competing needs of having a maximum number of differentiated recognition and behavioural classes on the one hand, and of having more sophisticated ones on the other. The price of insight is inaction.

It is assumed always that (a) learning is accompanied by changing patterns of connectivity; and usually that (b) synaptic efficacy changes are responsible. We can say that there is in principle a difference between the process of classification of sensory information and modification of the process (learning). This means that there are two sorts of measure of functional capacity—(a) the maximum number of classes that can be extracted from sensory information and hence the maximum number of output classes for behaviour; (b) the proportion of the classes than can be appropriately modified or rearranged. Even given knowledge of the number of nerve cells, it is not obvious how to derive these two parameters. In addition, since both maturation and learning may be expected to cause changes in connection pattern, it may be difficult to decide which is responsible in practice.

A non-specific decrease in the number of classifying cells will reduce the number of classes available; but I do not see why this should necessarily lead to less sophisticated or less appropriate classes. I therefore suggest it is unlikely that a developmental error of this type, provided it is not too dramatic, would be observed as mental retardation.

Evidence from Phylogeny

When we compare the scale of brains of animals of different species, we find that it alters with increased body size in at least three largely predictable ways:

(1) increased number of neurones
(2) decreased packing density of neurones
(3) increased volume of perikarya.

Von Bonin (1937) and Jerison (1963) have shown, over a 10,000-fold range, a striking relationship between the brain weight (W) and body weight (P) in adult mammals of different species.

$$W \propto P^{0.66} \qquad (1)$$

Thus brain weight increases less than body weight. Furthermore, Tower (1954) has shown that, over a similar range, the packing density of neurones (number of nerve cells per unit volume of cerebral cortex) goes down with increasing brain weight.

$$\text{number/unit volume} \propto W^{-0.32} \qquad (2)$$

or,

$$\propto P^{-0.32} \qquad (3)$$

substituting, a relationship is obtained between total number (n) of nerve cells (packing density x brain weight) and body weight (P).

$$n \propto P^{0.45} \qquad (4)$$

From Shariff's (1953) data, we can calculate that mean cell body volume is inversely proportional to the square root of packing density.

Simple though these relationships are, it is not clear what the significance of them is, nor how they constrain intelligence. This may be partly due to a difficulty in comparing the intelligence of, say, a mouse and a hippopotamus. Hodos (1970) has made a start in this direction by comparing the acquisition of a learning set for a number of mammals. In Table 1, column 1, the species from his data are arranged in descending order of ability. In column 2, the same species are ranked in groups by brain weight. While these observations are uncritical and inconclusive, they suggest a strategy for testing, within a taxonomic group, the hypothesis that increased brain size, *per se*, leads to increased intelligence. Von Bonin (1937) also has tables of a size-invariant parameter[1] which he calls the encephalisation coefficient (k). These too can be compared with Hodos' data (column 3). More sophisticated indices have been constructed, using parts of the brain (e.g. Stephan, Bauchot and Andy, 1970).

Thus the number of nerve cells in the brain can be thought of as being determined largely by the size of the species and in part by a species-specific (or an individual-specific) factor (Jerison, 1963). It remains the task of comparative psychology to decide how these influence brain function.

Evidence from Ontogeny

The justification for the construction of equation 4 is that the exponents measured in equations 1 and 2, being measures of scale obtained by a similar procedure from a large number of animals at similar stages of development, are probably accurate and representative of the scale of the whole nervous system. Indeed, if one takes the packing densities from three different areas of cortex (Shariff, 1953) and plots them against log. brain weight, the same exponent is obtained each time, despite a five-fold variation in absolute magnitude. What errors are present will be reflected in the proportionality constant, which is not used. These conditions are broken if they are applied to the growth of the brain during ontogeny. Data relating packing density of circumscribed groups of neurones to age, brain or body weight are available for several mammals, including humans, but because the brain does not develop synchronously, they cannot be taken as representative of the scale of whole brain, but only of the precise region from which they are taken. Hence we cannot by this method determine the changes

[1] Von Bonin's table contains errors in the data for *Felis domestica, Tupaja javanica,* and *Myrmecophaga jubata.*

in total nerve cell number during ontogeny, or senescence. Count (1947) has assembled the tables of brain weight against body weight, and shows that in the foetal period the slope of the log/log line is nearly 1, but decreases considerably soon after birth. In this connection, it is important to point out that higher vertebrates are specialised in that many other groups of animals are able to continue growing throughout life both in body and brain (e.g. fish, cephalopods). A third approach can be made by measuring total brain DNA (Dobbing and Sands, 1970). This also is indirect, giving total cell number, rather than total nerve cell number, but it has the significant advantages of using biochemical techniques.

On the Number of Neurones Within a Group

Why Have Many Nerve Cells Doing a Similar Function When One Might Do?

In certain situations, such as giant nerve cells of lower vertebrates, and in many invertebrate nervous systems, one nerve cell does do. In general, though, higher vertebrate nervous systems use many nerve cells for each function. The advantages depend upon the job: for instances, the set of retinal ganglion cells carries place information, the convergence of many rods onto each of them giving increased sensitivity; the motor neurone pool to one muscle is arranged by thresholds to give graded contraction (Henneman, Somjen and Carpenter, 1965) and the larger the number of spindle afferents from each muscle the more information is conveyed about muscle length (Stein, 1970). These advantages however are not infinitely augmented by unlimited increase in number, and so there exists a control problem.

What Controls the Number of Adult Nerve Cells Within a Group?

We can divide the control process into four.

(a) control of cell division
(b) control of migration
(c) control of selective differentiation
(d) control of cell death.

(a) *control of cell division.* Largely due to the introduction of tritiated thymidine autoradiography, it is now clear that the pattern of cell division in the embryonic nervous system is exquisitely controlled in time. In this technique (for a recent description, see Sidman, 1970) a pulse of tritium-labelled thymidine is given to the developing organism, either directly or via the mother, and this is incorporated into those cells undergoing DNA synthesis prior to mitosis. At intervals afterwards, the animals are killed and autoradiographs made to reveal which neurones are labelled. The thymidine is available for a matter of hours at the most, and is only retained to any extent in those cells that do not divide again, so the technique is tuned to determining the time of the final mitoses for any cell group. The extensive studies made all show that each particular population of neurones originates from the neural epithelium at a characteristic stage in ontogeny. These have been referred to as 'neuronal birthdays'.

As an example of this, we can take the well-known inside-out development of cerebral cortex. The earliest cells to cease mitosis and differentiate move out from the ventricular layer (for terminology, see Angevine *et al.*, 1970); later cells differentiating migrate through the earlier ones and thus the layered structure reflects a temporal sequence of birthdays.

It is also clear that the pattern of cell division is controlled spatially. It was recognised very early on that mitoses occurred, not randomly, but in predictable places at certain times; but the connection between locus of cell division and type of neurone subsequently differentiating had to wait for grafts, explants and cell cultures. From these experiments, it seems that the regional character of neurones is determined at the neural plate stage, that is, many generations before any differentiation into recognisable nerve cells. This indicates that some of the controlled processes must be hereditable through mitosis.

It is regrettable that the nature of these control processes in time and space is obscure. It seems certain that a suitable endocrine environment is required; but this hardly provides the richness of texture that must be demanded. One clue comes from studies on lower vertebrates which possess some powers of regeneration. For example, the retina of adult newt continues to grow by adding cells to all three cell layers at the ciliary margin, but very slowly. After section of the optic nerve, the retina degenerates, and extensive cell division at the margin subsequently restores the three layers (Gaze and Watson, 1968) right across the retina. There is evidence here of an on/off switch controlling mitosis, which may be susceptible to physiological analysis.

(b) *control of migration.* After final mitosis, the immature neurone migrates to its final location. An example of this in cerebral cortex has already been given. In some cases, the distance covered may be very large: the neurones destined for the nucleus griseum pontis arise in the rhombic lip and migrate as a well-defined sheet of cells forming the corpus pontobulbare. These cells are distributed along the surface of the embryonic brain stem from the rhombic lip to the base of the pons (Taber Pierce, 1966). Another interesting situation is found in the cerebellum, where granule cells, arising in the external granular layer, migrate downwards through the dendrites of the Purkinje cells, spinning out their axons behind them (Miale and Sidman, 1961).

The mechanism of this migration and its control is, once again, unclear. Cell migration has been intensively studied *in vitro* and the importance of the geometry of the mechanical substrate and its chemical nature repeatedly emphasised. *In vivo,* it can be studied by the use of lesions or, more profitably, of mutants (such as reeler; Sidman, 1968).

(c) *control of selective differentiation.* Cell differentiation is not an all-or-none event, but a gradual restriction of developmental potentialities together with expression of some of them. The factors responsible for each step may be varied. After the immature neurone has left the dividing population, it is already partially restricted, though most of its differentiation is not yet overt. It is possible that cells at this stage still possess some flexibility in being able to differentiate into alternative types of neurones. However, in at least one situation, they do not. Jacobson (1968) has shown that retinal ganglion cells lose their last vestige of pluripotency (that of being nasal or temporal, ventral or dorsal) at about the time the earliest cell ceases mitosis and starts overt differentiation.

(d) *control of cell death.* It has been recognised since Glücksmann's (1951) classic review that cell death (synonymous with degeneration) is a common feature of differentiating systems, both within and outside the nervous system. Some of this may be associated with morphogenetic modelling, but there remains the consistent observation that large numbers of cells die during histogenesis. This is concluded both from the presence of pycnotic nuclei seen with the light microscope and also decreases in cell number counted in serial sections. For example, the total number of mouse motor neurones declines from 10^5 at 11 days to 2.5×10^4 at 15 days gestation (Flanagan, 1969). A major bar to understanding the significance of the histology is that techniques for recording cell death are so rudimentary. In the same way that counts of numbers of visible mitoses by themselves give little information on rates of cell division, so too do counts of dying cells, unless the duration of death (as observed) is known for that tissue at that stage. Counts of the total numbers of nerve cells can only give net changes, and not the absolute amounts from the contributing factors.

The heading 'control of cell death' implies perhaps that there is positive control, but this has not been proved in the nervous system. It is easier to think that control is exerted by the presence or absence of the necessary conditions for cell survival; and the simplest hypothesis on function incorporates this idea by postulating that cell death is the negative term in a control process that optimises the number of neurones present to do the job. It thus acts as a damper on over-production. Put forward originally by Hamburger and Levi-Montalcini (1949), this hypothesis has been readily accepted, perhaps because it is difficult to see how it could be otherwise. The questions at issue go beyond. Is it essential to have neurones dying? We have not been able to do the experiment of prevention. Are there any other advantages to be gained by over-production and redundancy? We can only speculate. How does this control operate, and at what stages in differentiation?

There is a little evidence on these last questions (reviewed by Prestige, 1970). The concept of over-production implies that there is a threshold number of nerve cells which, if exceeded, causes the excess to die. This threshold can be tentatively identified with the set of synaptic or junctional sites available for the particular population of neurones to make contact with. This, for motor neurones, will be the appropriate muscle mass; and for inferior olive cells, will be the Purkinje cells in the cerebellum. For these, and other examples both centrally and peripherally, it can be shown that after final division and migration, the immature nerve cell becomes dependent on the successful termination of its axon in an appropriate locus. If by surgery or congenital defect this is totally prevented, the cell dies. The only exceptions *in vivo* that I know of to this generalisation are the cells of spinal ganglia, which do not require to innervate the spinal cord. In a characteristic note, Sherrington (1894) describes how he found in an amyelous foetus that these cells and their axons were present. Instead they have an absolute requirement for their fibres to terminate peripherally.

The concept of threshold comes from the results of increasing or decreasing the mass of tissue to be innervated, leading to increased or decreased numbers of innervating neurones. This has been demonstrated most clearly for sensory nerve cells, less so for motor neurones; for intracentral neurones, only the experiment of decreasing the post-synaptic field has been attempted.

By varying the time of the interruption of normal relationships between motor nerve and muscle, it is possible to investigate the time course of this interaction. It has been found that motor neurones are most susceptible at about the time function first appears, but that thereafter they become progressively less so (Prestige, 1967). The action of muscle cell on nerve fibre thus antedates the reverse influence of neurone on muscle.

Apart from ischaemia there are three other conditions recognised which may lead to death of neurones—transneuronal degeneration, disuse and senescence. Whether they have physiological as well as pathological functions is not known.

ACKNOWLEDGEMENTS

I am indebted to the Medical Research Council for support, and to Miss Margaret Gregson for her skills.

TABLE 1

Three ways of ranking brain function of different species: (1) by the rate of acquisition of a learning set (Hodos, 1970), (2) by brain weight, (3) by the encephalisation coefficient (k) (Von Bonin, 1937).

1	*2*	*3*
chimpanzee	donkey	chimpanzee
gorilla	gorilla	cebus monkey
rhesus monkey	chimpanzee	spider monkey
mangabey	rhesus monkey	squirrel monkey
mink	spider monkey	rhesus monkey
ferret	mangabey	mangabey
spider monkey	cebus monkey	gorilla
cebus monkey	cat	marmoset
skunk	squirrel monkey	squirrel
marmoset	marmoset	tree shrew
cat	squirrel	donkey
squirrel monkey	tree shrew	
rat	rat, ferret,	skunk, ferret, rat, mink,
squirrel	skunk and mink–	cat–not available.
tree shrew	not available.	See footnote 1

REFERENCES

Angevine, J. B., Jr., Bodian, D., Coulombre, A. J., Edds, M. V., Jr., Hamburger, V., Jacobson, M., Lyser, K. M., Prestige, M. C., Sidman, R. L., Varon, S. and Weiss, P. A. (1970). *Anat. Rec.* **166**, 257.
von Bonin, G. (1937). *J. Gen. Psychol.* **16**, 379.
Count, E. W. (1947). *Ann. N.Y. Acad. Sci.* **46**, 993.
Dobbing, J. and Sands, J. (1970). *Nature* **226**, 639.
Flanagan, A. E. H. (1969). *J. Morph.* **129**, 281.
Gaze, R. M. and Watson, W. E. (1968). In Wolstenholme, G. E. W. and O'Connor, M. (Eds) 'Growth of the Nervous System'. London, Churchill, p. 53.
Glücksmann, A. (1951). *Biol. Rev.* **26**, 59.
Hamburger, V. and Levi-Montalcini, R. (1949). *J. exp. Zool.* **111**, 457.
Henneman, E., Somjen, G. and Carpenter, D. O. (1965). *J. Neurophysiol.* **28**, 560.
Herrick, C. J. (1926). 'Brains of Rats and Men'. Chicago: University of Chicago.

Hodos, W. (1970). In 'The Neurosciences: Second Study Program' (ed. F. O. Schmitt), p. 26. New York: Rockefeller University.
Jacobson, M. (1968). *Dev. Biol.* **17**, 219.
Jerison, H. J. (1963). *Human Biol.* **35**, 263.
Miale, I. L. and Sidman, R. L. (1961). *Exp. Neurol.* **4**, 277.
Prestige, M. C. (1967). *J. Embryol. exp. Morph.* **18**, 359.
Prestige, M. C. (1970). In 'The Neurosciences: Second Study Program' (ed. F. O. Schmitt), p. 73. New York: Rockefeller University.
Shariff, G. A. (1953). *J. comp. Neurol.* **98**, 381.
Sherrington, C. S. (1894). *J. Physiol. Lond.* **17**, 211.
Sidman, R. L. (1968). In 'Physiological and Biochemical Aspects of Nervous Integration' (ed. F. D. Carlson), p. 163. New Jersey: Prentice-Hall.
Sidman, R. L. (1970). In 'Contemporary Research Techniques in Neuroanatomy' (eds S. O. E. Ebbeson and W. J. H. Nauta). New York: Springer-Verlag.
Stein, R. B. (1970). In 'The Neurosciences: Second Study Program' (ed. F. O. Schmitt), p. 597. New York: Rockefeller University.
Stephan, H., Bauchot, R. and Andy, O. J. (1970). *Adv. Primatol.* **1**, 289.
Taber Pierce, E. (1966). *J. comp. Neurol.* **126**, 219.
Tower, D. B. (1954). *J. comp. Neurol.* **101**, 19.

DISCUSSION

Richter: Biochemists have been regarded as crude for making homogenates and mixing up the nerve cells, but doing total nerve cell counts one has to start somewhere. Is there much information about the different types of cells?

Prestige: Counting situations are absolutely defined by the ability to recognise consistent criteria. Once one gets away from a set of nerve cells of distinctive morphology throughout their life time, then it is very difficult to do precise counts.

Hanefeld: In the role of contact, is it of any importance what type of cell contact is made? For instance in tissue culture with neurones and kidney cells?

Prestige: Tissue culture is a very difficult situation to analyse because in culture neurones seem to survive without any termination requirements. On the other hand, we are not sure what the mechanism of contact is and neurones only grow successfully in media containing a lot of serum and embryo extract. Since we have no idea what is achieved at contact, it may be that the protein or glycolipid material normally present in sera is relevant.

Dobbing: Dr. Prestige has concentrated upon nerve cell number, but it is obviously trite to suggest that there are other features about nerve cells than their number. Prof. Eayrs has demonstrated a deficit of connectivity and complexity. This adds great complexity to these matters.

Laurence: The disordered integration, I would have thought, would be at least as important in connection with mental retardation disorders as loss of abolute numbers. Mental retardation is most associated with a normal sized brain containing presumably normal numbers of neurones, than small brains with reduced neurones.

Prestige: I accept this.

Balázs: I take your point that reduction in number does not necessarily mean reduction in sophistication, and also Dr. Dobbing's point that it is probably the connections which have an important bearing on the operation of the system, but one has to bring in the type of cells as well, because it will make a very great difference to the function of the animals whether it is basket cells or granule cells which are deleted. Since there is a very marked difference in the 'birthday' of the different types of cells, therefore it is important for the insult, and its consequences, as to what type of cell will be defective. This will depend upon the time of the insult.

Kirman: It is a naive point but *à propos* of Dr. Laurence's remark, I was wondering what we are talking about. Are we talking about severe subnormality with an I.Q. below 50 or about those well above that? Dr. Crome's work shows that many of the former do have a reduction in brain weight and I wonder if we have enough evidence on the mildly retarded to justify Dr. Laurence's statement. Also if the brain cell is structurally abnormal, is it on its way out or is this state static?

Crome: There is no question that in the severely subnormal the brain weight and volumes are reduced in the majority, and when not reduced there are other changes which suggest that the total population of nerve cells is reduced. But what happens in the borderline cases is difficult to say. I know of no evidence that the principle that the number of cells is related to intelligence is disturbed. There is some E.M. work of Gonatas which supports that synaptic connections are very important, and he has shown that where nerve cell numbers and brain weight seem normal, there are certain abnormalities in the synaptic connections of nerve cells.

Sensitivity of the Developing Nervous System

A. GIROUD

The nervous system begins its development after the blastogenic stage and sometimes only finishes it after birth. During this time it remains very sensitive to all environmental factors. The processes involved in its evolution vary continually as do also the results of any injuries.

The main anatomical structures are formed first of all, histological details being gradually achieved towards the end of development. The consequences of this evolution is that the repercussions of the various factors vary considerably depending on the time at which they act. Thus, the final results, in the case of early injuries, may be death at birth or soon after and, in later injuries, a physiologically deficient cerebrum or cerebellum.

Because of these variations the evolution of the nervous system may be subdivided in two parts (Fig. 1): on the one hand the embryonic stage where anatomical differentiation predominates, and on the other hand, the foetal and post-foetal stages, where histological differentiation predominate.

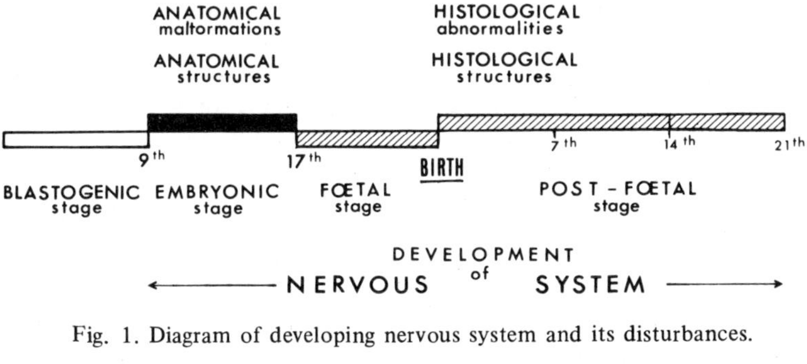

Fig. 1. Diagram of developing nervous system and its disturbances.

The Embryonic Stage and its Disturbances

The embryonic stage begins after the blastogenic stage and is considered to end when the morphological type of the species is achieved. During this stage the fundamental anatomical structures of the nervous system are formed.

Many factors may disturb its development at this stage inducing essentially anatomical malformations, such as anencephaly and its minor forms (encephalomeningocoele, meningocoele), cyclocephaly, hydrocephaly, as well as spina bifida and its minor forms.

(i) Physical Factors

Among the physical teratogenic factors, X-rays are the most important; they have been used at various periods throughout development. They do not induce malformations during the blastogenic stage, but only during the embryonic stage. Other alterations (histological) may be produced during the subsequent stages.

The first result of irradiation is the death of cells, especially neuroblasts. Various types of regeneration may follow. Some are localised, such as vegetations (rosettes) which invade the wall of the nervous system: their development may be the cause of heteropias. Some are diffuse in type: the result is a morphologically normal brain, but of small size (microcephaly).

(ii) Chemical Factors

Formerly, chemicals were used to disturb early development in order to understand its mechanism (Lehmann, 1933 and 1937; Pasteels, 1945). Some were discovered while investigating the cause of certain malformations, such was the case of Veratrin contained in the food of ewes, which induced cyclopia (Binns *et al.*, 1960).

Numerous investigations have been undertaken to find out the potential noxiousness of therapeutic drugs. Many of them have been found to be teratogenic to the nervous system of laboratory animals, particularly the case of anti-tumour agents. Antibodies, too, may be teratogenic. Brent (1964; 1967), and David *et al.* (1965) injected anti-kidney antibodies and obtained malformations of the nervous system. An indirect action was thought probable, such as disturbances in the yolk sac function or in maternal metabolism. Nevertheless, experiments *in vitro* on chick embryo leads one to suppose a direct action.

(iii) Infectious Factors

Certain infections are also teratogenic. Exencephaly and microcephaly have been observed with H 1 and RV virus (Ferm and Kilham, 1963), hydrocephaly with mumps virus (Johnson *et al.*, 1967) and absence of optic nerve in toxoplasmosis (Giroud *et al.*, 1966).

(iv) Nutritional Factors

Experiments demonstrate that a correct balance between nutrients is absolutely necessary; deficiency or excess of a certain nutrient may be teratogenic. Zinc deficiency induces nervous malformations (Hurley, 1969). Some vitamin deficiencies frequently produce nervous malformations. Such is the case of folic acid and cyanocobalamin deficiencies which induce hydrocephaly (Giroud and Lefebvres, 1951; Nelson *et al.*, 1952; Stempack, 1965), and pantothenic acid and α-tocopherol deficiencies also lead to nervous malformations. Vitamin A deficiency produces eye abnormalities (Warkany and Schraffenberger, 1944; Roux *et al.*, 1962), but its excess frequently causes anencephaly and spina bifida (Cohlan, 1953; Giroud and Martinet, 1955).

Hypercholesterolaemic or hypocholesterolaemic drugs (Tuchmann-Duplessis and Mercier-Parot, 1964; Roux, 1964) may cause nervous malformations. Deficiency or excess of amino-acids may also be dangerous. Excess of leucine in the rat has led to nervous malformations (Persaud, 1969).

At the embryonic stage, food restrictions have no effect. But there is one exception for in some strains of mice fasting during one day has induced malformations (Runner, 1959).

General Considerations

During the embryonic stage the most important results of injuries are the anatomical malformations, many of them being followed by death *in utero,* more or less early on, if not at birth.

Experiments have established that there is no specific teratogenic action of a given factor, and there are very few exceptions. Malformations are produced during the embryonic stage i.e. during the organisation period, and especially early in this period. The type of malformation depends essentially on the organisation process involved at the time of injury, and they are the result of a disturbance in the various organisation processes. Just as these processes vary with time, so do malformations similarly vary. This fact has been well illustrated

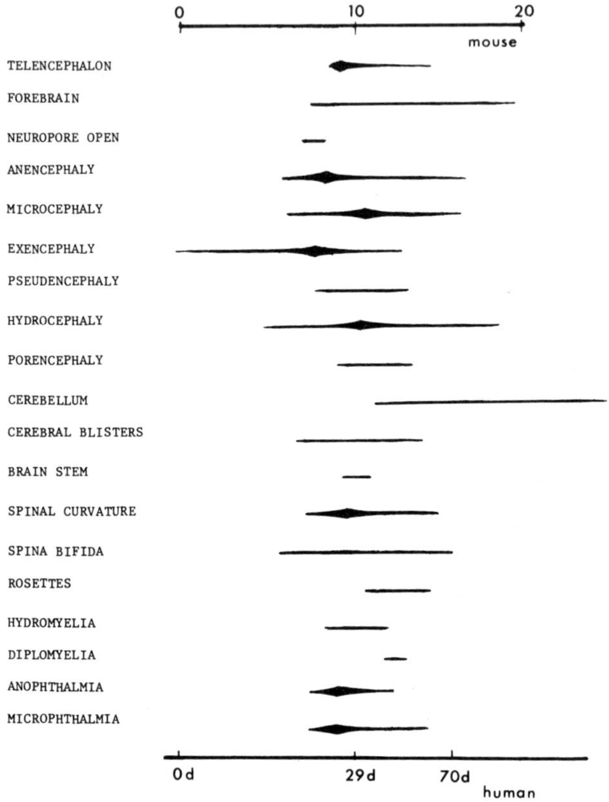

Fig. 2. Teratogenic stages in X-ray experiments. According to Rugh (modified).

from studies with X-rays. Russel (1950), Hicks (1953) and Rugh (1958) have given this time table (Fig. 2). Perhaps, as in the case of cleft palate, each date may be subdivided into two close dates. Two peaks of frequency were found in some cases by Murakami *et al.* (1969).

Teratogenic action does not need a factor of strong intensity. Five röntgen of X-rays are enough (Rugh, 1965), and drugs may be noxious at a dose 100 times less than in the adult (Murphy, 1960). Even unapparent infections may be teratogenic, and the same holds for very minor vitamin deficiencies (Giroud *et al.*, 1953).

Teratogenic activity depends on the genetic background. That it varies with the animal species or strains has been clearly demonstrated by experiments with drugs and with vitamin deficiencies which have been performed on a large scale in various species or strains. As a recent example, an antibiotic *rifampicin,* very frequently induces spina bifida in rats (22%) and in mice (16%), but not in rabbits (0%) (Tuchmann-Duplessis and Mercier-Parot, 1969).

Teratogenic action is direct on the embryo. This has been well demonstrated with X-rays: the embryo being shielded remained normal (Wilson and Karr, 1951). An indirect action has been suggested for trypan blue and for antibodies, but experiments on amphibians and on birds suggest the possibility of a direct action.

All these investigations have made it possible to establish some notions concerning the mechanisms of malformations of the nervous system.

The intervention of chromosomal alterations, which are a frequent result of irradiations, has been considered. But this is debatable since changes in chromosomes take place at all times with X-rays, whereas malformations are induced only at definite times (Tamboise and Tamboise, 1969). Perhaps, this hypothesis would be of value to explain the rare cases of exencephaly induced during the blastogenic stage (Rugh and Grupp, 1959). A reduction of the mitotic activity after X-rays has been noted (Fränz, 1971). Investigators working with X-rays, however, are of the opinion that above all, malformations are the result of massive necrosis of neuroblasts as an outcome of an inhibition of their enzymatic system by oxidising substances (Russel and Russel, 1954; Hicks, 1954; Wegner, 1966). Electron microscopical changes have been noted (Meissier, 1969).

Nevertheless, it seems that physiological disturbances of cells are often sufficient to induce malformations. This is particularly the case of vitamin deficiencies, since many cell enzymes are influenced by these vitamins. Similar disturbances may occur with chemicals, e.g. folic acid antagonists (aminopterine and α-methylfolic acid), which induce nervous malformations, inhibit the function of folic acid in nucleic acid metabolism and hence protein synthesis. Actinomycin D, which produces exencephaly and encephalocoele (Tuchmann-Duplessis and Mercier-Parot, 1958), inhibits the synthesis of mRNA; thus the genetic information required for embryonic differentiation is suppressed.

Hence, in the early stages, if there are functional disorders in the competent cells the induction processes may be disturbed and malformations produced. Later on, if nerve cells do not react to the migratory stimulation, malformations may occur: this is the case of abnormal migration of nervous fibres with subsequent absence of an optic nerve or of the olfactory bulb (Giroud *et al.*, 1966; 1968).

Foetal and Post-Foetal Stages and Their Disturbances

The development of the nervous system is not finished at birth, it continues after birth during a period which can be called the post-foetal stage. This lasts a few weeks in the rat, and several months in humans.

It is during the foetal and post-foetal stages that considerable histological and biochemical differentiation occurs. Birth has no correlation with the evolution of the nervous system: thus, depending on the species, the 'brain growth-spurt' (Dobbing, 1970) may take place in the foetal stage (guinea pig) and in the post-foetal stage (rat) or in both (man, pig).

During these stages there are no new anatomical structures except the formation of the corpus callosum and foliation of the cerebellum. Two fundamental processes take place during these stages: growth and differentiation (Fig. 3). They have been specially studied in the cerebellum and in the brain.

Winick and Noble (1966) demonstrated that brain growth results from two consecutive processes, namely cell multiplication as reflected by DNA content, and increase in cell size as estimated by the protein

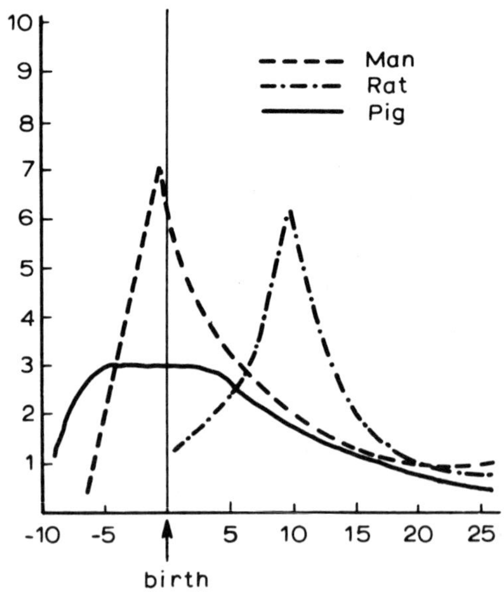

Fig. 3a. Variations of the dates of brain growth-spurt in various species. According to Dobbing.

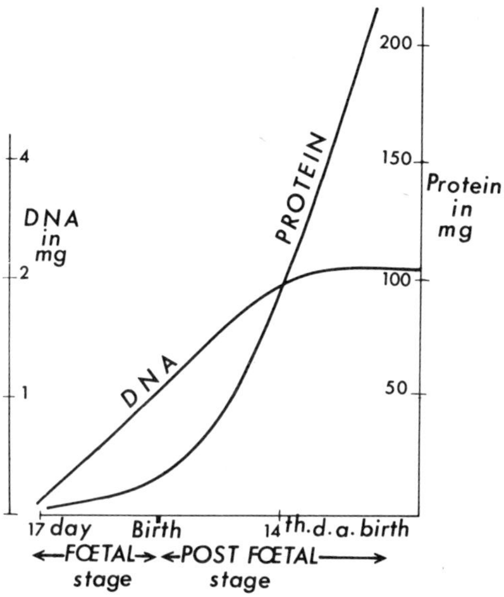

Fig. 3b. The two processes in growth of rat brain: cell multiplication (DNA), cell size increase (protein). According to Winick and Noble.

content. Dobbing and Sands (1970) emphasised that the neurological tissue occupies a predominant place in the last part of the brain growth-spurt time.

Histologically, there is a multiplication of neuroblasts followed by their migration and their progressive differentiation into neurons. The process of myelination takes place a little later.

During these stages there is also biochemical differentiation. There is at first an increase of metabolism (Flexner, 1955). An increased protein synthesis has been evidenced by the rapid influx of glucose ^{14}C into amino-acids (Pitts and Quick, 1967). According to Vos *et al.* (1967), a great activity of many enzymes occurs at the rapid growth period, such as γ-aminobutyric acid, and γ-aminobutyric transaminase.

Disturbances During the Foetal and Post-Foetal Stages and Their Causes

As in the embryonic stage, many factors may disturb development during the foetal and post-foetal stages, but the results are very different. There are very few anatomical malformations, but many histological alterations.

(i) Physical Factors

X-rays on the 18-19th day in the rat hampered the formation of the corpus callosum and foliation of cerebellum. In the early phase of the foetal stage cases of microcephaly may be induced.

The formation of glial cells may be affected and myelination altered (Vernadakis *et al.*, 1968). The external layer of the cerebellum is altered from the 18th day until more than a week after birth (Hicks, 1953). Physiological tests have revealed alteration of the brain (Hicks and D'Amato, 1966).

(ii) Chemical Factors

Various chemicals may be noxious.

Thyroid hormones play a considerable role, as it has been previously observed. Eayrs (1964) demonstrated its influence on the post-foetal nervous system. Thyroidectomy at birth results in a paucity of axodendritic connections and in disturbances in the development of electrical and behavioural activities. Sokoloff (1967) found that thyroxine stimulates protein synthesis in the immature brain.

Hatotani and Timiras (1967) confirm new facts by physiological tests. Thiouracil causes a chemical thyroidectomy and a cretinoid conditions in the rat (Barrnett, 1950). It seems possible that antithyroid antibodies may induce cases of cretinism by damage of the thyroid in the infant (Sutherland *et al.*, 1960).

Bilirubin is able to become fixed in some place inducing neurological damage. In cultures of newborn rat cerebellum, Silberberg *et al.* (1970) has seen swelling of neurons and myelin degeneration.

The antibiotic, isoniazid, causes a disturbance to pyridoxine metabolism and consecutively alters the evolution of the brain (Körner and Nowak, 1971).

Some substances electively alter the cerebellum. Cycasin injected into newborn mice and hamsters leads to necrosis of the external granular layer with locomotor disorders (Hirono *et al.*, 1969). Methylazoxymethanol injected on the 13-15th day of gestation in the hamster induces similar necrosis followed by regeneration, but injected soon after birth it also causes degeneration, but now followed by abnormal layering and physiological disturbances (Shimada and Langman, 1970).

During the foetal and post-foetal stages antibodies may disturb the developing brain. Auroux *et al.* (1967) in the rat observed (Fig. 4) that if antibrain antibodies are injected during the last stage of gestation, the young at two months have inferior performances on testing. The same result is noted when the injection is performed immediately after birth.

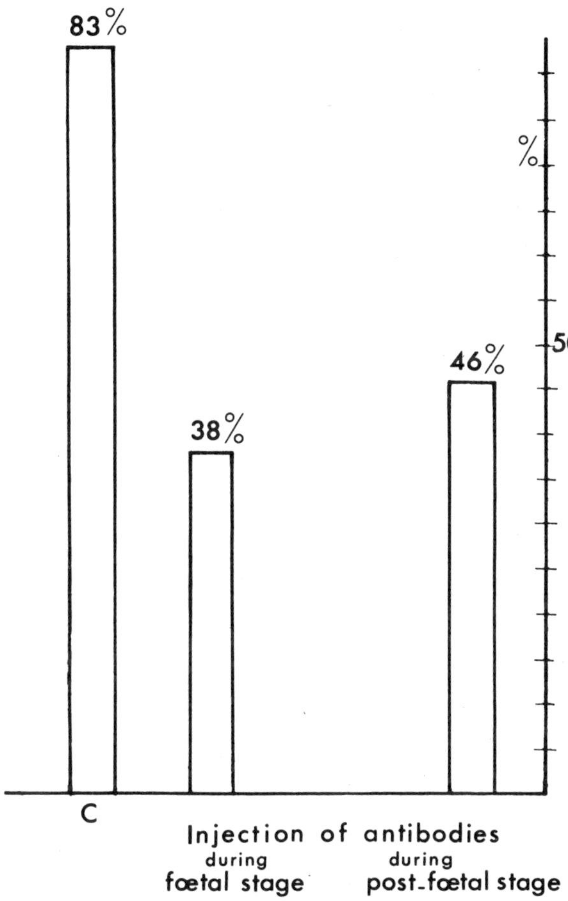

Fig. 4. Influence of antibrain antibodies on the evolution of the brain. The performance of treated are reduced. Frequency of positive results of tests in young rats; from left to right: normal treated before birth, treated after birth. According to Auroux.

(iii) Infectious Factors

Toxoplasmosis leads to localised degenerations in human brains. In sheep, the vaccine for blue tongue disease produces brain hypoplasia (Shulz and DeLay, 1955), and in rat, *Rickettsia burneti* produces a degeneration of ganglionic cells and of the optic nerve (Giroud *et al.*, 1968).

In various species many viruses are active: the viruses of mucous diarrhoea and of swine fever, the mitolytic DNA virus and the attentuated cholera virus (Kahrs *et al.*, 1970; Kilham and Margolis, 1966; Done and Harding, 1966) induce hypoplasia of the cerebellum with degeneration of the granularis externa.

(iv) Nutritional Factors

During the foetal and post-foetal stages the question of quantitative requirements becomes important, in relation to the growth of the brain.

Restriction of food has deleterious effects on the rat brain (Winick and Noble, 1966). A restriction from birth to weaning reduces cell multiplication; there is no recovery. Later it affects the protein content and recovery is possible. Restricted diet about the time of weaning reduces the brain weight and it is not corrected by refeeding (Dobbing, 1964). There is also an alteration of myelination (Davison and Dobbing, 1966). The activities in the brain of some enzymes such as creatine phosphokinase and isocitric dehydrogenase are reduced (Swaiman *et al.*, 1970).

Moreover, in the foetal and post-foetal stages a correct balance between nutrients always remains necessary.

The noxious influence of iodine deficiency is well known. Copper deficiency induces demyelination in the spinal cord of sheep (Innes, 1934) and brain alterations in the rat (Carleton and Kelly, 1969). Excess molybdenum disturbs myelination (Mills and Fells, 1960).

In the rat, vitamin A deficiency during the last two weeks of pregnancy and pursued for three months afterwards alters the myelination (Clausen, 1969). In mice, excess of vitamin A near the end of pregnancy affects the number of neurons and their differentiation (Langman and Welch, 1967).

Pyridoxine plays an important part in protein synthesis. Thus pyridoxine deficiency during gestation, and continued until weaning, causes chemical, e.g. γ-aminobutyric acid, glutamate decarboxylase and dopa-decarboxylase, and physiological disturbances in the brain (reduced performances) (Körner and Nowak, 1971).

(v) Proteins

With the growth of the foetus the requirements in proteins, containing all the essential amino-acids, are increased and a sufficient supply must be ensured to allow the synthesis of new proteins.

The results of protein-restricted diet are significant. Platt and Stewart (1968) have seen that bitches on a deficient protein diet for a long period of time give birth to young with neurological disorders. If such a diet is continued after weaning the results become worse, and recovery is imperfect. Rats on a poor protein diet from the 11th day of gestation give birth to young which have bad performances (Caldwell and Churchill, 1967). On a similar diet newborns have a reduced number of cells in the brain (Zamenhof *et al.*, 1968) and if it is continued into the post-foetal stage the brain contains only 40% of the expected number of cells (Winick, 1969) (Fig. 5).

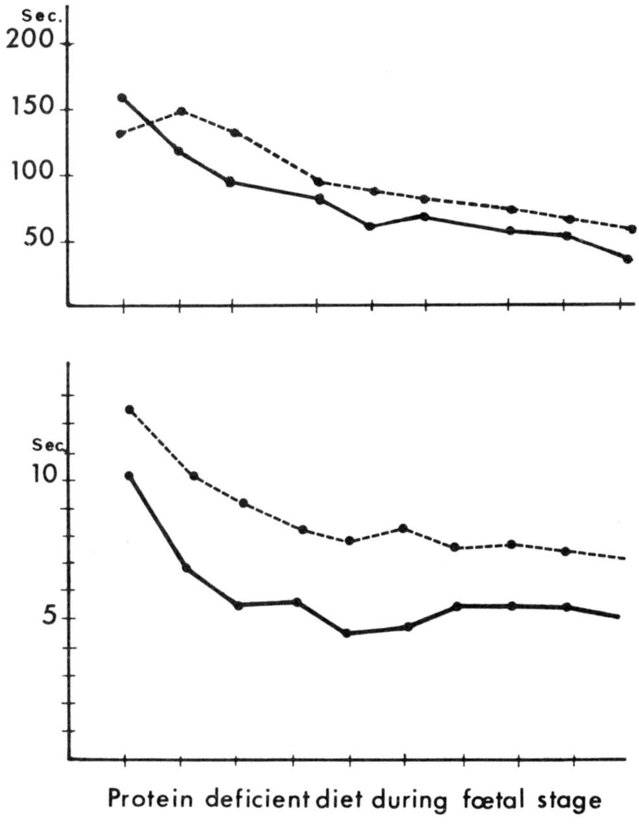

Fig. 5. Influence of a protein deficient diet on the development of the brain. The performance of the young rats on protein deficient diet (dotted line) are reduced. On the top, mean latency to traverse the Lashley III maze: on the bottom, mean latency on the pole jump avoidance test. According to Caldwell and Churchill.

Deficiency of a single amino-acid must have the same results, but an excess can also be detrimental. The last fact is well established for phenylalanine. If an excess is given to rats during gestation, the young have behaviour and intelligence disorders (Wooley and Van Der Hoven, 1964). It is the same in monkeys (Kerr *et al.*, 1968). Similar conditions, correlated to a maternal error in metabolism are well known in humans.

All these facts demonstrate that the terminal development of the brain may be particularly disturbed by an inadequate protein or amino-acid intake (see Giroud, 1970).

Conclusion

Thus, the developing nervous system appears to be very sensitive to various factors, but the repercussions of injuries vary with time, depending on the types of processes involved.

At the beginning (embryonic stage), when anatomical structures are being built up, the results of injuries are essentially anatomical malformations. Many of them are frequently followed by death at birth, or more or less later on.

In the last period (foetal and post-foetal stage) there are essentially histological and biochemical differentiation processes. This period is very important since these processes particularly involve the cerebellum and above all the cerebral cortex.

Many factors may disturb the evolution of the brain. In a few cases infectious or chemical factors produce some degeneration of the already existing structures, just as in adult pathology. Essentially, disturbances in the histological and biochemical differentiation are specially important during the 'brain growth-spurt'. The influence of nutritional factors appears predominant. At these stages the quantitative requirements become greater and greater, and restricted feeding has a noxious influence on the brain. Nevertheless, the qualitative requirements remain essential and a correct equilibrium between nutrients must be ensured: deficiency and excess are both dangerous. The effects of Iodine and Copper deficiency are well known. Vitamin B_6 deficiency alters the developing brain by reduction of protein synthesis. Nevertheless, the importance of protein and amino-acid intake remains fundamental. A restricted protein diet impedes the growth, the differentiation and the function of the cerebral cortex. The lack of an essential amino-acid or its excess (phenylalanine) are equally detrimental.

Some of these disturbances are permanent, while some may be corrected: it depends on the time of injury. Thus, such repercussions may be extremely serious in humans, for the newborn survive but remain mentally deficient.

REFERENCES

Auroux, M., Alnot, M. O. and Jouvensal, C. (1967). *C.R. Soc. Biol.* **161,** 1917.
Barnett, R. J. (1950). *Yale J. Biol. Med.* **22,** 313.
Binns, W., Anderson, W. A. and Sullivan, D. J. (1960). *J. Amer. Vet. Med. Assoc.* **137,** 515.
Brent, R. L. (1964). *Amer. J. Anat.* **115,** 525.
Brent, R. L. (1967). *Proc. Soc. Exp. Biol. Med.* **125,** 1024.
Caldwell, D. F. and Churchill, J. A. (1967). *Neurology* **17,** 95.
Carleton, W. W. and Kelly, W. A. (1969). *J. Nutrit.* **97,** 42.
Clausen, J. (1969). *European J. Biochem.* **7,** 575.
Cohlan, S. Q. (1953). *Science* **117,** 535.
David, G., Mercier-Parot, L. and Tuchmann-Duplessis, H. (1965). *C.R. Soc. Biol.* **157,** 939.
Davison, A. N. and Dobbing, J. (1966). *Brit. Med. Bull.* **22,** 40.
Dobbing, J. (1964). *Proc. Roy. Soc. Lond.* **159,** 503.
Dobbing, J. (1970). *Amer. J. Dis. Child.* **120,** 411.
Dobbing, J. and Sands, J. (1970). *Nature* **226,** 639.
Done, J. T. and Harding, J. D. J. (1966). *Proc. Roy. Soc. Med.* **59,** 1083.
Eayrs, J. T. (1964). *Arch. Biol. (Liège)* **75,** 529.
Ferm, V. H. and Kilham, L. (1963). *J. Embryol. Exp. Morph.* **2,** 659.
Flexner, L. B. (1955). In 'Biochemistry of the Developing Nervous System' (ed. Waelsch), p. 281. London: Academic Press.
Fränz, J. (1971). In 'Malformation Congénitales des Mammifères' (Colloque Pfizer), p. 151. Paris: Amboise, Masson.
Giroud, A. (1970). 'Nutrition of the Embryo'. Springfield: C. C. Thomas.
Giroud, A. and Lefebvres, J. (1951). *Arch. Franc. Pediat.* **8,** 648.
Giroud, A. and Martinet, M. (1955). *Rev. Internat. Vitaminol.* **26,** 10.
Giroud, A., Martinet, M. and Deluchat, C. (1965). *Arch. Anat. Histol. Embryol.* **48,** 205.
Giroud, A., Martinet, M. and Deluchat, C. (1966). *Bull. Soc. Opthalm. Fr.* 19th March, **3,** 1.
Giroud, A., Levy, G., Lefebvres-Boisselot, J. and Depuis, R. (1953). *Arch. Franc. Pediat.* **10,** 55.
Giroud, A., Giroud, P., Martinet, M. and Deluchat, C. (1968). *Teratology* **1,** 257.
Hatotani, N. and Timiras, P. S. (1967). *Neuroendocrinol.* **2,** 147.
Hicks, S. P. (1953). *Amer. J. Roentgenol.* **49,** 272.
Hicks, S. P. and D'Amato, C. J. (1966). In 'Advances in Teratology' (ed. Woollam), p. 196. London: Academic Press.
Hirono, I., Shibuya, C. and Hayashi, K. (1969). *Proc. Soc. Exp. Biol. Med.* **131,** 593.
Hurley, L. S. (1969). *Amer. J. Clin. Nutrit.* **22,** 1332.
Innes, J. R. M. (1934). *Cambridge Univ. Inst. Anim. Path. Rep. Dir.* **35,** 227.
Johnson, R. T., Johnson, K. P. and Edmonds, C. J. (1967). *Science* **157,** 1066.
Kahrs, R. F., Scott, F. W. and de Lahunta, A. (1970). *Teratology* **3,** 181.
Kerr, G. R., Chamove, A. S., Harlow, H. F. and Waissman, H. A. (1968). *Pediatrics* **42,** 27.
Kilham, L. and Margolis, G. (1966). *Amer. J. Path.* **49,** 457.
Körner, W. F. and Nowak, H. (1971). In 'Malformations Congénitales des Mammifères' (Colloque Pfizer), p. 243. Paris: Amboise, Masson.
Langman, J. and Welch, G. W. (1967). *J. Compar. Neurol.* **131,** 15.
Lehmann, F. E. (1933). *Rev. Suisse Zool.* **40,** 18.
Lehmann, F. E. (1937). *Arch. f. Entwickl. Mech.* **136,** 112.

Meissier, P. E. (1969). *J. Embryol. Exp. Morph.* **21,** 309.
Mills, C. F. and Fells, B. F. (1960). *Nature* **185,** 20.
Murakami, U., Kameyama, Y. and Hoshino, K. (1969). Proc. 9th Annual Handford Biology Symp., Washington, May 5-8th, p. 755.
Murphy, M. L. (1960). *Ciba Found. Symp.* **78,** 114.
Nelson, M. M., Asling, C. W. and Evans, H. M. (1952). *J. Nutrit.* **48,** 61.
Pasteels, J. (1945). *Arch. Biol.* **56,** 105.
Persaud, T. V. N. (1969). *Naturwissenschaften* **56,** 37.
Pitts, F. N. and Quick, C. (1967). *J. Neurochem.* **14,** 561.
Platt, B. S. and Stewart, R. J. C. (1968). *Develop. Med. Child. Neurol.* **10,** 3.
Roux, Ch., Fournier, P., Dupuis, Y. and Dupuis, R. (1962). *Biol. Neonat.* **4,** 371.
Rugh, R. (1958). *J. Pediat.* 1952, 531.
Rugh, R. (1965). *Excerpta Medica Int. Congr. Ser. No. 105,* 1356.
Rugh, R. and Grupp, E. (1959). *J. Neuropath. Exp. Neurol.* **18,** 468.
Runner, M. N. (1959). *Pediatrics* **23,** 245.
Russel, L. B. (1950). *J. Exp. Zool.* **114,** 545.
Russel, L. B. and Russel, W. L. (1954). *J. Cell. Compar. Physiol.* **43,** 103.
Shimada, M. and Langman, J. (1970). *Teratology* **3,** 119.
Schultz, G. and DeLay, P. D. (1955). *J. Amer. Vet. Med. Assoc.* **127,** 224.
Silberberg, D. H., Johnson, L. and Ritter, L. (1970). *J. Pediat.* **77,** 386.
Sokoloff, L. (1967). *Amer. J. Dis. Child.* **114,** 488.
Stempak, J. G. (1965). *Anat. Rec.* **151,** 287.
Sutherland, J. M., Esselborn, V. M., Burket, R. L., Skillman, T. B. and Benson, J. T. (1960). *New Engl. J. Med.* **263,** 336.
Swaiman, K. F., Daleiden, J. M. and Wolfe, R. N. (1970). *J. Neurochem.* **17,** 1387.
Tamboise, E. and Tamboise, A. (1969). *Bull. Soc. Anat,* **143,** 1625.
Tuchmann-Duplessis, H. and Mercier-Parot, L. (1958). *C.R. Acad. Sci.* **247,** 2200.
Tuchmann-Duplessis, H. and Mercier-Parot, L. (1964). *Bull. Acad. Nat. Med.* **148,** 392.
Tuchmann-Duplessis, H. and Mercier-Parot, L. (1969). *C.R. Acad. Sci.* **269,** 2147.
Vernadakis, A., Casper, R. and Timiras, P. S. (1968). *Experientia* **24,** 237.
Vos, J., Schade, J. P. and Van Der Helm, H. J. (1967). In 'Developmental Neurology' (eds Bernhard and Schade), p. 193. Elsevier: Amsterdam.
Warkany, J. and Schraffenberger, E. (1944). *Proc. Soc. Exp. Biol. Med.* **57,** 49.
Wegner, G. (1966). Autoradiographische Untersuchungen des DNS-Synthese. Habilitationsschrift, Freiburg-im-Breisgau, Universität.
Wilson, J. G. and Karr, J. W. (1951). *Amer. J. Anat.* **88,** 1.
Winick, M. (1969). *Pediatrics* **74,** 667.
Winick, M. and Noble, A. (1966). *J. Nutrit.* **89,** 300.
Wooley, D. W. and Van Der Hoeven, T. (1964). *Science* **144,** 883.
Zamenhof, S., Van Marthens, E. and Margolis, F. L. (1968). *Science* **160,** 322.

DISCUSSION

Magee: I wonder if Prof. Giroud can give us some views on the best species or methods for assaying chemicals and drugs for their teratogenic action?
Giroud: It is certainly useful to study the noxious effects of various

chemicals on the brain during the foetal and post-foetal stages, and the possible recovery. It is interesting to note at birth or at weaning the morphological and biochemical changes, but it is necessary, as in the case of lack of nutrients, to see if later there is recovery, by doing chemical and physiological tests on the young. Now, the results of such experiments are not always in accord, but the variable timing of these experiments is probably the explanation. In some cases there is no recovery: thus in vitamin B_6 deficiency in the rat, if the vitamin is given before weaning there is recovery but if this is done after this time there is no further recovery.

Dobbing: Might I suggest to Dr. Magee that if one takes into account the different timing of the events in relation to birth in the different species, it does not too much matter which species one uses, and one should be guided by which is the most convenient. Might I also suggest that we should be looking, in this drug testing, not only at the more obvious teratological anomalies, but also at the animal's performance induced by changes too slight to be normally discernible.

Richter: Could I suggest that these differences might come from their ability to detoxicate some of the compounds?

Giroud: There is some discussion about the definitive results because the timing of experiments is not always the same in each case and timing is very important. Usually we distinguish between two consecutive phenomena, but between them there are also the complex cellular differentiation. The results must depend on the timing of the action of various external factors. So the question is complicated and it is necessary to study the results of such timing not only at birth and at weaning, but afterwards to know whether there is recovery, and how much agreement there is about these findings.

Kirman: I have long been intrigued by brain antibodies, can someone tell me of clinical work in this area?

Giroud: There are few cases of antibodies having an action in human foetuses. Nevertheless, it must be noted that women having high circulatory levels of antithyroid antibodies may give birth to cretinoid children (Sutherland, J. M., Esselborn, V. M., Burket, R. L., Skillman, T. B. and Benson, J. T., *New Engl. Med. J.*, 1960, **263**, 336-341).

Zlotnik: I have the impression that with antibodies and the brain one has to be cautious. In those reactions with brain damage a cell mediated immunity is more important, and humoral antibodies do not act at all. This has been shown by using immuno-suppressants and giving a virus peripherally. In such a situation an antibody complex may take part in the damage, but circulating antibodies do not seem to play the same part in the brain.

Kirman: What about maternal antibodies?

Zlotnik: I have got the impression that maternal antibodies do not reach the brain. How could they reach the brain? Generally, even a virus very seldom penetrates to the foetus.

Kirman: What I meant was a similar mechanism as is thought to apply to the thyroid, suppressing thyroid growth by antithyroid antibodies in the mother.

Wigglesworth: How specific are cerebral antibodies?

Stern: Caspary and Field have done some work on circulating antibodies in a variety of neurological diseases, and so possibly one could see if any damaged infant has been reported in mothers where these are present.

Zlotnik: I do not think they apply to neonatal life.

Stern: Their cases are applicable to adult patients. If any of those mothers subsequently have children, you would have evidence whether or not this is true.

Zlotnik: I don't agree. Even with infections where antibodies can be demonstrated in a foetus or immediately after birth, you find that if you deprive this animal of its colostrum it has no antibodies. Such has been shown in louping-ill. This can also be shown by removing the lamb by Caesarian section the day before birth; this lamb has no antibodies while the mother has a very high level. Complete protection occurs after 24 hours from antibodies in the colostrum. I do not think antibodies can penetrate the placenta.

Davison: Isn't it true that a high proportion of normal people have circulating antimyelin antibodies? There is no evidence at all that antibodies produce an effect in the foetus.

Kirman: I'm still not clear whether a situation like that which produces experimental encephalomyelitis in the adult might not apply to the foetus.

Richter: Taylor and Levine (*Biol. Psychiat.* 1970, **2**, 279-283) have recently reported the birth of brain-damaged and stillborn offspring to mothers who developed prepartum 'process schizophrenia' within the first three months of gestation. The evidence suggests a foetal antibody response but other interpretations are also possible.

Woollam: I have been interested in teratology for 15 to 20 years and I've taken the view that one ought to give the insult to the mother about the 9th or 12th day in the rat. Recently, we have found that we can attack the blastocyst with an insult like hypovitaminosis A to the mother. If you look at this with the E.M. about a day after this insult you do get very large numbers of dead cells and an unusual-looking blastocyst. If you leave it for two or three days afterwards then it looks pretty normal and will go on to term. I get the impression that the nervous system is a good deal more labile at the very earliest stages than later on.

Giroud: According to Rugh x-rays may induce some cases of exencephaly during the blastogenic stage and perhaps it was the result of chromosome alteration. Usually no malformations are produced at this stage; either the blastocyst dies completely or if some cells die the others regenerate and there is no malformation. Whether they were without later alterations was not stated, since the foetuses were killed at birth.

Another question concerns the date of the detrimental action which occurs in some cases of mental retardation with small anatomical malformations; experiments show that anatomical malformations are induced during the embryonic stage, and that the histological changes arise later. The development of nervous system being a continuum of linked events, it is possible that mental retardation has its origin in such primary disturbances.

General Discussion

INTRODUCED BY J. DOBBING

I suppose the question we have been addressing ourselves to can be stated in general terms, thus: Are there interferences which one can impose on the developing brain which outlast all attempts at rehabilitation? I suppose it's perfectly natural that we should have been talking most of our time about the things we know most about, namely the teratology of the problem, which is only one example of permanent effects of early interference. The essential feature of teratology, which we have been reiterating, is the timing of the insults, and this period in human terms is during the first trimester. Now it is possible, although I believe none of us have any evidence, that during this time lesser degrees of damage also have permanent effects that could conceivably account for the unclassified cases of mental retardation. But it would be as well to remember that we are now finding evidence that the third human trimester and beyond is also a period in which permanent detectable anatomical, behavioural and neurochemical changes occur in the brain which are not obvious to the ordinary morbid anatomist. In the third trimester as Prof. Giroud has shown there occurs in the human a brain growth spurt. Let us say about the vulnerability of the brain growth spurt that we now know that during this time there need be only very mild restrictions of environment, and despite all efforts at rehabilitation traces of these can be detected in the adult brain. Although by necessity only rather crude estimates can be made, the brain is ultimately smaller, if you mildly restrict the total diet of the animal during the brain growth spurt. But it is not just a reduction in size. There is also a distortion of the proper architecture both anatomically and biochemically. Moreover, perhaps more significantly, one produces a brain that is too small for the size of the animal: it is small in particular regions, and the cerebellum is specifically and grossly reduced in the long term. Here I might take issue with the suggestion that has been made that a small deficit in the number of cells probably does not reduce sophistication. You can reduce the number of cells by

10-15% in the adult by this means, and since they are regional focal and not diffuse losses, this becomes a matter of significance. It is likely that much less than a 10% loss when confined to certain areas of the brain is going to produce some functional consequences. Not only do distortions of the lipid pattern of the brain show themselves, but also evidence of distortions of enzymic pattern are accumulating, and behavioural studies are beginning to yield information particularly in relation to the cerebellum.

I am particularly looking forward to the contribution by Dr. Drillien on long term effects of slower intrauterine growth. I hope we will discuss the finding that babies who have not grown well during the last trimester, or premature babies badly cared for or growing badly after birth, are showing permanent deficits in the only thing you can measure about the brain, the head circumference.

Davison: In Phenylketonuria, as a well-defined condition producing mental retardation, is it not true that children born to an untreated case develop normal mental functions, whereas a child born with phenylketonuria is retarded? If true, does this not suggest that the postnatal development is critical to intellectual development? Women with marked phenylketonuria may not, I believe, give rise to intellectually retarded children.

Clayton: From untreated mothers the chances of a severely damaged child are very high. Fifty-eight very badly damaged infants are known in the literature out of 62 recorded. The question is how early in pregnancy do you have to lower the blood level in the mother in order to get a normal infant. Microcephaly is very common and also other congenital abnormalities, e.g. dwarfism, congenital hearts and so on.

Stern: If the levels of phenylalanine are below 15-20 mg/100 ml, the chances of having a child not too badly damaged or normal are reasonably good. If the level is over 15-20 mg/100 ml then nearly always you get the syndrome. But there is probably no absolutely safe upper level because of the multifactorial nature of the problem.

There may be a slight risk even to the child of a heterozygous mother, because the placenta concentrates phenylalanine.

Dobbing: And there are examples where normal infants mistakenly treated with a low phenylalanine diet have ended with I.Q. levels of 80 without any other apparent cause than the diet.

Davison: Evidence suggests that it is around birth and for a period after birth that whatever changes are occurring are critical for mental development.

Crome: The brain changes in children born to phenylketonuric mothers seem to be quite different from the disease itself. The reason is unclear.

Cremer: In fairly mild nutritional deficiency what period is irrecoverable and at what stage on restoration to full nutrition does the animal recover completely?

Dobbing: It is said that you must cover the whole growth period by nutritional restriction, but it is known that the restriction needs to be less the closer one is to the growth spurt. It is alleged that if nutrition is restricted during the first one-quarter or so of the growth spurt and then rehabilitated that in crude quantitative terms there is apparently full recovery. But it is difficult to believe that you would recover from specific anatomical derangements inflicted in the first quarter, although the number of cells may recover.

Balázs: It was surprising to me when I began to work in this field to find that the early postnatal development may be so important to future development.

Due to their dramatic effects, people were previously inclined to place undue emphasis upon genetic factors and embryonic life as very important determinants for future interaction and behavioural performance. Now it seems that man resembles in many respects the smaller experimental animals, usually called 'nest' animals, although man in an evolutionary sense is not a 'nest' animal, although he has become one in a functional sense. This is reflected in the way cell formation and neuronal differentiation carries on after birth. It would probably, therefore, be advisable to re-evaluate some of the ideas as to the vulnerability of cerebral functions, for it seems likely that the early postnatal period is playing a much more important role than we hitherto thought.

Dobbing: The events of normal birth is of no importance at all for brain development, unlike many other organs.

Magee: Could I ask Dr. Prestige more about cell death? This may be due to failure of vascular supply, according to Dr. Woollam. How far has this been studied in detail?

Prestige: The evidence for cell death is the presence of pyknotic nuclei, and that the numbers go down. But the rate of degeneration cannot be decided from the presence of pyknotic nuclei, unless you know how long each cell takes in that phase. The quantitative data are somewhat restricted in interpretation.

Zlotnik: How much can you trust the presence of pyknosis? Certain manipulations at death can increase pyknotic nuclei.

Jellinger: This is the old problem of the so-called 'dark neurone'.

Zlotnik: The method of fixation and handling is very important.

Prestige: The rate of decline of cell number produces a curve that follows the curve of the number of pyknotic nuclei, and it is difficult to get away from the conclusion that there is cell loss.

Zlotnik: I would like to know whether multiplication of neurones takes place in tissue culture. It seems that usually they only survive, not multiply.

Prestige: Sidman has shown that cultures of human cells show evidence on H^3-thymidine labelling that uptake occurs in the neurones in these cultures.

Sylvester: May I ask Dr. Dobbing about learning in the postnatal period? Is there any evidence that stimulation of any sort helps the brain to grow?

Dobbing: There is all this work on 'gentling' and the brain growing bigger. How much is somatic and how much is regional is not clear. There is the work of Rosensweig and Krech who brought rats up in an enriched environment compared with restricted animals, claiming that this does specifically lead to an enlargement of parts of the cortex. Much of this is *sub-judice.*

Drillien: It has been suggested that prematurely delivered infants who are in the light when they should be in the dark are in fact advanced visually. Taking the post-conceptual age they fix and focus at an earlier age than infants who have spent the full 40 weeks in the dark.

Richter: It is reported that myelination of the central nervous system is more advanced in a seven-month-old baby than in an ordinary nine-month-old baby, suggesting that the axons at birth can affect the brain to some extent.

Dobbing: It has always been a big puzzle to me why the guinea pig foetus which is a prenatal-brain developer, opens its eyes a good two weeks before it is born.

Balázs: Giving cortisone to rats, which open their eyes late, somehow you trigger epithelial growth and the eye opens around 9-10 days. None the less, the morphological development of the neurones in the visual cortex are not advanced, so that although the eyes open the system does not operate.

Crome: May I ask Dr. Balázs whether we are born with a full complement of neurones or not? I understood him to say we are not. What is the evidence for this?

Balázs: What I want to establish by future research is whether or not we are born with a full complement of neurones. I think there is evidence that the cerebellum in man does not contain at birth the full complement of nerve cells. I am making the analogy that the microneurones of the cerebellum are formed at the same time as other microneurones in the cerebrum, e.g. in the hippocampus, in a number of other species. Why should man be different? This is work for morphologists, however.

Crome: To return to Dr. Zlotnik's interesting point about antibodies penetrating into the brain, in a recent symposium (Brent, R. L., 1966, in 'Advances in Teratology', ed. D. H. M. Woollam, Vol. I, p. 81, Logos Press, New York), it was suggested from experimental work that antibodies might be a cause of teratological defects in man. He said that they do not pass the placenta. What is the evidence?

Zlotnik: Virological studies do not provide any evidence that antibodies can get into the brain, and there is no specific method by which you can show that antibodies have entered the brain.

Giroud: Experiments on isolated neural tissues have demonstrated that antibodies may disturb their evolution. *In vivo* it has been suggested that malformations produced by antibodies may be the result of an indirect action: a disturbance in the placental function or in the mother's metabolism.

Kirman: There has been a lot of work with regard to the sympathetic system and antibodies. It was suggested that inhibition of growth of the parasympathetic nervous system could be achieved by specific antibodies.

Zlotnik: It is possible that they might have a peripheral effect rather than central one. But the immunity mechanisms are very different in the brain. If a mouse or hamster is given an attenuated strain of Western encephalitis virus, s/c or i/p, and at the same time given cyclophosphamide, then when challenged four days later with virulent virus they will die, because no antibodies are formed due to immuno-suppression. If, on the other hand, the attenuated strain is given intracerebrally and immuno-suppression caused by cyclophosphamide, then on challenge four days later the animals remain healthy. The suppression of all immune responses did not affect the brain. This work is not yet published, but it definitely shows that immune mechanisms are different in the brain from any other part of the body. One has to be very careful.

Kirman: Professor Giroud mentioned soft water as a cause. Is there more to this, or is it just speculation?

Giroud: Some years ago Penrose (1957, *J. Ment. Defic. Res.* **1**, 11), suggested that there was a noxious influence in some water. The recent observations of Lowe *et al.* (1971, *Brit. Med. J.* **2**, 35) have given clearer evidence concerning the influence of soft water on the appearance of anencephaly and spina bifida: the lack of a trace element other than calcium being envisaged. The necessity of various trace elements appear more and more important. Recently Hurley and Swenerton (1971, *Nutrition* **101**, 599) have demonstrated that even a very short deficiency of zinc is sufficient to induce malformations. There are stores in the body, but they are difficult to mobilise. I think that the lack of trace elements in water may be an explanation for the appearance of some malformations, perhaps in association with other causes, since we know that frequently the genetic background plays a role, and also other factors, as indicated by seasonal variations.

Zlotnik: The analogy in animals is the disease swayback, occurring in sheep on copper-deficient soils. It has not been produced experimentally in animals.

Harris: Can I make a general point? We all know from clinical experience that certain children appear to be at risk to become mentally defective, but yet in fact do very well. It might be helpful to look at children in vulnerable situations who have yet withstood the onslaught subjected to and have developed normally.

Laurence: If you look at perinatal deaths where there is an obvious anoxic episode more often than not no brain damage is found in survivors.

Richter: The method of screening is not always easy. A group of children with encephalitis have been followed up, and those with no neurological damage, none the less, showed a statistically greater list of abnormalities in their school reports, not at any other level.

Stern: Work done on children with severe malnutrition showed that without stimulation the right diet was ineffective, and vice versa. Psychological stimulation was therefore also needed as well as correction of the diet.

Dobbing: There is an even more telling account of this by Dr. Elsie Widdowson (1951, *Lancet* **i**, 1316) in relation to groups of German children soon after the War. Two groups were quite fortuitously differently stimulated and differently fed, and then the treatments were crossed over; good growth depended upon the stimulation not the nutrition.

2

Biochemical Aspects of the Developing Brain

The Effects of Pre-natal Growth Inhibition on Brain Composition

J. S. WIGGLESWORTH

Clinical and Experimental Background

Foetal Growth Retardation

Considerable variations of intrauterine growth rate have long been recognised in litter-bearing animals, such as guinea-pigs and rabbits, where there has been shown to be an inverse relationship between litter size and birth weight of individuals within the litter (Ibsen, 1928; Hammond, 1934). The idea that intrauterine growth of the human foetus also might in certain circumstances be impaired, with resultant short or long term effects on physical and mental development, is a surprisingly recent one, dating from the description by McBurney (1947). The recognition of the variability of human foetal growth rate was long delayed by the description of all babies below 2500 g as 'premature', irrespective of the supposed length of gestation, so that the variations in outcome of different groups of low birth weight babies went unrecognised. Over the past 10 years, however, it has been increasingly realised that impairment of human intrauterine growth is an important and frequent phenomenon.

Early experiments carried out on several animal species showed that impairment of maternal nutrition in pregnancy could also cause retardation of foetal growth in animals such as rats (Barry, 1920) and sheep (Wallace, 1948). Anatomical studies of the retarded foetuses produced in these experiments showed that there was considerable reduction in growth of muscle tissue and certain body organs, including liver, but relatively little overall weight reduction in the CNS. The effects of intrauterine starvation on growth of the foetus seemed similar to the effects of starvation on weight of the different organs in the adult, with sparing of the CNS until the final stages of inanition.

When it became recognised that the human foetus also could suffer from growth impairment, interest was soon aroused in the long term effects that this might have on physical and mental development. Some early studies indicated that the outlook was very poor, e.g. Warkany *et al.* (1961), whereas others suggested that it might be relatively favourable (Pick, 1954). More recently it has become apparent that type and timing of action of growth inhibitory influences may be important in determining the ultimate effect. Naeye (1965a & b) pointed out on the basis of quantitative histological studies on organs other than the brain that decrease in size might, in general terms, be associated with predominant decrease either in cell size or in cell population. He found that decreased *cell numbers* were the more characteristic feature of babies with malformations, particularly those with minor cardiac malformations, whereas decreased *cell size* was the major feature of organs from growth retarded babies whose mothers had toxaemia. There was always some decrease in cell population, in liver parenchyma and exocrine cells of the pancreas for instance, even in the toxaemia group. The inference to be drawn from this work was that there might well be variations in cell populations in the brain in different types of intrauterine growth retardation.

Biochemical Approach to Cell Population of Organs

The concept that in any species all diploid cell nuclei contain the same quantity of DNA enables an estimate of the cell population of any tissue to be made on the basis of its total DNA content, a far less tedious approach than is involved in assessment of cell populations by morphometric techniques. If additional measurements of weight, total protein and RNA are also made, it is possible to compute averages for cell size and protein and RNA content. This approach was first utilised in the study of organ growth in the rat by Enesco and Leblond (1962) but has been extensively exploited by Winick and his colleagues in New York (e.g. Winick and Noble, 1966; Winick, 1969) and used also by Dobbing and others.

For each organ Winick has defined three phases of growth, an initial phase of increase in cell number, followed by a phase of increase in both number and size of cells and, finally, a phase of increase in cell size alone. The transition from one phase to another depends on slowing down and finally cessation of DNA synthesis. In the whole rat brain DNA synthesis stops at 17 days but protein continues to increase until 3 months age. Malnutrition of the rat occurring from birth interferes with cell division so that the animal is left with a permanent deficit in cell numbers in the brain and other organs even after refeeding. Malnutrition imposed after 21 days age has no effect on cell number in the brain but prevents normal increase in protein with a consequent decreased 'cell size'. The latter change is reversible with rehabilitation.

Here, clearly might be an explanation for the finding that some small-for-dates infants develop well after birth but others do poorly. This is not a simple problem as the time course of cell proliferation may vary from one organ to another, and indeed, from one cell type to another. In Winick's experiments (Winick, 1969) if the rat brains were divided into different regions each showed its own pattern of response to malnutrition. In rats malnourished from birth, the cerebellum showed a reduced DNA content by six days of age but the cerebral cortex remained unaffected until 14 days. The time course of brain development in man is very different from that in the rat. Dobbing has shown that there is a growth spurt, apparently in the neurones, at the end of the first trimester in man and that the growth spurt in the glia occurs over a longer period from early in the 3rd trimester until several months post-natal age (Dobbing and Sands, 1970).

If Winick's findings in the rat are applicable also to man, the variation in brain cell numbers and variation in post-natal brain growth might be related to the time course of action of growth inhibiting influences in intrauterine life. In the experimental animal the most severe reduction in brain cell population as well as in growth potential generally is seen in doubly deprived animals, that is animals subjected to malnutrition both *in utero* and after birth. It would seem that pre-natal malnutrition renders an animal unduly susceptible to the growth retarding effects of neonatal malnutrition.

Winick and Rosso (1969) have shown that perinatal malnutrition in man is indeed associated with reduction in brain cell population. The brains of Chilean children who had died of malnutrition in the first year of life all had lower total DNA levels than normal and in several the figure was down to 40% of the expected value. Comparison of head circumference with brain weight and biochemical measurements indicated that brain weight and protein content were decreased in proportion to the decrease in head circumference, whereas DNA was reduced to an even greater extent. These findings not only confirm that low brain cell population occurs in man in association with impairment in perinatal nutrition, but also that measurements of head circumference in the young child may genuinely reflect the adequacy of brain growth.

The use of total organ DNA as a measure of cell population in the brain or any other organ is of course a remarkably crude procedure, since the structure of two brains with the same total cell population could differ very considerably. The ideal method of study of cellular growth would be to combine this approach with morphometric studies of the relative numbers of different cell types.

Biochemical Changes other than Variations in Cell Population

There is no reason to expect that efficiency of brain function will be related in any straightforward way to cell population. A lowered cell population is, however, an indication of the action of some growth inhibiting influence and is likely to be associated with other biochemical changes which may be more directly related to impaired brain function. One such possible factor is impairment in myelination. Myelin is a complex and stable lipid which contains a high proportion of the total brain cholesterol. It has been shown that malnutrition during the phase of most rapid myelination in the rat and in the pig causes reduction in brain cholesterol which persists despite rehabilitation (Davison and Dobbing, 1966). This effect might be due to reduction in the number of cells available for myelin synthesis, but there is some evidence that lowered activity of enzymes involved in myelin synthesis may be partly responsible (Chase *et al.*, 1967). Myelination like brain cell multiplication is a 'once only' process which has to be completed within its set time scale.

Other biochemical changes involving lowering of enzyme levels may well prove to be of equal importance.

Specific Growth Inhibition in Man

Quite apart from the effects of malnutrition there is evidence that small-for-dates infants may be born with low organ cell populations as a result of the action of a number of growth inhibitors *in utero.* Intrauterine infection with the rubella virus is one obvious example (Naeye, 1965b). Affected infants are born with low head circumference so that, although no brain DNA measurements have to my knowledge been made on such infants, we can reasonably conclude that they are likely to have low brain cell populations. Many teratogenic agents are known to inhibit mitotic activity and indeed many malformed babies are small-for-dates. At necropsy such infants show reduction in brain size in proportion to the overall reduction in body size. It seems logical to postulate that a growth inhibiting influence which impairs differentiation in one organ may suppress a generation of cell divisions in all organs with resultant limitation in growth potential.

Experimental Studies on Foetal Growth Retardation in the Rat

Introduction

My own studies on foetal growth retardation have not been directed specifically at investigation of brain development but have involved study of the conditions under which foetal growth can be inhibited experimentally, the effects on different organs, including the brain, and the modifying effects of varying timing and severity of growth retarding stress.

The rat has been used for cheapness and convenience although it is arguable that this is not the ideal species for studies on intrauterine brain development in foetal growth retardation.

We have used several models of foetal growth retardation including uterine vessel ligation, maternal starvation, and administration of specific chemical growth inhibitors. Because of a variety of difficulties associated with long term studies most of the experiments have involved killing the animals at term.

Uterine Vessel Ligation

In the early uterine vessel ligation experiments (Wigglesworth, 1964) studies on the brain concerned only the effects on brain weight, in absolute terms and relative to body weight. Following unilateral vessel ligation on day 16 of pregnancy the organs of foetuses killed on day 20 (24 hours before delivery was expected) showed changes resembling those of the human infant of a mother with toxaemia, or the foetus of an animal starved in pregnancy with considerable reduction in birth weight, namely marked reduction in weight of internal organs such as liver, but minor reduction in weight of the brain.

More recently we have returned to this particular growth retardation model to see how variations in severity of growth retardation were related to changes in size and cell population of different organs (Keith and Wigglesworth, in preparation). Laparotomy was performed under ether anaesthesia on day 16 of pregnancy (date of finding sperms in vagina is day 0) and the number of viable conceptuses counted in each uterine horn. Provided that there were four or more implantations in each horn unilateral ligation of the uterine vessels was performed as described previously (Wigglesworth, 1964) ligating the more, or less, crowded horn in alternate animals. The rats were killed on day 21 and the foetuses removed, weighed and decapitated. Two foetuses were selected for sampling from each animal. From the ligated horn the survivor nearest to the site of ligature was selected and from the control horn the foetus whose weight was closest to the mean for the horn was sampled. As there was no consistent association between foetal weight and position in the control horn and a variable number of foetuses might have died following operation in the ligated horn, the foetuses sampled from each horn might come from any horn position. Brains, livers, kidneys, hearts and placentae were weighed and the larger organs analysed for DNA, RNA and protein content.

For each animal organ weight variations and biochemical parameters were expressed in relation to the degree of growth retardation of the foetus from the ligated horn as compared to the foetus from the control horn. There was a straight line relationship between the reduction in body weight and the reduction in weight of brain, liver and kidneys. The reduction in brain weight was, however, very much less than that of liver and kidneys: the most severely retarded foetus, with a body weight 45% below that of its control, had a brain weight reduction of 15% and 60% reduction in weight of liver and kidneys. Total brain DNA was reduced by no more than 8% although that of the liver and kidneys was reduced by 50%.

The changes in the brain although less marked than those in other organs were highly significant and indicated a reduction both in cell population and average cell mass in proportion to the degree of body weight reduction. Although total brain RNA and protein were reduced there was no constant change in the concentration of protein or RNA per cell. The change in average cell mass may be a genuine phenomenon or it may be due to selective loss of large cells within the brain as we have not performed morphometric studies on these foetuses.

One possibility that we considered was that the changes in organ weight and structure in the retarded foetuses might just be an accentuation of changes seen in foetuses of varying weight within the control uterine horn. By an analysis of covariance procedure we could show that this was not so for brain weight or average cell mass but it remained a possibility as far as changes in cell number were concerned.

Inhibition of DNA and Protein Synthesis

A separate series of experiments performed by Dr. B. Klionsky involved the administration of chemical growth inhibitors to pregnant rats (Klionsky and Wigglesworth, 1970).

Most of the work carried out with growth inhibitors in pregnancy has been concerned with the interruption of pregnancy or with the teratogenic activities of these substances. There has been very little study of their effects on foetal growth and development if given after the period of organogenesis. The drugs we used were hydroxyurea and cycloheximide. Hydroxyurea prevents DNA synthesis by inhibiting conversion of ribonucleotides to desoxyribonucleotides (Chaube and Murphy, 1966). It is rapidly equilibrated in body water and may be excreted unchanged in the urine or actively metabolized to urea. The half life of the plasma concentration is only 30-60 min and the cytotoxic effects are limited to cells undergoing DNA synthesis. The drug does not damage cells which are not in division and allows growth and differentiation of existing cells to proceed normally (Gale, 1968). Cycloheximide inhibits protein synthesis at the ribosomal level without inhibiting RNA synthesis by preventing transfer of amino-acids from soluble (transfer) RNA to the forming polypeptide chain (Trakatellis *et al.*, 1966). The inhibitory effects begin soon after administration and reach a peak with 1-2 hours.

Each drug was given at two separate time intervals in pregnancy, either at 15 days or at 18 days. The time course of pregnancy in the rat is such that 15 days is just after the completion of organogenesis and 18 days is about the latest time for treatment if a significant effect on foetal growth is to be produced by the time of delivery (22 days).

Following preliminary trials, doses of each drug were selected to result in foetuses retarded by two or more standard deviations in weight below the mean of control foetuses at term. Administration of either drug produced growth retarded foetuses who differed little in their external appearances.

When either drug was given at 15 days the brain weights were reduced in proportion to the reduction in body weight, this reduction being of the order of 20-25%. In the hydroxyurea group the reduction in total brain DNA was similar to that of brain weight, whereas in the cycloheximide group it was rather less.

Administration of either drug on day 18 resulted in reduction of brain weight by only 5-10%; a relative sparing of brain weight as compared to body weight. Brain DNA was reduced by about 10% in the hydroxyurea group but was not significantly affected by cycloheximide. Changes in RNA and protein concentration were not significant. The livers of these animals showed a similar pattern of changes to that seen in the brain with decrease in DNA more readily produced by drug administration on day 15 than on day 18, and more readily produced by hydroxyurea than cycloheximide.

Significance of Animal Experiments in Relation to Foetal Growth Retardation in Man

These experiments are, of course, of very limited significance as far as human problems of mental retardation are concerned, and indeed are very crude even as studies on brain composition. They do, however, illustrate a number of points which may be relevant to any discussion on the brain composition of the growth-retarded human infant. They demonstrate that even in the foetal rat with a relatively immature brain there is wide variation in the extent to which brain weight, brain cell population and average cell size can be altered by different forms of growth inhibiting stress. In addition, the experiments confirm that timing is important in determining the effects of any growth retarding influence. The foetal rat is rather resistant to alterations in brain cell population in the last three days of pregnancy compared to the preceding three days. This may well be due to the foetus having passed the time of maximum growth spurt among the neurones but not having commenced the growth spurt among the glia. Certainly, judging by the result of malnutrition experiments, the rat appears to be at greater risk of cerebral growth impairment in the neonatal period than in the last three days of pre-natal life. Each type of growth retarding stress produces a characteristic pattern of changes at a particular stage in pregnancy but there may be a wide range in the severity of the changes.

Finally, although I have not made any biochemical studies on the brains of growth retarded human infants, I have looked at the way in which the weight of the brain is affected by varying degrees of growth retardation. The group I studied were babies who died during or just after birth with morphological features which indicated that they were mature, and in the absence of malformations.

As compared to the mean weight for gestation (from the data of Gruenwald, 1963) the brains of growth retarded infants may be reduced in weight by up to 30% and, as in the rats, there is a correlation between the severity of body weight reduction and the reduction in brain weight.

The sparing of brain growth at the expense of other tissues is true only in relative terms: there is a reduction in brain mass in absolute terms which must be associated with considerable disturbances in chemical composition.

I would forecast that detailed biochemical studies of these brains would show a similar wide range of variation in brain composition to that found in the growth retarded rat foetus.

REFERENCES

Barry, L. W. (1920). *Contr. Embryol.* **11**, 91.
Chase, H. P., Dorsey, J. and McKhann, G. M. (1967). *Pediatrics* **40**, 551.
Chaube, S. and Murphy, M. L. (1966). *Cancer Res.* **26**, 1448.
Davison, A. N. and Dobbing, J. (1966). *Brit. Med. Bull.* **22**, 40.
Dobbing, J. and Sands, J. (1970). *Nature* **226**, 639.
Enesco, M. and Leblond, C. (1962). *J. Embryol. Exp. Morph.* **10**, 530.

Gale, G. R. (1968). *Experientia* **24,** 57.
Gruenwald, P. (1963). *Biol. Neonat.* **5,** 215.
Hammond, J. (1934). *J. Exp. Biol.* **11,** 140.
Ibsen, H. L. (1928). *J. Exp. Zool.* **51,** 51.
Klionsky, B. and Wigglesworth, J. S. (1970). *Brit. J. Exp. Path.* **51,** 361.
McBurney, R. D. (1947). *West. J. Surg.* **55,** 363.
Naeye, R. L. (1965a). *Arch. Path.* **79,** 284.
Naeye, R. L. (1965b). *Am. J. Path.* **47,** 905.
Pick, W. (1954). *New Eng. J. Med.* **250,** 905.
Trakatellis, A. C., Montjar, M. and Axelrod, A. E. (1966). *Biochemistry* **4,** 2065.
Wallace, L. R. (1948). *J. Agric. Sci.* **38,** 93, 243, 367.
Warkany, J., Monroe, B. B. and Sutherland, B. S. (1961). *Amer. J. Dis. Child.* **102,** 2, 127.
Wigglesworth, J. S. (1964). *J. Path. Bact.* **88,** 1.
Winick, M. and Noble, A. (1966). *J. Nutr.* **89,** 300.
Winick, M. (1969). *J. Pediat.* **74,** 667.
Winick, M. and Rosso, P. (1969). *J. Pediat.* **74,** 774.

DISCUSSION

Kleihues: How did you determine cell weight?

Wigglesworth: This is mean cell weight or average weight per cell, i.e. the number of cells divided by the net weight. When looking at total protein or total RNA, that is to say the sort of indices by which one would assess cell mass, although there were reductions with body weight, there were no significant reductions in relation to DNA.

Kleihues: Were the changes in cell weight due to water uptake or to protein increase? In some experiments described with alkylating agents there is an effect called 'growth dissociation'. This is where cell division is arrested, such as with hydroxyurea, and although protein synthesis is going on, there is no increase in DNA.

Wigglesworth: Although we thought that the increase in 'average cell weight' seen in the livers of one group of animals treated with hydroxyurea was due to loss of haemopoietic cells, we might be getting such a 'growth dissociation' effect in addition. There was some suggestion that this was also occurring in the brain, but without morphometric studies we could not really say whether there had been any increase in cell cytoplasm.

Laurence: How did you weigh your brains, and how did you allow for possible oedema? Many infants dying in the neonatal period have considerable brain oedema, adding perhaps 20% to the weight. Perhaps dry weight would be more useful to correlate with body weight, or better, body length?

Wigglesworth: Certainly in some cases there is obvious oedema, but not in most of ours. Certainly it occurs in resuscitated still-births.

Laurence: Nearly all the neonatal brains that I see are oedematous, as judged by convolutional flattening and compression of the ventricles, as well as obvious congestion.

Wigglesworth: This is certainly true for a proportion, but certainly not all.

Balázs: When cell formation is blocked by cortisone in liver cells of young rats or in adults after hepatectomy, the liver weight increases due to cell enlargement with proteolipids and glycogen. In your experiments you may have produced a stress and some of the effects may have been mediated this way.

Wigglesworth: The effects of hydroxyurea in the mother were minimal. This is a very potent teratogenic agent on the foetus, but it has a remarkably little effect upon the adult.

Cremer: How well do the foetuses survive?

Wigglesworth: They seem to do very well, but remain very grossly retarded. We didn't follow them more than a week or so.

Kleihues: Hydroxyurea can be given in a dose that just inhibits DNA synthesis, but does not cause cytotoxic effects. Were your doeses in this range, or was there death of proliferating cells?

Wigglesworth: We might have caused death of proliferating cells with our double dosage scheme, but we did not look closely at this.

Prestige: This varies with the cell population. In some there is no stage where you can block DNA synthesis without some cell damage.

Drillien: Within the small-for-dates group there is a significant group where small birth weight is appropriate for them. They turn out to be perfectly normal individuals, but with small heads. They are short in stature, and their small brains seem to be perfectly adequate for all the purposes related to intelligence. This bothers me when we talk about head size. I am at present measuring the weights and head sizes of student midwives. This is a group of girls with good intelligence and their head sizes appear to correlate with stature rather than to their intelligence. I would deny rather strongly that women are less intelligent just on the grounds that they have smaller heads.

Dobbing: Per gram wet weight they are more efficient! This is an important point of confusion. What do we mean by microcephaly?

Kirman: Dr. Williams and I were interested in this. We were using for our purposes three standard deviations below Westropp and Barber's (1956, *J. Neurol. Neurosurg. Psychiat.* **19**, 52) figures and below figures for U.C. students and various convicts for adults, taking age and sex into account (Penrose, unpubl. data). The question is whether there is not a qualitative difference when you get beyond three standard deviations below the normal. I think there probably is, although we could not find any adequate norms for small people to check this point. I have not found, however, an exception amongst the clinical material to this criterion of three standard deviations that below which means microcephaly with reduction in intelligence.

Dobbing: Can Dr. Wigglesworth add to this definition from his babies? Do you take body weight and size into account?

Wigglesworth: I think the only way to do it is by the degree below the normal for the age.

Dobbing: It is surely a brain inappropriately small for the baby size.

Holt: A few years ago Illingworth (1965, *Arch. Dis. Childh.* **40**, 672) stressed the need to related head circumference to body weight rather than length because the latter is a difficult parameter to measure.

Wigglesworth: Paediatricians in practice are interested more in rate of change and growth.

Crome: It should be stressed that many microcephalics are not so at birth, when they have normal head size, the microcephaly becoming evident later.

Kirman: Also a few very early hydrocephalics end up with heads three standard deviations below the mean. Especially if there is early brain damage.

Rundle: I think one has got to be very careful of relating head-circumference or cephalic index to stature, and trying to argue from normals to young potentially mentally retarded patients. A positive correlation was found between head circumference and stature in normal adults, but when we carried out a large number of measurements in young mentally retarded cases, the head measurements were least adequately correlated with any other parameters. There are dangers inherent in drawing conclusions from such correlations.

Kirman: It is a question of the order of the change, I think. In gross mental retardation, of course, the correlations are fairly gross.

Dobbing: The definition of microcephaly is undoubtedly a source of great difficulty among doctors, which we sometimes rather take for granted.

Hormonal Aspects of Brain Development

ROBERT BALÁZS

Hormones are known to affect behaviour: reversible mental changes have been observed in patients receiving adrenocortical therapy, and mental changes are frequently associated with the dysfunction of endocrine glands. In the adult, normal behaviour may be restored by remedial treatment of the endocrine disorder. On the other hand, the behavioural anomalies appear to be permanent when they result from hormonal imbalance occurring during certain periods of the development of the CNS (cf. Harris, 1964; Barraclough, 1967; Phoenix *et al.*, 1967; Levine and Mullins, 1968; Eayrs, 1968: Howard and Granoff, 1968). There is evidence that the altered behaviour is associated with permanent changes in terms of the morphology and the biochemistry of the CNS (cf. Eayrs, 1968; Balázs, 1971). In the studies reviewed, extreme experimental conditions have sometimes been used, but similar anomalies with variable severity may also occur in pathological conditions. The experimental animals used in most of the studies reviewed were rats or mice, which are relatively immature at birth: the effects of hormones on brain development could therefore be studied with relative ease. The experimental observations can be related to those in man which, as a 'mother-clinging' animal in the evolutionary sense, 'has become a sort of nest animal' (Robinson and Tizard, 1966).

Effect of Thyroid State

The effects of thyroid state on brain development have recently been reviewed (Eayrs, 1968; Balázs, 1971). Therefore the results which are most pertinent for the following discussion will only be briefly summarised.

It appears that thyroid hormones are involved in the regulation of post-natal cell formation in the brain. Cell number was estimated in terms of DNA content; within certain limitations this gives a good approximation to cell number (cf. Balázs *et al.*, 1971). Figure 1 shows that cell formation is appreciable in the rat brain after birth, and that the development of the cerebellum is delayed in comparison with that

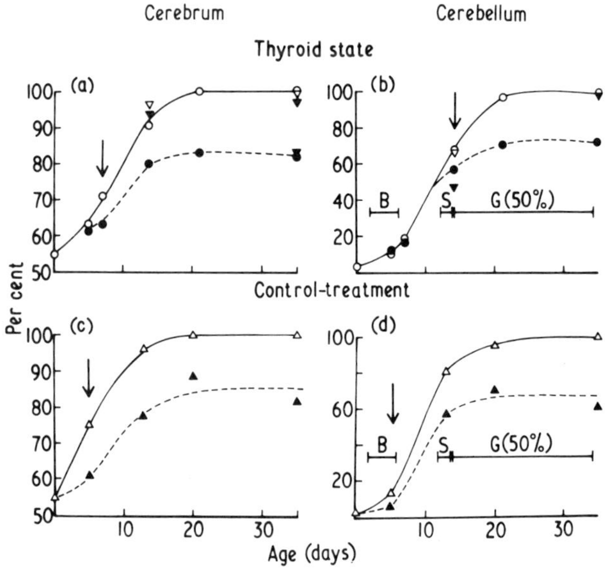

Fig. 1. The post-natal inrease in the DNA content of whole cerebrum (a, c) and cerebellum (b, d) respectively is expressed as a percentage of the adult values observed in 35- to 50-day-old rats. The data are taken from the following references: ○–treatment with thyroid hormone (25 μg T_3 at birth followed by 0.5-1.5 μg every second day), Balázs *et al.*, 1971; ▽–neonatal thyroidectomy (150 μC ^{131}I s.c. at birth), Balázs *et al.*, 1968; △–treatment with cortisol (0.2 mg per day from the first to the fourth day after birth), Cotterell, 1971; Cotterell, Balázs and Johnson (1971). ○, ▽, △–Controls; ●, ▼, ▲–experimental animals. The differences between control and experimental animals become significant from the age indicated by the arrow.

The dating of neurone differentiation in the cerebellar cortex is also indicated. The data are taken from Altman (1970). The period is shown when the formation of basket cells (B) and stellate cells (S) is maximal; the period is also indicated when about 50% of the granule cells (G) are formed.

of the cerebrum. The rate of DNA deposition was retarded in the cerebellum of thyroid deficient rats although at 35 days the normal level was reached. On the other hand treatment with thyroid hormone (triiodothyronine, T_3) in early life resulted in a permanent deficit in cell number in the brain. T_3 affected cell formation rather than cell destruction, since the rate of DNA synthesis measured by the incorporation [^{14}C] thymidine into DNA was less than in controls (Kovács *et al.*, 1969). The reduction was more marked towards the end of the period of massive cell proliferation (50%) than at the peak of cell multiplication (10-20%).

The results indicated that T_3 treatment caused a premature termination of cell proliferation which is associated with an advancement of the maturation of the CNS. The biochemical differentiation was accelerated as shown by the age curves of the conversion of glucose carbon into amino acids (Fig. 2) and of the

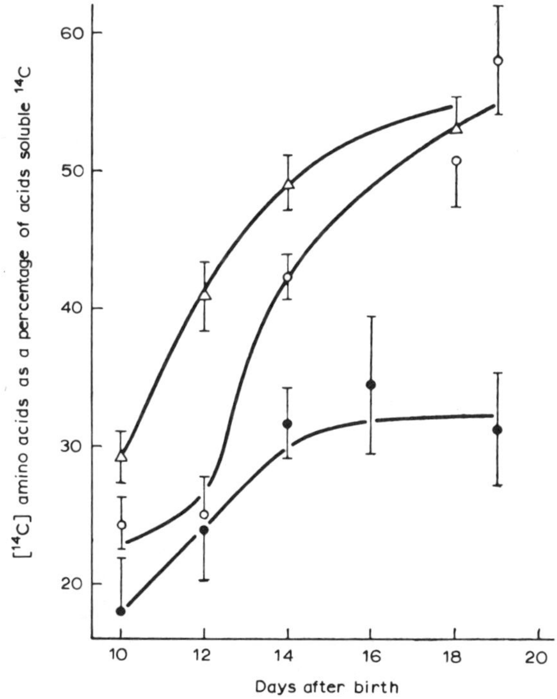

Fig. 2. Conversion of glucose carbon into amino acids in rat cerebrum at 20 min after the i.p. injection of 10-20 μC of [U-^{14}C] glucose per 100 g body wt. The amino acids of the acid soluble fraction of brain tissue were separated by ion exchange chromatography. The age curves for the experimental animals differed significantly from those of controls. The results are taken from Cocks *et al.* (1970). ○–Control; ●–thyroid deficient, and △–T_3 treated rats.

metabolic compartmentation of glutamate (Patel and Balázs, 1971). The functional development was also advanced as indicated by the time of appearance of innately organised behaviour (Eayrs, 1968). However, Eayrs (1968) has previously observed that when T_3 treated animals grow up their performance in tests of adaptive behaviour is impaired in comparison with controls. In the rat post-natal cell proliferation involves not only glial cells, but also microneurones in certain regions of the brain, such as the hippocampus and cerebellum (Altman, 1970). Altman (1970) has suggested that microneurones formed after birth may modify the structural and functional organisation of the developing nervous system to an extent depending on environmental influences. It would therefore appear that the impairment of adaptive behaviour caused by treatment with thyroid hormone in early life may be related to the resulting deficit of microneurones in certain regions of the brain. Other factors which may also be involved have previously been discussed (Balázs, 1971).

The influence of thyroid hormones on the maturation of the CNS is also shown by the effects of thyroid deficiency, in that the appearance of the various manifestations of the differentiation of nervous tissue is retarded. The biochemical effects (cf. Fig. 2) are associated with a reduction in both the axonal and dendritic components of the neuropil (Eayrs, 1968). Adaptive behaviour is permanently impaired, as is known to occur in cretins (Eayrs, 1968).

Effect of Treatment with Corticosteroids

Howard (1968) observed that treatment of mice with corticosterone during the first few days after birth caused a permanent deficit in the total number of cells in the brain. Cotterrell (1971) and Cotterrell, Balázs and Johnson (1971) have investigated the effects of cortisol administration in the first few days of life on brain development in the rat. They found that the final deficit in cell number was similar to that in the brain of rats treated with thyroid hormone (Fig. 1). The reduction in DNA content resulted from a depression of cell proliferation: the rate of DNA synthesis was severely inhibited, especially during the period of cortisol administration (Fig. 3). It is known that corticosteroids also influence cell reproduction in organs other than brain and the effect depends on the cell type (cf. Balázs and Richter, 1971).

In spite of the marked interference with post-natal cell formation the biochemical differentiation of the brain was only little affected by cortisol treatment. The age curve for the conversion of glucose carbon into amino acids in the brain was not significantly different from

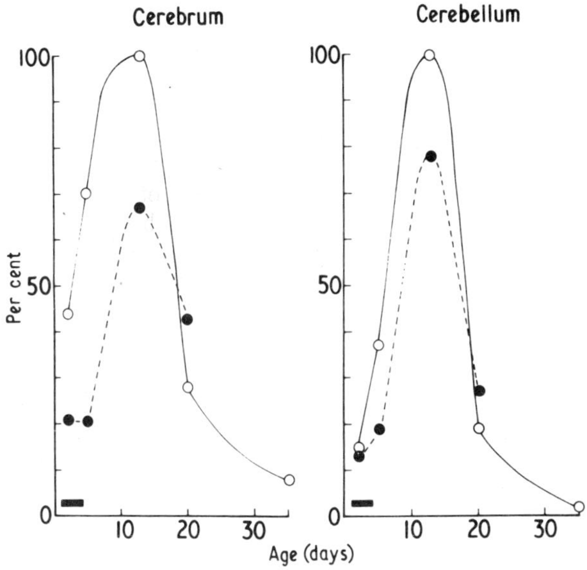

Fig. 3. The incorporation of [2-^{14}C] thymidine into brain DNA of control and cortisol-treated rats at 1 hour after injection (20 μC per 100 g body wt., s.c.) is expressed as a percentage of the maximum in the normal cerebrum and cerebellum respectively. The results were analysed by analysis of variance; the age curves for the experimental animals differed significantly from those of controls. The solid bars indicate the period of cortisol administration. The results were taken from Cotterrell, 1971 and Cotterrell and Balázs, 1971. ○–Control; ●–treatment with cortisol.

controls, although a slight retardation was noted at 14 days after birth (Cotterrell, 1971). At about the same age a transient retardation in spine formation on cortical neurones has also been reported (Schapiro, 1968). These changes are associated with a retardation of the maturation of evoked cortical potential responses (Schapiro *et al.*, 1970), and a delay in the development of seizure patterns characteristic of the adult animal (Woodbury and Vernadakis, 1967).

Hormones and the Development of Behaviour

It must be emphasised that any attempt to approach the understanding of behaviour by comparing the effects of different hormonal states on the biochemical and morphological manifestations of brain development has serious limitations. Correlations between different factors do not necessarily imply a causal relationship, although they may help to limit the number of possibilities that need to be considered. More meaningful is the observation of the dissociation of an apparent correlation when the development of the CNS is disturbed by various means. Difficulties of interpretation also arise in comparing results derived from experiments varying in respect of conditions such as species, type of hormone, dosage and timing of administration. The evidence described is not entirely free from such objections, but it is worth mentioning that rat and mouse, the two species which are mainly compared, have much in common in terms of the post-natal development of the CNS. Furthermore, in the experiments which are considered below the mice and rats were both exposed to high levels of corticosteroids at about the same time after birth (cf. Howard and Granoff, 1968, and Cotterrell, 1971). Moreover, preliminary studies from our laboratory indicate that brain growth is depressed in a similar wa by an effective dose of either cortisol or corticosterone, and the results are not greatly affected by the route by which the hormone is administered.

Keeping the above limitations in mind, it appears that the behavioural effects of corticosteroid treatment in early life are different from those observed after treatment with thyroid hormones. In contrast to the effects of T_3-treatment, there is a retardation of certain features of innately organised behaviour, such as swimming (Schapiro *et al.;* 1970). It has also been reported that although, in comparison with controls, the animals treated with corticosteroids are emotionally more labile and that their ability to perform tasks requiring fine motor coordination is impaired, their performance in tests of adaptive behaviour remains unchanged (Howard and Granoff, 1968). Thus, the proposal mentioned earlier for explaining the impairment of adaptive behaviour of thyroid treated animals, based simply on a reduction in cell number, and specifically in microneurones, cannot account for all the functional consequences of corticosteroid treatment in early life.

A lead for the understanding of the behavioural consequences of hormonal imbalances in early life appears to be provided by the analysis of the effects of treatment with either thyroid hormone or corticosteroids on post-natal cell formation in the brain. The timing of the effect was different under the conditions of the respective treatments. Corticosteroids inhibited cell multiplication mainly during the period of the treatment (Figs. 1 and 3): the rate of DNA deposition was relatively little affected after the treatment was terminated (Fig. 1), and the observations indicated that the rate of cell proliferation exceeded that in controls during the third week of life (Fig. 3). Nevertheless, massive cell proliferation ceased at about the same age as in the brain of untreated animals (Fig. 1). On the other hand, thyroid hormone affected cell formation mainly after a delay of one to two weeks after the start of treatment, depending on the region of the brain concerned (Fig. 1). It is known that the types of nerve cells formed in various parts of the CNS differ at different times during development. Thus in the cerebellum the peak of the differentiation of the basket cells takes place at 2-6 days, and that of the stellate cells at 13 days, whereas about half of the granule cells develop during the third week after birth (cf. Fig. 1) (Altman, 1970). It is also known that the functions of the various types of 'microneurones' in the cerebellum are different (Eccles *et al.*, 1967). It is proposed therefore that the different behavioural effects produced by corticosteroids and thyroid hormones may depend on the cell types affected by the respective treatments in different parts of the brain. This hypothesis may be applicable also to other conditions, such as the effects of malnutrition (Winick, 1969) and amino acid imbalance (Chase and O'Brien, 1970) which interfere with cell formation in the brain after birth. Recent work has shown that post-natal cell formation is appreciable also in the human brain (Winick, 1969; Dobbing, 1970): cell number increases from birth until over a year by about 3-fold in the cerebrum and the rise is approximately 6-fold in the cerebellum (Dobbing, personal communication). It is not yet known whether post-natal cell formation in the human brain involves microneurones. However, the features of post-natal cell formation in man, a functional 'nest animal', have apparently much in common with those observed, for example, in the brain in rat, a nest animal in the evolutionary sense. In contrast to the foetus which is protected by the mother, the regulatory mechanisms in the infant are not yet fully developed. Hence it is possible that in man, as in experimental animals, various insults after birth will affect neurogenesis in the brain in such a way as to cause an impairment later in brain function.

Although the cerebellum is not the critical part of the CNS with respect to adaptive behaviour, it offers certain advantages as a *model* to test the above hypothesis. Since the time of formation and the functions of the different types of 'microneurones' in the cerebellum are well established, it can therefore be ascertained whether or not a deficit in a specific cell type is produced by interfering with cell formation at different times after birth. The cerebellum may also serve as a marker for determining retrospectively the stage of development when an insult had affected the CNS. In man, as in the rat, the cerebellum is a part of the CNS that develops late. Thus, it may be expected that insults affecting the CNS after birth will retard the growth of the cerebellum more than that of the cerebrum. The ratio of cerebellar to cerebral weight is therefore an index which may help in assessing the importance of post-natal damage in patients with behavioural disorders. Furthermore, impairment of fine motor coordination ('clumsy' child) may be taken as suggestive of CNS damage occurring during the period of extensive neurogenesis in the cerebellum, and thus microneurone formation in general.

There is general agreement that, apart from the cerebellum, microneurone formation is relatively extensive in the hippocampus which is part of the limbic system (Altman, 1970). Howard and Granoff (1968) have suggested that the emotional lability of corticosterone-treated mice is attributable to changes in the development of the limbic system. It has recently been reported that corticosteroids are retained in specific regions of the CNS. The highest retention was observed in some parts of the limbic system, and in these structures the hormone was relatively concentrated in the cell nuclei (McEwen *et al.*, 1969). A mechanism of this kind, if operative, may result in a certain specificity in the action of corticosteroids in early life. It is known that corticosteroids are involved in nervous tissues in the control of the synthesis of certain enzymes (cf. Balázs and Richter, 1971), including some enzymes which are critical in the pathways of formation of neurotransmitter substances such as 5HT (Azmitia and McEwen, 1969). The induction of tyrosine by hydroxylase has also been reported in peripheral and central adrenergic neurones in rats exposed to stress (Thoenen, 1970), and the involvement of the neuroendocrine system in regulating the synthesis of the enzymes of catecholamine metabolism has also been documented (Axelrod *et al.*, 1970). Therefore, at a critical time during the differentiation of the cells, corticosteroids and possibly other hormones, may influence the genetic expression in terms of the enzyme systems concerned in neurotransmitter synthesis. It is generally accepted that the same transmitter is liberated at all the synaptic terminals of a neurone (Dale's principle). Furthermore, there is ample evidence that the response of a given nerve cell to different neurotransmitters is specific in terms of excitation, inhibition or no response. Thus, hormones may change permanently the genetic plan of 'wiring pattern' in the affected region.

It appears therefore that adverse influences during the early post-natal period may affect the development of brain functions, not only by interfering with the formation of microneurones, but also by influencing the differentiation of certain nerve cells. A part of the CNS whose functional modification would have wide-ranging consequences is the hypothalamus. Evidence suggests that treatment with thyroid hormones in early life results in some chronic impairment of the functioning of the hypothalamo-pituitary-thyroid axis (Eayrs, 1968).

Kovács *et al.* (1969) have observed that the maturation of the hypothalamus is advanced by thyroid treatment: in comparison with controls, the rate of protein synthesis reached its peak about a week earlier, followed by a premature fall. As a consequence the rate of synthesis was about 30% less than in controls during the period 21 to 35 days of age. In the untreated rats the rate of protein synthesis was still increasing during this period in the pituitary; the progressive rise did not occur in the experimental animals, so that there was a permanent depression of pituitary protein synthesis.

The administration of corticosteroids in early life has also a permanent effect on the development of the hypothalamo-pituitary system: in the pituitary of adult experimental animals the amount of growth hormone is decreased, and this is associated with a marked reduction in the content of growth hormone releasing factor in the hypothalamus (Sawano *et al.*, 1969). The releasing factors are produced by specific neurosecretory nerve cells in the hypothalamus; thus, there is independent evidence that hormone treatment in early life can interfere with the development of particular neurones at certain sites in the CNS. The interference may result in qualitative changes, e.g. the defective differentiation of a cell involved in the synthesis of a specific neurosecretory product. Alternatively, the change may be quantitative in affecting the rate of neurohormone production.

The effect of sex hormones is a well known example of hormonal interference with the differentiation of certain parts of the CNS. It seems that the basic mechanisms involved in reproductive activity and sexual behaviour are of the female type; they are altered to the male type by androgen action at certain stages of development, which in the rat extend from about 18th day of gestation till the 10th day after birth (Donovan, 1970). It is assumed that androgens affect sexual behaviour by influencing the neuronal organisation of the hypothalamus (Harris, 1964; Barraclough, 1967; Phoenix *et al.*, 1967; Levine and Mullins, 1968). The organisation of a system, such as the CNS, that is built up from fixed units may be permanently affected by (1) deleting certain units (cf. above; deficit in microneurones as a result of treatment with thyroid hormone or corticosteroids), (2) reducing the probability of interaction between different unit (cf. retardation of dendritic arborisation and formation of nerve terminals in the brain of thyroid deficient rats, cf. Eayrs, 1968) and (3) introducing at the time of the assembly units which are different from those in the original genetic plan. It appears that androgenisation operates according to the last mechanism. Androgens may change the character of certain nerve cells by affecting their differentiation in terms of receptors, both hormonal and neurotransmitter, and of neurotransmitter production.

They may thus specify the hormonal-neuronal pathway in which the affected nerve cells participate. The biochemical effects of androgenisation have, until recently, received less attention than the effects for example on behaviour. However, there are observations which are consistent with the above assumptions. The oestrogen-binding capacity is substantially reduced in hypothalamic areas of adult androgen-sterilised female rats; in the untreated female these areas are the sites of the neuronal organisation concerned in reproductive activity and sexual behaviour, and they are rich in oestrogen receptors (Flerko *et al.*, 1969; Vértes and King, 1971). It has also been reported that androgenisation depresses the developmental rise at 12 days after birth, which is characteristic of the female rat, in the concentration of 5HT in the brain (Ladosky and Gaziri, 1970). There is evidence indicating that 5HT, which is localised only in certain nerve cells, is involved in neurotransmission in the CNS. It is also generally accepted that neurones are specific in terms of the neurotransmitter they produce. The low concentration of brain 5HT at birth, and the developmental rise in the concentration of 5HT, indicate that the nerve cells, which in the adult synthesise 5HT, are at birth not yet differentiated in terms of the enzyme systems needed for 5HT formation. The effect of androgenisation on the age-curve of 5HT concentration suggests therefore, that androgens suppress the differentiation of certain neurones into cells producing 5HT as the neurotransmitter. Alternative explanations are also possible involving a change in the formation or utilisation fluxes of 5HT. Androgens could operate by modifying genetic expressions in terms of the rate limiting enzyme of 5HT formation, tryptophan hydroxylase, which is known to be controlled by steroid hormones (cf. above). Alternatively, they could act by affecting the development of the tryptophan-transport system, so influencing 5HT production by affecting the concentration of free tryptophan in the relevant neuronal structures (cf. Graham-Smith, 1971).

SUMMARY

Evidence has been presented that transient changes in hormonal balance during development can influence the organisation of the CNS in a way that produces permanent changes in brain function. In animals which are relatively immature at birth, brain development is especially vulnerable during the early post-natal period when the regulatory mechanisms of the infant are not yet fully developed: this applies also to man.

Adverse influences may operate by inhibiting the formation of certain types of nerve cells ('microneurones') in specific parts of the brain. It appears that the behavioural consequences depend on the timing of the event in relation to the state of post-natal neurogenesis.

There is also evidence that hormones can affect the differentiation of nerve cells in the CNS. The dendritic and axonal growth of nerve cells is retarded after neonatal thyroidectomy. Excess thyroid and adrenocortical hormones alter permanently the function of specific neurosecretory nerve cells in the hypothalamus. The effects of androgens at certain stages of development on the neurological 'organisation' of the hypothalamus can be attributed to their influencing the differentiation of certain nerve cells associated with sexual behaviour by modifying hormone-receptor (trigger) and/or neurotransmitter production mechanisms.

It appears, therefore, that anomalous hormonal states can influence both the formation and differentiation of certain nerve cells and thus lead to permanent changes in behaviour as a result of alterations in the 'wiring pattern' of certain parts of the CNS. It is suggested that the cerebellum may serve both as a model to test this hypothesis, and as one of the markers for determining the stage of development when insults had affected the CNS.

REFERENCES

Altman, J. (1970). In 'Developmental Neurobiology' (ed. W. A. Himwich), p. 197. Springfield, Ill.: C. C. Thomas.

Azmitia, E. C., Jr. and McEwen, B. S. (1969). *Science* **166**, 1274.

Axelrod, J., Müeller, R. A. and Thoenen, H. (1970). In 'New Aspects of Storage and Release Mechanisms of Catecholamines' (Bayer Symposium No. 2), p. 212. Berlin: Springer-Verlag.

Balázs, R. (1971). In 'Cellular Aspects of Neural Growth and Differentiation' (ed. D. C. Pease),p. 273. Los Angeles: Univ. Calif. Press.

Balázs, R., Kovács, S., Teichgräber, P., Cocks, W. A. and Eayrs, J. T. (1968). *J. Neurochem.* **15**, 1335.

Balázs, R., Kovács, S., Cocks, W. A., Johnson, A. L. and Eayrs, J. T. (1971). *Brain Res.* **25**, 555.

Balázs, R. and Richter, D. (1971). In 'Biochemistry of the Developing Brain' (ed. W. A. Himwich). New York: M. Dekker (in press).

Barraclough, C. A. (1967). In 'Neuroendocrinology', vol. 2 (eds L. Martini and W. F. Ganong), p. 62. New York: Academic Press.

Chase, H. P. and O'Brien, D. (1970). *Pediat. Res.* **4**, 96.

Cocks, J. A., Balázs, R., Johnson, A. and Eayrs, J. T. (1970). *J. Neurochem.* **17**, 1275.

Cotterrell, M. (1971). M.Sc. Thesis (in preparation).

Cotterrell, M. and Balázs, R. (1971) (in preparation).

Dobbing, J. (1970). *Am. J. Dis. Child.* **120**, 411.

Donovan, B. T. (1970). 'Mammalian Neuroendocrinology', New York: McGraw-Hill.

Eayrs, J. T. (1968). In 'Endocrinology and Human Behaviour' (R. Michael), p. 239. London: Oxford Univ. Press.

Eccles, J. C., Ito, M. and Szentágothai, J. (1967). 'The Cerebellum as a Neuronal Machine'. Berlin: Springer.

Flerko, B., Mess, B. and Illei-Donhoffer, A. (1969). *Neuroendocrinology,* **4**, 164.

Graham-Smith, G. D. (1971). In 'Metabolic Compartmentation in Brain' (eds R. Balázs and J. E. Cremer). London: Macmillan (in press).

Harris, G. W. (1964). *Endocrinology,* **75**, 627.

Howard, E. (1968). *Exp. Neurol.* **22**, 191.

Howard, E. and Granoff, D. M. (1968). *Exp. Neurol.* **22**, 661.

Kovács, S., Cocks, W. A. and Balázs, R. (1969). *Biochem. J.* **114**, 60P.

Kovács, S., Cocks, W. A. and Balázs, R. (1969). *J. Endocr.* **45**, IX.

Ladosky, W. and Gaziri, L. C. J. (1970). *Neuroendocrinology,* **6**, 168.

Levine, S. and Mullins, R. F., Jr. (1968). In 'Early Experience and Behaviour' (eds G. Newton and S. Levine), p. 168. Springfield, Ill.: C. C. Thomas.

McEwen, B. S., Weiss, J. M. and Schwartz, L. S. (1970). *Brain Res.* **17**, 471.

Patel, A. J. and Balázs, R. (1971). *Biochem. J.* **121**, 469.

Phoenix, C. H., Goy, R. W. and Young, W. C. (1967). In 'Neuroendocrinology', vol. 2 (eds L. Martini and W. F. Ganong), p. 163. New York: Academic Press.

Robinson, R. J. and Tizard, J. P. M. (1966). *Br. med. Bull.* **22**, 49.

Sawano, S., Arimura, A., Schally, A. V., Redding, T. W. and Schapiro, S. (1969). *Acta Endocrin.* **61**, 57.

Schapiro, S. (1968). *Gen. Comp. Endocr.* **10**, 214.

Schapiro, S., Salas, M. and Vukovich, K. (1970). *Science,* **168**, 147.

Thoenen, H. (1970). *Nature,* **228**, 861.

Vértes, M. and King, R. J. B. (1971). *J. Endocr.* (in press).

Winick, M. (1969). *J. Pediat.* **74**, 667.

Woodbury, D. M. and Vernadakis, A. (1967). In 'Neuroendocrinology', vol. 2 (eds L. Martini and W. F. Ganong), p. 335. New York: Academic Press.

ACKNOWLEDGEMENTS

The author acknowledges the collaboration of Mrs. W. A. Cocks, Mr. J. A. Cocks, Prof. J. T. Eayrs, Mr. A. L. Johnson, Drs S. Kovács and A. J. Patel. The collaboration of Mrs. M. Cotterrell is acknowledged in the yet unpublished studies reported in the present communication. Thanks are expressed also to Drs L. Crome, B. W. L. Brooksbank, B. T. Donovan, R. J. B. King and J. Stern for helpful discussions and to Drs M. Vértes and R. J. B. King for the preview of their paper before publication. Gratitude is expressed to Dr. D. Richter for his encouragement and help in the preparation of the manuscript.

DISCUSSION

Holt: Were these pharmacological doses of hormones or physiological variations?

Balázs: We use Eayrs' treatment, namely 2.5 μg of T_3 at birth and from then on 0.5-1.5 μg every second day; injections were stopped if severe hypothyroidism developed. Cortisol (0.2 mg per day) was given from first to fourth day after birth, but no effects occurred below 0.18 mg/animal. These doses are relatively high so that the experiments must be considered as model systems.

Harris: Moving from rats to humans Dr. della Rovere, Dr. Prior and myself (Harris, R., della Rovere, M. and Prior, P. F. (1965) *Arch. Dis. Childh.* **40**, 612) looked at the EEG's of hypothyroid children particularly in relation to treatment and it was interesting that they all had abnormal EEG's. They were small babies and very young children and their EEG's had a quality of rhythmic activity that one would expect for their age. After treatment it was never less than three weeks before one began to see more normal rhythmic activity. We felt that this fitted in with Eayrs' work on the maturation of the neurones. We ultimately got reasonably normal EEG's even though they remained quite mentally retarded.

Crome: This problem has also a bearing on public health. The influence of hormones is a very topical question in view of the 'Pill' and the oestrogens used. And also, of course, because of the progesterones used in other conditions. We are not yet certain as to the long-term effects of these on pregnant women. In addition, we have not until now discussed specific maldevelopments of certain brain regions. The cerebellum is an important organ in undifferentiated mental retardation for the cerebellum is often reduced in size and not the cerebrum, and sometimes the reverse occurs. It is very constant in mongolism for the cerebellum and the frontal lobes to be small.

Dobbing: The cerebellum is differentially susceptible in almost any growth retardation as well as in specific processes. Could it be used as an index of such having taken place?

Richter: Dr. Woollam asked whether in cretinism the reduced blood supply is primary or secondary. I wonder if these experiments on thyroid deficiency show that retardation of growth of nerve cells is the first effect and that this must limit the growth of the blood supply.

Woollam: It was Prof. Eayrs that suggested that the blood supply was responsible.

Zlotnik: How did Dr. Balázs exclude the glial cells from his calculations, if the growth was calculated on the DNA levels.

Balázs: I didn't, the DNA content gives an overall estimate of cell number. I was speculating about the implications of the experiment. We are currently trying to identify the cell types that may be deleted. In the cerebellum we are sure that the neurones must be involved, because of the magnitude of the effects of hormone treatment.

Hanefeld: You have shown that cortisone reduces the final number of neurones. We use cortisone to treat infantile spasms and in young babies it stops the fits. Most of the children are retarded. Could this be due to your kind of cortisone effect? The theory of the action of cortisone and ACTH in this case is that they lift the neurones to a higher level of maturation, and maturation is advanced thereby.

Balázs: I am glad to hear of this. We have until now only considered the rat. Of course, I'm prejudiced, but I would say yes. On the basis of animal experiments, however, I would rather doubt whether cortisone advances neuronal maturity.

Kleihues: The main reason for the reduction in DNA content seems to have been inhibition of DNA synthesis. Is this a general effect or specific to the cerebellum?

Balázs: Cortisol seems to affect some cells but not others (Balázs, R. and Richter, D. (1971) *loc. cit.*). Some cells (e.g. ileal epithelium) are not affected, while in others (e.g. basal loop of maxillary incisor) cell replication is accelerated. It is inhibited in lymphoid tissue, liver, and in brain cells. It is not known for sure how it works, but it is very specific to certain stages of the G1 phase.

Magee: You mentioned oestrogen receptors in nerve cells. Are these comparable to the protein factors you get in the uterus?

Balázs: The protein factors seem to be very similar to oestrogen receptors in the uterus; they are involved in binding the hormone, translocating it into the nucleus and they are probably also cleaved in the nucleus. They have the same 9.5 S sedimentation constant, so most likely it is a very similar type of protein to that observed in the uterus (Toft, D. and Gorski, J. (1966) *Proc. Nat. Acad. Sci.* **55**, 1574; Hensen, E. V., Suzuki, T., Kawashima, T., Stumpf, W. E., Jungblut, P. W. T., Heinreichs, W. L. and Herrmann, W. L. (1969) *Nature* **223**, 313; Vertés, M. and King, R. J. B. (1971) *J. Endocrinol.* (in press). Similar receptors which are specific for glucocorticoids have recently been identified in target cells (Wira, C. and Munck, A. (1971) *J. biol. Chem.* **245**, 3436; Baxter, J. D. and Tomkins, G. M. (1970) *Proc. Nat. Acad. Sci.* **65**, 709; Melnykovych, G. and Bishop, C. F. (1971) *Endocrinology* **88**, 450). A similar type of receptor exists for cortisone.

Harris: To return to infantile spasms and ACTH, there have been enough children now treated with ACTH or steroids, and not treated in this way, to show that there is really no difference between them in their ultimate outcome.

Richter: A point about nomenclature. We use the word 'retarded', but do we not sometimes mean a qualitative change? Another word might be better.

Holt: The meaning may be different in different parts of the country. In some parts it means a child who is going to catch up, in other parts of the country it means a very badly damaged child.

Kirman: It is a matter of education perhaps. This is the correct word, since we are dealing with a child at an earlier stage than it should be. We are not in a position to detect by psychometric tests whether there is any qualitative difference.

Holt: I would support this strongly for I think that if we can introduce other terms to signify not only delayed development, but also deviant development, this would be very helpful.

Kirman: In the majority of our unclassified cases, we are unable to do that. The exception perhaps in classified cases is Down's syndrome, in which there is a perhaps quite specific cerebellum syndrome. In most cases, however, we are dealing with an all-round retardation. There are discrepancies within the group, but we are not really in a position to show a relationship between aetiology and the qualitative substrate within the brain on the one hand, and the pattern of psychometrics on the other.

O'Connor: It seemed to me this morning, as a psychologist, that I was getting nowhere very much, because the brain was being treated as an undifferentiated mass. This afternoon it has been differentiated a little more. So far as the people called 'subnormal' are concerned, the notable feature of their maldevelopment is that it is uniformly maldevelopment, at least as far as psychometrics goes. If we are talking about brain injury we would normally mean a specific deficit, such as in neurologically damaged adults, where one part of the cortex will have been damaged where localisation of function takes place. The last paper gets closer to pointing out possible functional approaches to such a situation, and I thought also that Dr. Wigglesworth's paper also might give me, as a psychologist, a possible lead to talk about the difference between say learning deficits in cases where the cell population is reduced, or in cases where the cell constitution is affected. Now, I do not know whether one can speculate about these possibilities, but in the past at least the recalcitrant part of physiology and neurochemistry of maldevelopment for the psychologist has been that he cannot latch on to anything that would help him to differentiate a deficit of memory, a deficit of learning, a deficit of transfer, or something of that kind. None of the functions that we have been able to deal with have so far been localisable in mental defect. If you have a cerebellar defect that is a different matter, but most of the time we are hamstrung by our colleagues in neurochemistry, except this afternoon, who have not given me much opportunity to see how we can develop further.

Dobbing: There is no doubt that this is one of the central issues of the problem.

Richter: I feel there are qualitative differences besides the quantitative ones in development and this requires to be brought out, and I wonder if the hyperkinetic child is one where there are very distinct qualitative differences associated with mental changes. The terminology should enable us to express that difference.

Changes in Enzyme Activity and the Developing Brain

JILL E. CREMER

There has been a steadily accumulating inventory of the activity of enzymes and amounts of DNA and protein in developing brain. This is particularly so for rat brain. Not only is the rat a convenient experimental animal but the immaturity of its nervous system at birth allows a day-by-day examination of changes accompanying maturation.

Changes in the Amount of DNA and Protein in the Developing Rat Brain

Before considering the induction and repression of enzyme synthesis in the developing rat brain it is essential to take into account cell multiplication and cell growth. The morphological post-natal changes in the cerebral cortex of the rat were described by Sugita (1917). Starting at birth there is a period of rapid growth and during the first 10 days the weight of the brain increases almost four-fold. During the second phase from the 10th to the 20th day few new cells are formed in the cerebrum but there is an increase in the size of the existing cells with growth of axons and dendrites. Myelination begins on about the 14th day after birth, and in the rat continues into adult life.

Similar observations have been made on rat cerebellum where the phase of cell proliferation is delayed by several days and is maximal between the 5th and 15th day. The second phase, namely cell growth, occurs between the 15th and 50th day (Balázs, Kovács, Cocks, Johnson and Eayrs, 1971).

A quantitative assessment of the number of cells in the developing brain can be made by measuring the total content of DNA (see review article by Altman, 1969). For whole rat brain there is a virtually linear increase in the amount of DNA per brain from birth to 20 days of age when the adult level is reached (Mandel, Rein, Harth-Edel and Mardell, 1964).

Separate analyses of the cerebrum and cerebellum for their DNA content showed clearly the large and rapid increase in cell number in the cerebellum between the 5th and 20th day compared with the more gradual increase in the cerebrum starting from birth (Balázs *et al.*, 1971). When the DNA content is expressed per unit wet wt. of tissue then there is a continuous decline in the concentration of DNA from birth to 20 days in the cerebrum. In the cerebellum a peak is reached between 10 and 15 days and thereafter the value decreases until around 50 days (Pasquini, Kaplun, Garcia-Argiz and Gomez, 1967; Balázs *et al.*, 1971). A decrease in the concentration of DNA can be taken to represent an enlargement of cell size.

When the protein content of the whole brain is expressed in units per unit wet wt. of tissue (usually mg protein/g brain) there is a continuous increase in the value from birth to around 50 days of age. The increase in the ratio is far greater in the cerebellum than in the cortex. When expressed as mg protein/mg DNA there is a six-fold increase in the ratio in the cerebrum from 0 to 30 days. In the cerebellum the time-course of changes in the ratio is more complex due to the period of rapid cell proliferation between the 5th and 15th day. The greatest increase in the ratio of protein/DNA occurs after cell multiplication has ceased, that is from about the 21st to the 50th day (Pasquini *et al.*, 1967).

Patterns of Enzymic Activity During the Maturation of Rat Brain

From this brief account of cell proliferation and growth in the developing rat brain it is readily apparent that the activity of an enzyme expressed per unit weight of either fresh tissue, DNA or protein will be strongly influenced by the age of the animal and the area of the brain, such as the cerebral cortex or the cerebellum. The majority of enzymes will show an increase in activity when expressed per g wet wt. of brain since the protein content increases from 6.5 to 10.5% of the wet wt. during the main period of maturation (Clouet and Gaitonde, 1956).

It might be argued that the most informative method of expression of enzyme activity is in terms of units of DNA since this will show changes with the maturation of the cell. Perhaps the most commonly used method is as per mg of protein. If the composition of the total protein in a cell did not change but the amount of protein increased during development then no change would be observed in the activity of any enzyme when expressed in terms of weight of protein. For most of the enzymes studied so far changes have been observed and these will be considered further.

From a survey of the literature it has been possible to group together various enzymes under particular patterns exhibited when enzyme activity in the brain is plotted against the age of the animal. To enable a direct comparison between all the enzymes given in Fig. 1 their activities have been brought to a common term of expression. From the shapes of the curves it can be seen that many of the enzymes fall into pattern 1 (Fig. 1a) showing a fairly steep rise in activity from about the 5th to the 20th day after birth reaching adult, or near-adult values at about this age. It seems appropriate to pass comment on the metabolic pathways in which these enzymes are involved and their intracellular localisation. Enzymes of glycolysis are aldolase and lactate dehydrogenase, both are located in the cytosol. Malate dehydrogenase is located in both the cytosol and mitochondria. In the latter location it forms part of the tricarboxylate cycle in which both succinate dehydrogenase and cytochrome oxidase are involved. Two enzymes of the pathway forming γ-aminobutyrate, an amino acid of particular importance in nervous tissue are glutamate dehydrogenase, present in mitochondria and glutamate decarboxylase, present in the cytosol. Another enzyme of importance in amino acid metabolism is aspartateoxoglutarate amino transferase which is located in both the cytosol and mitochondria. The enzymes exhibiting pattern 1 as shown in Fig. 1a, are between them participant in various metabolic pathways and have at least two main sites of location within the cell.

Two enzymes, D-β-hydroxybutyrate dehydrogenase and 3-oxoacid CoA transferase, followed pattern 2, shown in Fig. 1b. Both these enzymes are required for ketone-body metabolism and are located in mitochondria. The distinguishing feature is the fall in activity after about the 25th day of age. One of these enzymes, β-hydroxybutyrate dehydrogenase, will be considered in more detail later.

Two enzymes, glucose-6-phosphate dehydrogenase, a cytosolic enzyme, and acetoacetyl-CoA thiolase located in mitochondria, showed virtually no change in activity during development, which represents pattern 3 in Fig. 1c.

Finally, one enzyme has been observed by several investigators to have a completely different profile of activity with age. This enzyme is NADP-isocitrate dehydrogenase which shows an unusually high activity at birth and falls fairly steadily during the brain developmental period. This has been shown as pattern 4 in Fig. 1d.

The enzyme activities grouped in Fig. 1 can be converted to activity per mg protein or DNA by reference to Table 1 which gives the changes with age in mg of protein and DNA per g wet wt. of whole brain. The precise shapes of the curves will alter but the enzymes can still be grouped under four distinctive patterns.

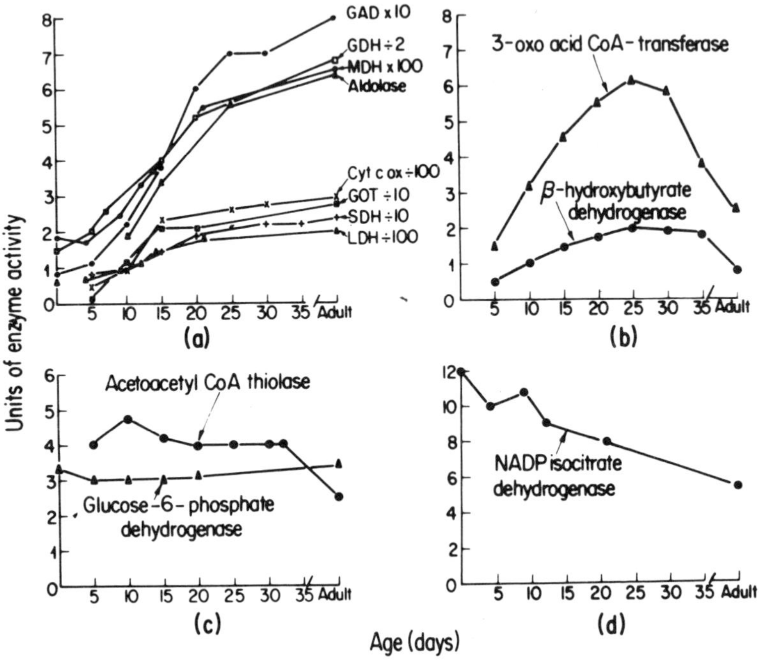

Fig. 1. Enzymic activity is expressed as μmol substrate changed/g wet wt. brain/min. Data have been obtained from the following sources:

(a) ● (GAD) glutamate decarboxylase (Van den Berg *et al.*, 1965; Sims and Pitts, 1970). □ (GDH) glutamate dehydrogenase (Kuhlman and Lowry, 1956). ○ (MDH) malate dehydrogenase (Robins and Lowe, 1961). △ Aldolase (Swaiman *et al.*, 1970). x (Cytc Ox) cytochrome c oxidase (Klee and Sokoloff, 1967). ■ (GOT) aspartate 2-oxoglutarate amino transferase (Bayer and McMurray, 1967). + (SDH) succinate dehydrogenase (García-Argiz *et al.*, 1967). ▲ (LDH) lactate dehydrogenase (Robins and Lowe, 1961).

(b) 3-oxoacid CoA transferase (Page *et al.*, 1971). β-hydroxybutyrate dehydrogenase (Page *et al.*, 1971; Pull and McIlwain, 1971; Cremer and Somogyi, unpublished observations).

(c) Acetoacetyl-CoA thiolase (Page *et al.*, 1971). Glucose-6-phosphate dehydrogenase (Kuhlman and Lowry, 1956).

(d) NADP-isocitrate dehydrogenase (Robins and Lowe, 1961).

TABLE 1

Content of Protein and DNA in the Developing Rat Brain

Age (days)	*Protein content mg/g wet wt. brain*	*DNA content mg/g wet wt. brain*
1-3	65	–
4-6	66	1.76
7-9	69	1.65
10-12	79	1.97
13-15	92	1.67
19-21	95	1.67
30-40	107	–
50	114	1.65
Adult	107	–

The values are averages for whole brain (or cortex plus cerebellum). Those for the protein content are taken from the data of Clouet and Gaitonde, 1956; Robins and Lowe, 1961; Garcia-Argiz *et al.*, 1967 and Balázs *et al.*, 1971. Those for the DNA content are taken from the data of Pasquini *et al.*, 1967 and Swaiman *et al.*, 1970.

Enzymic Activity in Relation to Metabolic Rate: A Consideration of Ketone-body Utilisation by the Young and Adult Rat Brain

Presumably, the activity of an enzyme will bear some relationship to the rate of the metabolic pathway in which it participates. Information is meagre on the quantitative aspects of metabolism in brain *in vivo.* In the author's laboratory attempts are being made to determine the rates of utilisation of certain substrates by the brains of young and adult rats.

Recently, there has been a considerable body of evidence to support the concept that the immature brain is capable of oxidising ketone bodies (β-hydroxybutyrate and acetoacetate) in sufficient amounts to contribute to the energy requirements of the tissue (see Hawkins, Williamson and Krebs, 1971). It has therefore been of considerable interest to follow the activity in the developing rat brain of those enzymes necessary for the initial steps in ketone-body metabolism and to relate their maximal activity to the rate of ketone body utilisation.

$$\beta\text{-hydroxybutyrate} + \text{NAD} \xrightleftharpoons{\beta\text{-hydroxybutyrate dehydrogenase}} \text{Acetoacetate} + \text{NADH} \quad (1)$$

$$\text{Acetoacetate} + \text{Succinyl CoA} \xrightleftharpoons{\text{3-oxoacid CoA-transferase}} \text{Acetoacetyl-CoA} + \text{Succinate} \quad (2)$$

$$\text{Acetoacetyl-CoA} + \text{CoA} \overset{\text{Acetoacetyl-CoA-thiolase}}{\rightleftarrows} \text{2-Acetyl-CoA} \quad (3)$$

Klee and Sokoloff (1967) were the first to describe the profile of activity with age for β-hydroxybutyrate dehydrogenase in the rat brain during maturation. The pattern has been confirmed by several other investigators (Page *et al.*, 1971; Pull and McIlwain, 1971; Cremer and Somogyi, unpublished observations, Fig. 2), although the absolute

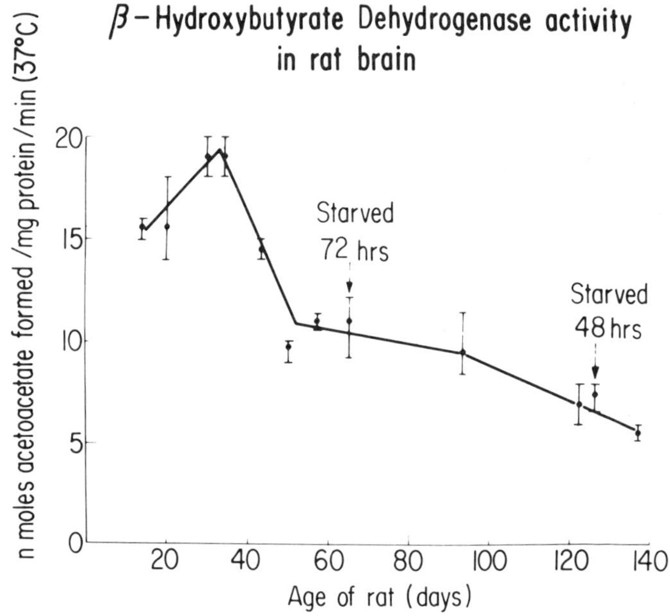

Fig. 2. Data are from Cremer, J. E. and Somogyi, J., previously unpublished.

activity of the enzyme was found to be about three times higher than reported by Klee and Sokoloff. The striking finding was the sharp decline in activity following the maximum peak reached between 25 to 30 days (Fig. 1b). This fall is most clearly seen when the enzyme activity is expressed per mg protein (Fig. 2). Page *et al.* (1971) have shown that the enzyme for step 2 in ketone-body metabolism, 3-oxoacid CoA-transferase, has a very similar profile (Fig. 1b). The enzyme for step 3, acetoacetyl-CoA thiolase, is not the same although it also shows a low activity in adult brain compared with the maximum reached in the developing brain (Fig. 1c). All three enzymes involved in the initial steps of ketone-body metabolism have profiles different from those of the majority of enzymes studied which are involved in the metabolism of glucose and oxidation reactions in the tricarboxylate cycle (see for example aldolase and cytochrome c oxidase in Fig. 1a).

Having shown that the enzymes necessary for ketone-body utilisation are present in the brains of young rats and that they are in particularly high amounts between 15 and 30 days, it became of interest to establish whether a sufficient supply of ketone-bodies was available to the brain during this time. Drahota *et al.* (1964) showed that neonatal rats are ketotic. That is to say, the blood concentrations of acetoacetate in 1- to 23-day-old rats are as high as in adult-starved rats. A more complete analysis of the blood content of metabolites during post-natal development of the rat has been made by Page *et al.* (1971). They confirm and extend the original findings of Drahota *et al.* (1964) leaving no doubt that in normal suckling rats the concentrations of acetoacetate and β-hydroxybutyrate in the circulating blood are high.

The first quantitative data on the utilisation of ketone-bodies by the suckling rat brain *in vivo* were reported recently by Hawkins *et al.* (1971). These authors measured arterio-venous differences across the brain of 16- to 22-day-old animals. They expressed the results as μmoles of substrate per ml of blood and showed that the uptake by the brain of ketone-bodies was directly proportional to their concentration in arterial blood. Similar experiments on adult rats showed that uptake values by the brain were three to four times less than in the young animals for a given concentration of blood ketone-bodies. For example, in 18-day-old rats with an arterial blood concentration of β-hydroxybutyrate of 1.69 mM the arterio-venous difference across the brain was 0.305 μmol per ml whereas in a 48 hour starved adult rat the values were 2.0 mM and 0.075 μmol respectively.

A different experimental approach has been made in the author's own laboratory for measuring ketone-body utilisation. The results have not been published previously so the information is given in some detail in Fig. 3. From radioactive tracer experiments using D-β-hydroxy [3-^{14}C] butyrate an approximate measure has been made of the rate of ketone-body utilisation expressed as μmol/g brain/min. A previous study (Cremer, 1971) has shown that in adult rat brain ^{14}C from injected D-β-hydroxy [3-^{14}C] butyrate accumulates to a great extent in glutamate and other amino acids in a manner very similar to that from ^{14}C glucose. Over a period of several minutes amino acids act as a trap for ^{14}C in the brain. Therefore, if the total radioactivity in this

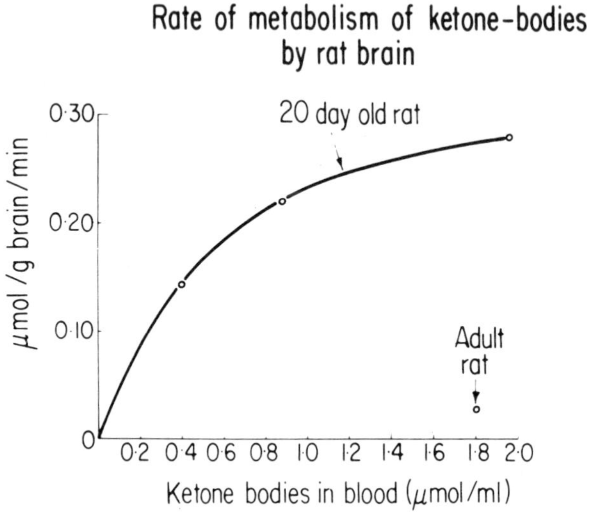

Fig. 3. Animals were given D-β-hydroxy [3-^{14}C] butyrate (1 μCi to young animals and 5 μCi to adults) by intraperitoneal injection and were killed between 2 and 10 min later. Blood samples were analysed for the amount and radioactivity of acetoacetate and β-hydroxybutyrate. The amino acid fraction from the brains was obtained as described by Cremer (1971) and the total radioactivity of this fraction was measured. The rate of ketone body metabolism by the brain was calculated as:

$$\frac{\Delta q/\text{g brain/min}}{\text{spec. activity of blood ketone-bodies (dpm}/\mu\text{mol)}}$$

where q is the total radioactivity in the amino acid fraction of the brain. The data will be given in full elsewhere.

amino acid fraction increases linearly with time while the specific radioactivity of the blood ketone-bodies remains constant then an approximate measure of the rate of utilisation of the blood ketone-bodies by the brain is given by:

$$\frac{\Delta q/\text{min}}{\text{sp. radioactivity of blood ketone-bodies (dpm}/\mu\text{mol)}}$$

where q = total dpm in amino acids/g of brain.

This formula was found to be applicable to the data obtained for both adult and 20-day-old rats given D-β-hydroxy [3-^{14}C] butyrate by intraperitoneal injection provided they were killed within the first 10 min following the injection. Results given in Fig. 3 show that the rates of utilisation of ketone-bodies for the brains of 20-day-old rats were proportional to the concentration of ketone-bodies in the blood. In the highest state of ketosis studied the rate was approximately 0.29 μmol/g brain/min.

In adult rats starved 48 hours (i.e. with a comparable concentration of ketone-bodies in the blood) the rate was very much less being approximately 0.03 μmol. The results support the findings of Hawkins *et al.* (1971) and show that there is a high rate of ketone-body utilisation in the brains of young rats at a time when the maximal activities of the necessary enzymes are high. The rates calculated from the radioactive experiments show that the slowest enzyme, β-hydroxybutyrate dehydrogenase, is present in about a six-fold excess in the 20-day-old rat brain. The lower value for this enzyme in the adult brain seems to correlate with the lower rate of ketone-body utilisation.

Drahota *et al.* (1964) pointed out that the high level of ketone bodies in the blood of suckling rats is almost certainly related to the high fat content of rats' milk (Dymsza *et al.*, 1964; see Table 3). At

TABLE 2

Composition of Various Milks

	Water %	*Protein* %	*Fat* %	*Lactose* %	*Minerals* %	*Cal/100 g*
Rat	72	8	12.3	3.0	1.5	159
Rabbit	73	11	12	2.0	2	–
Dog	76	8	9	3.1	0.9	125
Cow	87	3.5	3.7	4.9	0.7	66
Human	87	2.3	3.8	6.2	0.3	68

weaning rats are usually placed on a high carbohydrate diet and the concentrations of ketone-bodies in the blood fall almost immediately; in a normal adult rat they are very low. This raises the question as to whether the lack of provision of substrate is causally related to the decline in enzyme activity of β-hydroxybutyrate dehydrogenase and acetoacetyl-CoA thiolase, in the brain. Evidence in support of a direct relationship appeared in a report by Smith *et al.* (1969a) who stated that premature weaning of 10-day-old rats onto a high carbohydrate diet caused an earlier decline in blood β-hydroxybutyrate levels and brain β-hydroxybutyrate dehydrogenase activity whereas weaning at the usual age of 20 days onto a high fat (40%) diet maintained the relative ketosis and delayed the decline of the brain enzyme activity. These authors (1969b) also reported that in the adult rat brain β-hydroxybutyrate dehydrogenase was induced by a two- to three-day period of starvation, but other laboratories have not been able to substantiate this (Williamson, Bates, Page and Krebs, 1971; Pull and McIlwain, 1971; Cremer and Somogyi (unpubl.) in Fig. 2)

Concluding Remarks

The utilisation of ketone-bodies by the developing and mature rat brain has been considered here in some detail for two main reasons. Firstly, because the information is recent and provides evidence that a class of oxidisable substrates other than glucose is used in appreciable quantities by the young rat brain. Secondly, because the system appears to provide an example of adaptation by the brain to its environment through regulation of enzyme synthesis. However, almost nothing is known about the mechanisms controlling the rates of synthesis and removal of enzymes in brain cells. For instance, how far are changes in a developing cell's composition triggered off as a pre-determined invariant sequence of events and how far are they flexible to influences from the environment? Certain hormonal treatments seemingly affect both the number of cells in the developing brain and also their enzymic composition (García-Argiz *et al.*, 1967). Food deprivation from birth reduces the number of cells formed during maturation of rat brain (Winick and Noble, 1966) but alters only marginally the ratio of mg protein/mg DNA and the activity of several enzymes when expressed per mg DNA (Swaiman *et al.*, 1970). A limited food supply during development has been shown to result in functional impairment of the brain (Mourek *et al.*, 1967). In rats chronically starved during the 5th to 10th day after birth and then replaced on a normal diet longer latencies in the evoked cortical potentials to visual and auditory stimuli could be detected in animals 35 days after starvation had ended. The questions raised by Mourek *et al.* as to what are the limits of irreversible damage to the central nervous system and what are the limits of compensation are highly relevant to a consideration of mental retardation in relation to nutrient factors.

REFERENCES

Altman, J. (1969). In 'Handbook of Neurochemistry' (A. Lajtha, ed.), Vol. 2, p. 137. New York: Plenum Publishing Co.

Balázs, R., Kovács, S., Cocks, W. A., Johnson, A. L. and Eayrs, J. T. (1971). *Brain Res.* **25**, 555.

Bayer, S. M. and McMurray, W. C. (1967). *J. Neurochem.* **14**, 695.

Clouet, D. H. and Gaitonde, M. (1956). *J. Neurochem.* **1**, 126.

Cremer, J. E. (1971). *Biochem. J.* **122**, 135.

Drahota, Z., Hahn, P., Kleinzeller, A. and Kostolánská, A. (1964). *Biochem. J.* **93,** 61.
Dymsza, H. A., Czajka, D. M. and Miller, S. A. (1964). *J. Nutr.* **84,** 100.
Garcia-Argiz, C. A., Pasquini, J. M., Kaplun, B. and Gómez, C. J. (1967). *Brain Res.* **6,** 635.
Hawkins, R. A., Williamson, D. H. and Krebs, H. A. (1971). *Biochem. J.* **122,** 13.
Klee, C. B. and Sokoloff, L. (1967). *J. biol. Chem.* **242,** 3880.
Kuhlman, R. E. and Lowry, O. H. (1956). *J. Neurochem.* **1,** 173.
Mandel, P., Rein, H., Harth-Edel, S. and Mardell, R. (1964). In 'Comparative Neurochemistry' (D. Richter, ed.), p. 149. London: Pergamon.
Mourek, J., Himwich, W., Myslivec̆ek, J. and Callison, D. A. (1967). *Brain Res.* **6,** 241.
Page, A. M., Krebs, H. A. and Williamson, D. H. (1971). *Biochem. J.* **121,** 49.
Pasquini, J. M., Kaplun, B., Garcia-Argiz, C. A. and Gómez, C. J. (1967). *Brain Res.* **6,** 621.
Pull, I. and McIlwain, H. (1971). *J. Neurochem.* (in press).
Robins, E. and Lowe, I. P. (1961). *J. Neurochem.* **8,** 81.
Sims, K. L. and Pitts, F. N. (1970). *J. Neurochem.* **17,** 1607.
Smith, A. L., Satterthwaite, S. H. and Sokoloff, L. (1969a). In 'Second Int. Meeting. Int. Soc. Neurochem' (R. Paoletti, R. Fumagalli and D. Galli, eds), p. 371. Milan: Tamburini.
Smith, A. L., Satterthwaite, S. H. and Sokoloff, L. (1969b). *Science* **163,** 79.
Sugita, N. (1917). *J. Comp. Neurol.* **28,** 495.
Swaiman, K. F., Daleiden, J. M. and Wolfe, R. N. (1970). *J. Neurochem.* **17,** 1387.
Van den Berg, C. J., Van Kempen, G. M. J., Schadé, J. P. and Veldstra, H. (1965). *J. Neurochem.* **12,** 863.
Williamson, D. H., Bates, M. W., Page, A. M. and Krebs, H. A. (1971). *Biochem. J.* **121,** 41.
Winick, M. and Noble, A. (1966). *J. Nutr.* **89,** 300.

DISCUSSION

Giroud: The study of the evolution of the amino acids correlated with DNA is very interesting, since we know that protein synthesis which ensures expansive growth of neurites takes place largely in the perikaryon (Droz, B. and Leblond, C. P. (1963) J. comp. Neurol. **122,** 325).

Richter: I feel it is very valuable to know that weanling rats can utilise ketone bodies. Have you any clues as to why the adult gives up this capacity, seeing that already at 20 days when the cells are largely differentiated they do all this? Is this reversible in the adult?

Cremer: The original work by Prof. Sokoloff (Smith, A. L., Satterthwaite, S. H. and Sokoloff, L. (1969) loc. cit.) indicated that this was so. He was trying to relate the activity of β-hydroxybutyrate dehydrogenase with diet in the adult after a period of starvation when ketosis occurs. It did look as though the enzyme went up in activity again. Several laboratories have been unable to repeat this work, however. Nonetheless there may well be extreme conditions which we have not yet looked at where this does occur, particularly since the impetus for this work originated in observations on prolonged starvation in humans. They were virtually starved for 40 days and measurements of A-V differences across the brain showed that the brain was utilising ketone bodies. It may, therefore, come back again in the adult. Very recent information from Dr. Hawkins (personal communication) about these ketone body enzymes in human adult brain agree very well with those from the adult rat. Whether there was a time when they showed a high activity at any time we do not know.

Dobbing: It is certainly very surprising how little affected the adult brain is in composition by the most severe starvation. We did not look at the enzymes, but whatever is compensating it is doing it very efficiently.

Rundle: I was very interested in what Dr. Dobbing was saying earlier about species differences and particularly the critical nature of the post-natal period in humans. I wonder if there are any data about the switch-over of enzymes from the foetal to the adult state. For proteins we know that foetal haemoglobin in man continues for several months after birth. I wonder whether some of those species differences may be due to interference with the switch-over from foetal to adult form?

Kirman: I would like to ask a supplementary question. I wonder if the shapes of Dr. Cremer's curves helps us with the understanding of the effects of such point mutations as tuberous sclerosis and Apert's syndrome. Does it help us at all in looking at the question of unclassified mental retardation, that may have bits broken off into specific entities, if we can identify enzymes that are failing early on and so produce things like the de Lange syndrome or other things that are not properly identified yet?

Stern: One of the most remarkable studies in humans is the ketotic hypoglycaemia of Colle and Ulstrom (Colle, E. D. and Ulstrom, R. A. (1964) *J. Pediat.* **64**, 632). These children respond to carbohydrate starvation by ketosis and hypoglycaemia, but this is not recognised because no abnormality is found by routine testing. It is suggested that in these children the alternative pathways are less easily switched on.

Wigglesworth: Ketone body metabolism is obviously very important in relation to neonatal hypoglycaemia. Some babies seem to get hypoglycaemic symptoms more easily than others.

Magee: Can I ask about the stability of these enzymes? Is it reasonable to determine them in post-mortem material, or do you have to use operation material?

Cremer: I don't know.

Balázs: Once we did a silly experiment, putting a brain in formalin and then measuring the enzyme activity. You can do it if you get rid of the excess formalin with Sephadex. You do not get 100%, but you can get a base level.

Rundle: I have looked at enzymes on post-mortem brain, liver and kidney. You get very little change in pattern on starch-gel electrophoresis up to 2-3 months when kept in the deep-freeze, but it is a product of the number of times you thaw the tissue out. If the post-mortem is early enough and you cool the tissue rapidly, then the iso-enzyme patterns are little changed, but it varies with the enzyme. Transpeptidases lasted several months in the deep freeze, whereas some naphthyl-amidases were quite labile.

Davison: I think it is important that people are not put off from attempting to measure enzymes in post mortem brain material. There are several papers on the effects of room temperature on enzymes that show that even after a day or so they are still active. This is, of course, only true of some enzymes.

Clayton: I think there is a great danger in taking tissues a long time after death. Storage is the least problem. Autopsy samples for enzymes, in my experience, are extremely risky. It is terribly important to have control material.

Laurence: Tissue taken at operation is often quite severely traumatised.

Clayton: Whatever you do in man, it is never going to be perfect for control data, and it is worse in children.

Davison: But there is no reason why you shouldn't try, provided you are exceptionally careful about controls.

Dobbing: With stable substances such as DNA, and cholesterol, you can leave a rat brain a week on the bench and still get good answers.

Davison: With cytochrome oxidase its activity stayed constant. Succinic dehydrogenase tends to go off very slightly, but many remain unchanged.

Crome: It is in chromosomal anomalies where enzyme studies may help. Perhaps someone has some information on anomalies other than in Down's disease?

Dobbing: Dr. Adlard in my department has looked at certain enzymes during undernutrition and has found the usual variety of patterns. We thought this corresponded to the variety of patterns of development which we showed. Aldolase can be reduced by undernutrition during the first three weeks, but this catches up. ACh-ase is reduced also, but you end up with an increased amount per gram wet wt., which may be a concentration effect. As usual the cerebellum showed the grossest effects and the brain stem the least.

Sylvester: One difficulty in handling human material is not only time after death and destruction of possible enzyme patterns, but also the administration of drugs during life. I never know to what extent this may affect enzyme studies; I wonder if anyone could enlighten me on this?

Davison: It has certainly been ,shown for example that iproniazid affects monoamine oxidase after death and isoniazid affects the B_6-dependent enzymes.

Hanefeld: Anticonvulsants produce an increase in many enzymes, for example alkaline phosphatase is as high as in rickets if children are treated for a long time with anticonvulsants. It is thought that this is due to enzyme induction so that you metabolise vitamin B_6 faster.

Stern: Barbiturates generally stimulate microsomal enzymes. Certain anaesthetics, in association with hyperthermia, produce fantastic increases in creatine phosphokinase, so that if such a child died you would find very abnormal enzyme patterns. Chromosomal abnormalities and enzyme levels were discussed in Study Group No. 2 (1970) and the results have been rather disappointing. Work from Greece on the pattern of enzymes in red cells in Down's syndrome found this to be age-dependent, that is some enzymes were not significantly different from normal in the neonate with trisomy, but were raised subsequently. The only one which was consistently raised was phosphofructokinase. This is the key enzyme in the control of carbohydrate metabolism and it is affected by a very large number of factors, AMP, ADP, citrate, etc. (Lowry, D.H. and Passoneau, J. V. (1966) *J. biol. Chem.* **241**, 2268). There are thus many environmental reasons why this enzyme should be abnormal. No consistent pattern of abnormality, however, has emerged for the other trisomies.

Prestige: Do you feel sure that this ketosis is for energy production? Is there any histochemistry that can be done on these enzymes?

Cremer: From work in progress, in which we use radioactive precursors, we find that the ketone bodies follow the same pattern of C^{14} distribution into brain metabolites as glucose and we therefore assume from this that the behaviour of the two is very similar. The other types of precursors, e.g. acetate or glutamate, show a very different pattern. It is likely, therefore, that ketones are providing energy.

General Discussion

INTRODUCED BY A. N. DAVISON

It was Dr. O'Connor who asked the biochemist to provide more guide lines for advance for those interested in mental retardation. The papers this afternoon show some of the difficulties that face biochemists. Dr. Wigglesworth has spoken about techniques for producing damage to foetal brain, in particular the use of hydroxyurea. Dr. Balázs, in producing experimental hypothyroidism in rats, has most interesting results, and biochemists should make more use of this kind of procedure. It would be very interesting to try the effects of these various agents at different times during development in the hope of identifying some changes of cellular structural development which produces a common behavioural abnormality. In that way it might be possible to focus on the specific nature of the factors concerned with mental retardation.

I would also like to ask if it is safe to assume, in this group of mental retardations, that the damage is structural, affecting either cell number or cellular maturation, for example. Perhaps such diseases may be associated with structural changes of the enzyme protein and the activity may be reduced. Alternatively there may be a reversible effect on metabolism, such as, for example, that of 5-HT. All the papers this afternoon seem to indicate that structural changes are associated with mental retardation. The correctness of this view is particularly striking in cretinism, which becomes irreversible if treatment is delayed beyond three months, whereas mental aberrations develop much more slowly in adults with myxoedema. This argues that the retardation in the cretin is linked to a process of structural maturation. The same might be said for other diseased systems (e.g. aminoacidurias) that could produce mental retardation. In attempting to evaluate these possibilities, it is necessary to correlate changing biochemical parameters with developing changes in anatomical structure. In the human brain two critical periods are recognisable in cellular development, related to neuronal and glial proliferation respectively. The neuronal population is largely established pre-natally and glial multiplication perinatally. After birth

TABLE 1

Changes in Glycolipids, Succinic Dehydrogenase Activity and Brain Organelles of Rat Brain During Development

Mitochondria (mg./g wet wt.)	7.2 ± 2.0	39	15.9 ± 6.9	85	17.7 ± 8.5	95	18.7 ± 2.4
Succinic dehydrogenase activity (μmol. substrate/hour/g wet wt.)	24	5	329 ± 11	63	439 ± 71	91	481 ± 68
Synaptosomes (mg./g wet wt.)	8.1 ± 2.1	46	15.1 ± 5.8	85	17.6 ± 7.4	100	17.7 ± 2.0
Gangliosides (mγ NANA/g wet wt.)	450	33	1100	80	1400	100	1360
Myelin (mg. dry wt./g wet wt.)	0	–	4	17.5	8.5	37	23
Cerebroside (μmole/g wet wt.)	0	–	1.1	9	2.0	18	11.3
Wet weight of brain (g)	0.3 – 0.5	22	1.15 ± 0.15	65	1.3 ± 0.1	73	1.78 ± 0.3

(Data from Maccioni and Caputto (1968) and other sources.)

increased weight of the brain may be largely ascribed to growth of neuronal processes and deposition of myelin, while the adult proportions of most subcellular components is reached soon after birth (i.e. 2-3 weeks in the rat), deposition of myelin continues for a very prolonged period. In the human infant it is, therefore, probable that the process of myelination is particularly susceptible to the action of neurotoxic agents and to variations in substrate supply.

It would be valuable to have specific indices of brain anatomical structures, but very few stand up to critical evaluation. The use of differential and density gradient centrifugation has been of considerable

TABLE 2

Biochemical Correlates With Brain Structure

Cellular component	*Biochemical 'marker'*
Nucleus	DNA polymerase
Mitochondrion; outer membrane	Monoamine oxidase
inner membrane	Succinic dehydrogenase
	Cardiolipin
Synaptosomes	Gangliosides
External synaptic membranes	Acetylcholinesterase
Microsomes	Cytochrome P-450
Plasma membrane	5′-Nucleotidase
Lysosomes	β-Galactosidase
Myelin	Cerebrosides
	2′,3′ Cyclic-nucleotide 3′-phosphohydrolase
	Basic EAE protein
Glial cells	S-100 protein
	Cholinesterase
	Carbonic anhydrase
Neurones	Protein 14-3-2

help to biochemists in separation of cerebral organelles; great care must be taken, however, to obtain reproducible separations. It is important to decide if quantitative separations are necessary or if homogeneity is more desirable, for while pure mitochondria, nuclei and myelin can be obtained in doing so, it is not possible to avoid losses in purification. An example of data is shown in Table 1 where dry wt. (after complete removal of sucrose) determinations indicate the relative abundance of synaptosomes, mitochondria and myelin in the developing rat brain.

Besides fractionation techniques, estimation of specific substances, or 'markers' may indicate changes in cellular components (Table 2). Succinic dehydrogenase activity has been used as a 'marker' enzyme for mitochondrial inner membrane, gangliosides for synaptosomes, and cerebrosides for myelin.

For example, succinic dehydrogenase and cytochrome oxidase may give a clue during development to the multiplication of mitochondria within the nervous system (but see Gregson and Williams) (Gregson, N. and Williams, P. L. (1969) *J. Neurochem.* **16**, 617). Estimation of ganglioside, or of glutamate decarboxylase, gives a very approximate indication of the increase of nerve-ending particles. Estimation of cerebrosides and of proteolipid proteins in phenylketonuria and other aminoacidurias gives an index of the extent of myelination, and has been used to detect amyelination. Further advance in this field must await quantitative isolation of different cell types and the discovery of more specific analytical criteria (e.g. immunological reactions).

Finally, the field of genetics and inborn errors of brain metabolism must inevitably be a fruitful approach. The original concept of a mutation giving rise to a single enzyme deficiency has been amply confirmed in human disease (e.g. absence of uridyl-galactosyl transferase in galactosaemia), but more recently further possible effects of gene detection have been discovered. Thus, if the Jacob-Monod hypothesis applies to the mammalian nucleus, it would be expected that mutation of the operator gene would switch off all the cistrons in the gene operon leading to a regulatory defect.

In some cases of inherited metabolic disease multiple enzyme deficiencies have been noted (Auerbach, V. H. and Di George, A. M. (1965) *Amer. J. Med. Sci.* **249**, 718). Such a case may apply to orotic aciduria where two enzyme deficiencies have been observed. In other human disorders definite, though small amounts, of enzyme may remain (e.g. acatalasia) suggesting a structural gene abnormality while, on the other hand, more subtle changes may occur such as reduced affinity constants (K_m) of an enzyme. Another possible metabolic regulation of enzyme activity may be by repression of enzyme activity through excess substrate, for example in the Lesch-Nyhan syndrome where overproduction of 5-phosphoribosyl-1-pyrophosphate may stimulate uric acid biosynthesis. In the future it may be possible to supply missing enzymes in encapsulated form (e.g. liposomes) (Gregoriadis, Leathwood and Ryman (1971) *F.E.B.S. Letters* **14**, 95) or to induce specific enzyme activity. Alternatively, a new clone may be introduced into the body or, conceivably, a genetic deficiency might be corrected by supplying a virus carrying DNA for the relevant missing enzyme.

Hanefeld: In Switzerland people from Rossi's Hospital were able to correct metachromatic leucodystrophy in tissue-cultured cells by adding arylsulphatase.

Stern: It is true that the alteration of K_m (substrate affinity) in isolated cases has been corrected, for instance, in homocystinuria with Vitamin B_6, and one variant of maple sugar urine disease, methyl malonic acidaemia, responds to B_{12} and proprionicacidaemia responds to biotin. In each of these at least one case has been found responding to very large doses of these vitamins. Pauling, of course, suggested that this was the general cause of mental illness, namely abnormality of vitamin concentrations. What was wrong, he said, was that very high vitamin levels were necessary. He even thought that schizophrenia might be caused in this way.

Davison: Do you think that as regards the chemical pathological investigation of these diseases we ought not to go through them all looking at enzyme affinity constants rather than just absolute activities?

Stern: In citrullinuria the K_m is, in fact, at fault and, of course, in every one of the inborn errors there are several genetic variants. Also, with respect to regulator genes in Kreigler-Najjar syndrome, there is evidence that this is a defect in a regulator gene, because this enzyme could, in fact, be induced.

Balázs: However important it is to increase our collection of well-defined enzymes, I think the pattern is more important. For example, does the activity of phosphofructokinase by itself mean very much? It is definitely the critical enzyme in glycolysis, but I don't think it means much when you measure it under optimal conditions. It has so many modulators that its activity *in vivo* will be determined by the modulators rather than the enzyme protein. There are a number of rate-limiting enzymes which determine the pattern of the metabolism. And these are probably more important in dysfunction. In mental retardation, therefore, disturbance to function may not be shown up by the activity of the individual enzymes.

Dobbing: Since in the brain the question of structure versus function is determined by the structure itself, have people any views on the question of the withdrawal of treatment of inborn errors after the brain has grown under their regimen?

Clayton: The literature has a number of cases of phenylketonuria with withdrawn treatment, but often those are not the best cases anyway. At Great Ormond Street Hospital we withdrew the diet from a 12½-year-old girl who was one of the first to be treated early, having been treated from 3½ weeks of age. So far as we can tell she has remained well. In subsequent children we have withdrawn the diet at the age of eight years. Many experienced paediatricians will disagree strongly with withdrawing the diet at all, but how do you detect a slow, gradual mental deterioration if this should take place? Our impression is that the first 18 months on the diet is the really important time.

Dobbing: It depends entirely whether only the developing brain is affected by this change.

Davison: There are cases with high phenylalanine levels who are intellectually normal.

Clayton: And there are children with all the biochemical stigmata of phenylketonuria, who are of normal intelligence. But whether they achieve what they might otherwise have achieved is unknown.

Kirman: Is it possible to distinguish the different alleles by the kinetics of the different enzymes, and can you, therefore, distinguish hyperphenylalaninaemia from true phenylketonuria?

Clayton: Theoretically yes, but there is little information on the enzymes in either affected or in normal cases. We have yet to make this approach, but biopsies are a problem in such children. At present we are working on the enzymes in normal biopsy material and following back to abortion material from phenylketonurics.

Richter: Children are more irritable when off their diet for a time. Is that true and is this a toxic effect?

Clayton: It is true that they are temporarily disturbed but they settle down.

Richter: Does this imply a toxic effect?

Clayton: It implies a toxic effect of something, but of what, I do not know.

Hanefeld: Older children when detected late become easier to handle when on the diet, even though their intelligence is not improved.

Woollam: The technique of chromosome analysis is much less productive now in explaining disease entities than it was. Do biochemists still expect their subject *vis-à-vis* mental defect to go on expanding or will it follow chromosome analysis in this way?

Dobbing: I would have thought that their reservoir of untapped information is still vast.

Clayton: I agree. It is both lack of space and of people that holds one up from working on these children. You need trained staff for each child and this shortage is certainly very frustrating.

Kirman: But chromosome analysis is only one technique, while biochemists have hundreds of potentially available techniques. Leigh's encephalopathy (Editorial *Brit. Med. J. (1971)* 2, 238) is one such example, where the relevant enzyme defect is found in blood. With developing techniques the hope is that evidence outside the brain may be found.

Rundle: The only trouble about studying blood is that the more enzymes you estimate the wider becomes the picture and the more confusing it is. With increasing numbers a computer will be needed to handle the data.

Stern: Precisely this is happening in Norway. Prof. Eldjarn (Jellum, E., Stokke, O. and Eldjard, L. (1971) *Scand. J. Lab. clin. Med.* 27, 273) uses an I.B.M. computer linked to an automated system of gas chromatography and mass spectrometry for the study of urine from patients with mental retardation. He has detected new inborn errors both in amino acids and now in organic acid metabolism.

Rundle: But we need first more normal children.

O'Connor: Hearing about normal children prompts me to ask the question whether we have any useful information on the biochemistry of normality and its range? In mental retardation there are children with an I.Q. of 70 up to 80 or 85, which is perhaps within normal limits judged by certain criteria. One should be looking for deviations which might have the effect of arresting the I.Q. but still in a sense be normal.

Harris: The sheer economics of research in this field is evident in any mental subnormality hospital, where there is clearly barely enough money to maintain their daily care. If it is difficult at Great Ormond Street Hospital to get the necessary staff and equipment, this is only the tip of the iceberg.

Dobbing: If prevention is our main aim someone should calculate how much it costs to remain as we are at present.

Laurence: This is known for Down's syndrome. To do an amniocentesis on the pregnant population over the age of 30 would be a worthwhile investment, and certainly all pregnancies over 40 should be looked at. This would reduce the population of Down's syndrome by 20%. Going to 35 years, which would be 10% of the pregnant community, would halve the population of Down's syndrome. It costs at least £22,000 over a lifetime to care for a retarded child.

Davison: I wonder whether there is not a much greater unexplored field in terms of brain metabolism itself. Here our advance depends on basic knowledge, and for example about regulation of gene expression, the role of spermidine, histones and so on, in DNA control. A really big and major advance would be to look at brain tissue itself rather than the products of faulty metabolism in the body fluids. I would prefer to see more efforts in developmental neurobiology. There is a great need in this country for this effort.

Richter: Up till now we have considered only monogenic disturbances. There would seem to be an even greater field for the polygenic ones where two or more enzyme abnormalities exist. This raises the important question mentioned by Dr. O'Connor of the normal variation and its meaning.

Rundle: I think one is in danger if you think in terms of a clear-cut difference between the normal and the mentally sub-normal person. You get into difficulty if you take biochemical data and compare it with one or more cases. I was intrigued by the earlier remark on the effect of drugs on alkaline phosphatase. We are also interested in this, and although we have only done 500 or 600 estimations and we haven't yet correlated it with any specific anticonvulsant. What seems to be happening is that there is an equally great difference between a normal and a subnormal person not on anticonvulsant, as there is between subnormals and those on anticonvulsants. One has to look at differences within the mentally subnormal group as well as between these and the normal.

Kirman: There are very few of the classified entities that do not trespass into the territory of the normal. For instance, tuberous sclerosis like most of them provides examples with average intelligence. Similarly with phenylketonuria, or histoidinaemia and other errors which commonly determine mental retardation, these can exceptionally occur in average or above-average intelligence. There are relatively few exceptions to this rule.

O'Connor: I suppose you could grade these because one of the problems that psychologists have with undifferentiated subnormality is that it appears for them to be part of the normal curve whereas since Pearson and Jaederholm (Pearson, K. and Jaederholm, G. A. (1914) 'On the Continuity of Mental Defect'. Dulau and Co., London) in about 1870, the argument has been that a certain number fall beyond the range of this normal curve. I presume that the cases we are discussing today fall for the most part beyond that range or near the bottom end of it. Without disputing with Dr. Kirman, in mongolism for example one tends to get somewhat lower I.Q.'s than you would expect from the normal curve.

Kirman: This is an exception, of course, unless you include mosaics in this concept which provide a 'touch' of mongolism, as it were. I think, however, with a fairly large number of these entities, this is so. Looking at this problem in general one shouldn't allow one aspect of a phenomenon to influence too much one's looking at other aspects. For example, a distribution curve is only a mathematical expression of the findings, it doesn't necessarily carry any implication as to aetiology, when certain cases lie off the normal curve.

O'Connor: The hyperintelligent leave one with something of a problem, I suppose, unless you are prepared to account for normality as a disorder.

Magee: I would like to raise again the possible hazard from oral contraceptives for the offspring. What had you in mind when you raised this?

Kirman: Dr. Gal (Gal, I., Kirman, B. and Stern, J. (1967) *Nature, Lond.* **216**, 83; Gal, I., Parkinson, C. and Croft, I. (1971) *Brit. Med. J.* **2**, 426) did a study on the pregnancy test. It was only preliminary but it suggested that its use could influence abnormalities.

Laurence: This has been repeated, but not substantiated.

Dobbing: How much hard fact is there about the 'Pill'?

Crome: I know of at least two examples where pregnancy occurred in spite of the 'Pill' and the children were very good. I know of one example where the child was an idiot.

3

Mutagenic Agents and Their Effects on the Developing Brain

Virus Infection and Brain Development

I. ZLOTNIK

Introduction

The object of this communication is to draw attention to the hazards and long term effects of virus infection on the developing CNS. The immediate results of virus infections are more or less known as they usually lead to overt signs of disease and occasionally death. However, the damage that such infections may leave can be very serious, as the developing brain is very prone to such sequelae, much more so than the adult brain.

Newborn animals appear to be highly susceptible to experimental viral infections of the CNS and many viruses which produce only inapparent infections in adults will cause a fatal disease in immature animals (Doherty, 1969; Zlotnik *et al.*, 1971). Under natural conditions, however, the developing foetus is protected against many viral infections, while the newborn receives passive immunity against some infections from the maternal colostrum. On the other hand, there are some viruses which in the absence of maternal immunity can penetrate to the foetus and cause either death of the foetus and abortion, or give rise to congenital malformations. Since Gregg's (1941) account that rubella may produce a variety of foetal malformations in man, there is a general awareness of virus infections during the gestation period and a number of viruses were shown to give rise to foetal CNS damage.

In early post-natal life virus infection of the CNS may produce acute lethal diseases or may leave, after the recovery from the acute attack, sequelae which lead to mental retardation and neurological symptoms. While such sequelae may be permanent and impair the health of the individuals, they cannot be always related to the degree of the severity of the original infection.

In the present paper a review will be given of the existing evidence of human viral pre-natal and post-natal infections, followed by a description of hitherto unpublished experiments in small laboratory animals, aimed at producing pre-natal and post-natal infections.

Virus Infections in Man

Pre-natal Infections

There does not seem to be any doubt that *rubella* occupies a special place in maternal infections likely to cause the transmission of the disease to the foetus and to produce a variety of foetal malformations (Gregg, 1941; Greenberg *et al.,* 1957; Michaelis and Mellin, 1960; Lock *et al.,* 1961; Crome and Stern, 1967). The virus of rubella is capable of producing transplacental infections during the first 12 weeks of pregnancy, and it was isolated not only from many foetuses and organs of infants that died with rubella-syndrome defects, but also from the nasopharynx of survivors. The risk of maternal rubella to the foetus is estimated to be about 30%, giving rise to abortions (5%), stillbirth (4.5%), post-natal death under two years (6.9%) and finally survival with congenital defects (13.0%). The malformations vary over a very wide field from spina bifida, hydrocephalus, microcephaly, microgyria, microphthalmia, cataracts and perceptive deafness. Apart from CNS changes, rubella may cause congenital heart disease, thrombocytopenia, hepatosplenomegaly, myocardial necrosis and interstitial pneumonitis.

The second disease of importance is *cytomegalic inclusion disease* which is primarily an illness of infancy, but may be also involved in transuterine infections. The human salivary gland virus responsible for the disease, very often causes in adults clinically inapparent infections with intranuclear and intracytoplasmic inclusions in the salivary gland cells. The foetal CNS is not often affected, the order of preference of organs being kidneys, lung, liver, pancreas and salivary gland. In generalised forms of cytomegalic inclusion disease, the CNS may be involved in about 10% of cases. The changes in the nervous system consist of periventricular calcifications with inclusions in the subependymal glial cells (Haymaker *et al.,* 1954), microcephaly, internal hydrocephalus and chorioretinitis. Cytomegaly is found in the ganglion cells of the brain stem and caudate nucleus, while disseminated necrotising calcifications is seen in other cases (Crome and France, 1959). The disease was known to cause foetal infections during the fourth month of pregnancy (Diezel, 1954) and virus was isolated and propagated in tissue culture cells from the salivary gland of an infant showing typical inclusions and from the kidney of a baby that died as a result of the generalised disease (Smith, 1956).

Poliomyelitis may cause intrauterine infections, especially towards the end of pregnancy, but the incidence was thought to be rare. There is no evidence of teratogenic effects, but stillbirth and death of the infant are likely. Virus (type 1) was isolated from the CNS of both mother and infant (Swarts and Kercher, 1954), and from the placenta and foetus in another case (Shaeffer *et al.*, 1954).

A number of other viruses were reported to be capable of producing transplacental infections with CNS involvement, thus *Coxsackie B virus* was implicated, giving rise to both brain and heart lesions in the foetus (Kilbrick and Benirschke, 1958). In a further communication a case of congenital hydrocephalus was described in a newborn infant, the mother of whom suffered from *epidemic hepatitis* in the second and third months of pregnancy (Kass, 1951). Of 18 women affected with *measles* during pregnancy three gave birth to defective infants and one aborted. In the same report mention is made of six mothers with *mumps* and two with *chickenpox* producing defective babies (Swan *et al.*, 1946). Finally *western equine encephalitis* (WEE) was diagosed in twin girls on the fifth day after birth. The mother of the babies was believed to have been bitten by mosquitoes 11 days before delivery. Both infants recovered and retained antibodies to WEE (Shinefield and Townsend, 1953).

The question whether *influenza virus* in the mother can produce teratogenic effects in the foetus is not yet fully answered. Coffey and Jessop (1959) reported that in Dublin following an outbreak of influenza 3.6% of mothers with influenza produced abnormal infants as compared with 1.6% in unaffected controls. Ingalls (1960) confirmed that during the months of March to June 1958 after the severe influenza in Pennsylvania during October and November 1957, there was a very high incidence of abnormalities amongst newborn babies, ranging from haemangiomata, club foot, cleft lip and palate, mongolism and anencephalus. On the other hand, Doll *et al.* (1960) and Pasamanick and Knobloch (1960, 1962) could not find any increase in child abnormalities following the outbreak of Asian influenza in 1957-58. It was suggested that the rather convincing results obtained in Dublin were not entirely due to a specific effect of the influenza virus but to the severe febrile illness in a population that is by and large at a marginal economic and nutritonal level.

Post-natal Infections

Children as a whole are highly susceptible to all virus infections of the CNS. The disease in infancy tends to be more severe than in adults and very frequently it leaves sequelae that might impair the health and the mental stability of the individuals.

Acute encephalitis caused by the virus of *herpes simplex* is an uncommon infection in early infancy, but cases were reported even on the fifth and seventh day after birth. The lesions in such cases of herpes encephalitis were either confined to the CNS or were generalised affecting also the liver and the adrenals. The disease was usually very severe giving rise to widespread necrosis and the outcome was fatal (Wolf and Cowen, 1959).

Measles encephalitis is usually a reversible condition, but cases were reported of temporary and permanent sequelae following clinical recovery (Adams, 1968; Byers and Meyer, 1952). These consisted of easy fatigability of intellectual function, defects in attention, defects in perceptual and spatial organisation, and defects in learning capacity.

In addition to measles encephalitis, *S.S.P.E. (Subacute Sclerosing Panencephalitis)* may represent a serious hazard to the young (Dayan *et al.*, 1967). The disease usually starts with psychological disturbances and intellectual deterioration and leads relentlessly to death. The general concensus of opinion is that, although measles virus can be traced as the major aetiological factor of the disease, an antibody complex or a type of cell-mediated immunity is to be blamed for triggering off the disease (Zeman and Kolar, 1968; Berman *et al.*, 1968; Lennette *et al.*, 1968).

Poliomyelitis, Coxsackie B virus and *von Economo's encephalitis* were reported in young infants. Polio was diagnosed as early as six days after birth. Coxsackie B virus caused in all verified cases mild to moderate focal meningo-encephalitis with mononuclear cellular infiltrations. Following World War I, cases of encephalitis lethargica were recognised also in infants (Wolf and Cowen, 1959).

Of the more exotic diseases, western equine encephalitis, west Nile fever, eastern equine encephalitis, Japanese B encephalitis and St. Louis encephalitis are known to cause acute infections in infancy. Very young infants appear to be especially susceptible to western equine encephalitis virus (WEE) and recovery from the acute disease leads often to complications and sequelae (Platou, 1940. Davis, 1940; Noran and Baker, 1943 and 1945; Nisenbaum and Wallis, 1965; Noran, 1944; Lewis *et al.*, 1947). It appears that the real danger to children from WEE is caused by the tendency of the lesions to become progressively subacute, resulting in chronic forms of brain damage including cavitation. The chronic disease is usually accompanied by intellectual deterioration and neurological symptoms such as convulsions, muscular weakness and paralysis.

Experimental Viral Infections in Laboratory Animals

In order to study transplacental and neonatal virus infections in animals a number of experiments were initiated, using either attenuated, vaccine type viruses or viruses of low virulence for adult animals. The results of some of these experiments proved to be very promising, especially as chronic forms of brain damage were observed, which persisted for considerable periods after the cessation of the acute lesions.

Materials and Methods

Three viruses were used in the experiments described in this paper as follows: virulent Langat TP 21 virus, attentuated Langat virus–clone TP 21-9 (Price *et al.*, 1963) and the attenuated western equine encephalitis virus–WEE–Clone 15 (Johnson, 1963). These three viruses proved to be of low pathogenicity for adult hamsters in that inoculations by any route did not result in clinical signs of disease, while the two attenuated clones caused only inapparent infections in mice when inoculated by a peripheral route.

White Porton mice, three months old, were used for transplacental infections. In order to determine the date of mating and conception pairs of mice were kept in individual cages and every morning the female mice were examined for vaginal plugs. Once mating was established the males were removed and the females were inoculated intradermally with attenuated Langat virus or attenuated WEE virus in doses of 0.2 ml of 10^6 MLD_{50} of virus, either on the 5th, 10th or 15th day after mating. A sufficient number of control females remained uninoculated. After the birth of the litters samples of offspring were sacrificed at various intervals and brains examined for lesions and the presence of virus.

Syrian golden hamsters aged from 1 to 15 days were used for neonatal and suckling period infections. The inoculated animals in a litter remained with their mothers until weaning and were divided into two major groups, one receiving inoculations of virus intradermally the other intraperitoneally. Each group was further subdivided into three subgroups according to the dose of virus as follows: 10^5 MLD_{50}, 10^3 MLD_{50} and 10^1 MLD_{50}. All three viruses were used in the experiments, the dose for suckling hamsters being 0.05 ml for the intradermal route and 0.1 ml for intraperitoneal infections. Inoculated hamsters were observed for 12 weeks and those showing symptoms were destroyed and brains removed for examination. In addition groups of 2-4 hamsters not showing any symptoms were sacrificed weekly for 12 weeks and brains examined for histological changes and the presence of virus. The techniques used for histological preparations were those reported previously (Zlotnik, 1968), while virus assays were carried out by i.c. inoculations of 10-fold aliquots of supernates of brain homogenates into one-day-old suckling mice.

Results

VIRUS INOCULATIONS INTO PREGNANT MICE

Pregnant mice inoculated with attentuated WEE virus did not develop symptoms and gave birth to healthy litters, irrespective of the time of infection. A sample of inoculated mothers was sacrificed at various periods after infection. In all cases limited inflammatory lesions were found in the brain, and virus was isolated from the CNS between third and seventh day after infection. Examination of brains of newborn litters and of those destroyed weekly for four weeks after birth did not reveal any pathological changes or traces of virus. A number of four-week-old offspring of infected mothers and their mothers were then challenged with the highly virulent WEE + 4 i.p. While all the mothers remained unaffected as a result of acquired immunity the offspring died from the infection. Thus, in spite of maternal infection during pregnancy, the litters did not become infected with the attenuated strain during the gestation period.

Pregnant mice inoculated with the attenuated Langat virus, either 10 or 15 days after mating produced healthy litters that did not show any signs of disease, brain lesions or the presence of virus in their brains. At the same time the inoculated mothers had inflammatory changes and virus in their CNS. On the other hand only a proportion of mice inoculated five days after mating (20%), gave birth to normal litters, the remainder either did not produce litters or aborted, cannibalising the foetus.

EXPERIMENTAL INFECTION OF NEONATAL AND SUCKLING HAMSTERS

Hamsters were chosen for post-natal infections in preference to mice, because they were found less susceptible in their adult state to peripheral infections with the three viruses used in this study, and especially that even the virulent Langat TP 21 caused neither disease nor constant brain lesions in three-week-old hamsters as against 20% mortality and 100% brain lesions in three-week-old, weaned mice.

Attenuated western equine encephalitis virus (WEE). Newborn hamsters and those aged 4-12 days developed acute symptoms with paralysis and died between the third and ninth day after inoculation, irrespective of the dose of virus or route of infection. Examination of the brains revealed as follows: widespread haemorrhages, capillary proliferation, perivascular cuffings consisting of one layer of infiltrating mononuclear cells, microglial accumulations, severe degeneration of neurons and necrosis of large areas of the cerebral cortex, spongy degeneration of subcortical centres and finally a marked and diffuse astrocytosis throughout the brain.

Fifteen-day-old hamsters, as a rule survived inoculations with attenuated WEE virus and did not develop signs of disease. However, irrespective of the route and dose of virus they developed acute lesions of encephalitis at the same time virus could be isolated from their brain during the first week after infection. The acute lesions consisted of a scanty meningeal exudate, widespread perivascular mononuclear infiltrations, surrounded by zones of microglial proliferation, spongy degeneration, cerebellar glial shrubs, astrocytic hypertrophy and proliferation and finally focal necrotic centres throughout the cerebral cortex and thalamus.

Two weeks after infection the pathological process in the brain became subacute in character. Huge perivascular cuffings composed of several layers of cells, either caused occlusion or narrowing of vascular lumina. Microglial proliferations gave rise to the formation of large granulomatous accumulations of cells in many parts of the cortex or subcortical areas. Necrotic centres of various sizes became widespread and showed various degrees of calcification. The astrocytes around the necrotic lesions or granulomatous accumulations became greatly hypertrophied with the formation of very thick long processes. A similar picture to the above was still present after three weeks, but some of the granulomatous lesions began undergoing granular calcification (Fig. 1), while in the cerebellum, both glial shrubs and many Purkinje cells became calcified.

After four weeks the inflammatory reaction receded almost completely, but the necrotic and calcified foci remained very prominent. Astrocytic proliferation and hypertrophy although very marked became limited to the hippocampus in the vicinity of calcified foci, around some enlarged blood vessels and at the periphery of the cerebral cortex, giving rise to dense fibrous tangles and huge astrocytic cell bodies (Fig. 2). This picture remained static for a long time and after 12 weeks about 50% of the hamsters retained large calcified or necrotic centres, especially in the temporal cortex and in the thalamus. In some cases small cavities lined with calcified debris appeared in the brain very often surrounded by a very dense zone of astrocytic proliferation. The cerebellum was very often affected, showed very widespread calcification of Purkinje cells and numerous empty baskets.

Virulent Langat TP 21 virus. Newborn and 5-day-old suckling hamsters developed acute symptoms and died between the fourth and eighth day after inoculation with virulent Langat virus. The lesions in the brain of affected hamsters were characteristic of acute meningo-encephalitis. However, hamsters aged 10 to 15 days remained clinically unaffected for periods of 12 weeks. Examination of brains of 10-day-old hamsters destroyed one week after infection revealed in all cases very mild signs of encephalitis with a few perivascular cuffings, occasional microglial infiltrations and a moderate astrocytic proliferation. However, two weeks after infection the actute inflammatory process was found only in about 20% of brains, but while 60% had hardly any change a further 20% had a progressive extension of the inflammatory process especially in the hippocampus and occasionally in the frontal cortex and in the anterior colliculi of the midbrain. Many capillaries appeared surrounded by huge cuffs composed of either mononuclear cells or microglia. A diffuse microglial infiltrate appeared in the granule cell layer while the astrocytes showed very marked hypertrophy with the formation of very long tortuous processes.

Beginning from the third week after infection all hamsters inoculated intradermally had only very occasionally residual lesions in the brain consisting of a few glial knots or rosettes. However, in hamsters inoculated intraperitoneally about 20-25% showed consistently subacute lesions that became progressively chronic leading to gross deformity of the hippocampus and occasionally other parts. In the hippocampus of such i.p. inoculated animals there was at three weeks after infection a very dense microglial infiltration into the pyramidal and granule cell layers with the destruction of many neurones. While many glial cells showed 'stab' cell transformation other cells assumed a clear cytoplasm and their nuclei became round and formed accumulations or cell nests. Many of the capillaries were also surrounded by several layers of microglial cells while the astrocytes formed thick fibrous tangles and whorls either around the capillaries or the cell nests.

Four weeks after infection the hippocampal lesions in the i.p. inoculated hamsters proved to be always bilateral and caused progressive shrinkage of the whole organ. There was destruction of pyramidal and granule cell layers and dense microglial infiltration in the molecular layer. The microglial cell nests formed large egg-shaped foci surrounded by dense astrocytic proliferation and hypertrophy. These lesions progressed even further in animals destroyed between 6 and 12

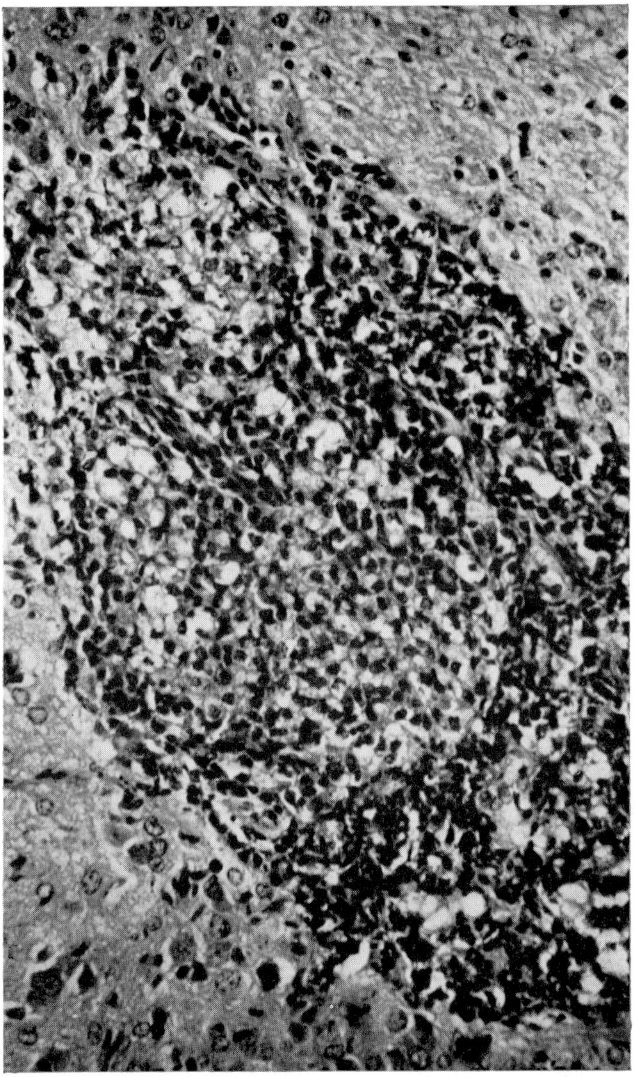

Fig. 1. Large granulomatous lesion, undergoing partial calcification in the frontal cortex. Fifteen-day-old hamster; 3 weeks after i.d. inoculation with the attenuated WEE virus. H & E × 330.

[*To face p. 110*

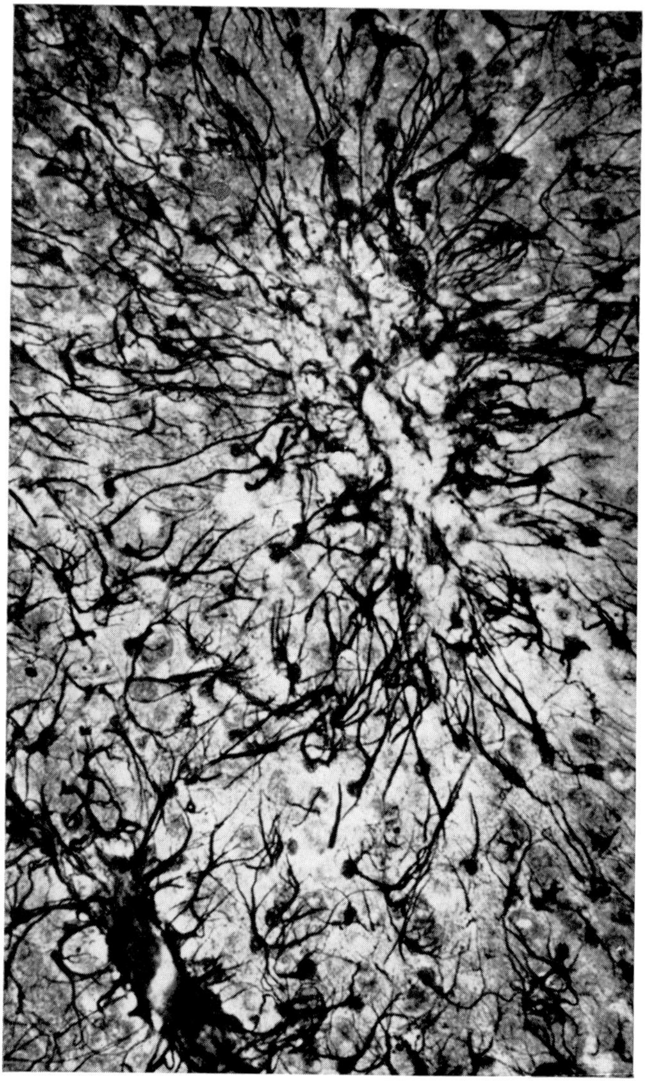

Fig. 2. Marked astrocytic reaction around a blood vessel in the temporal cerebral cortex. Fifteen-day-old hamster; 8 weeks after i.p. inoculation with the attenuated WEE virus. Cajal × 330.

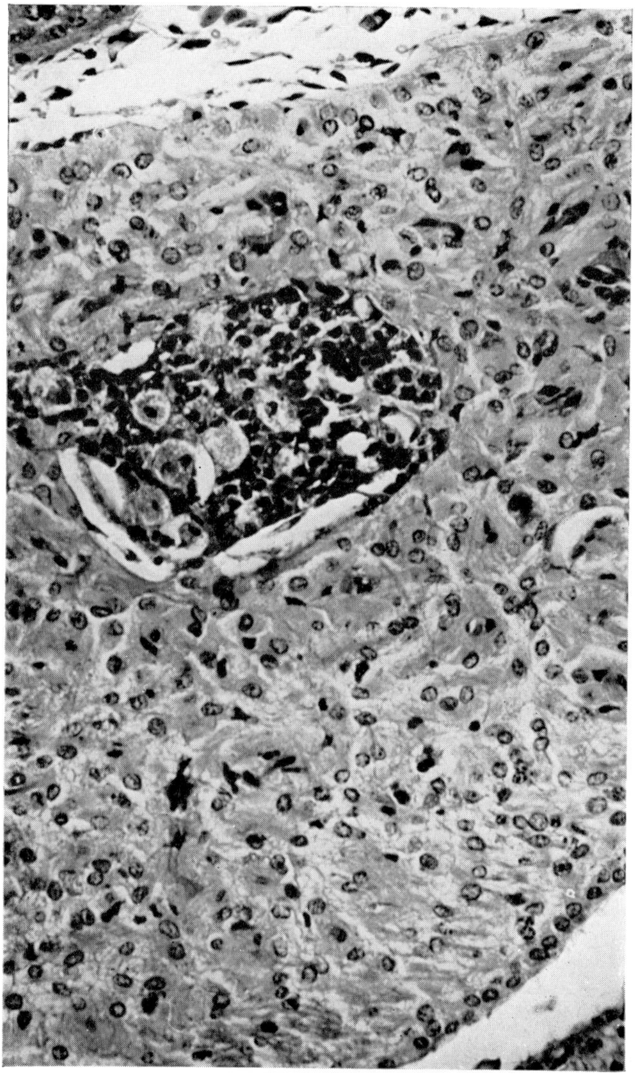

Fig. 3. Progressive changes in the hippocampus of a ten-day-old hamster infected with the virulent Langat virus. Note: Astrocytic proliferation, microglial cell nest and shrinkage of the hippocampus (6 weeks after i.p. inoculation). H & E × 330.

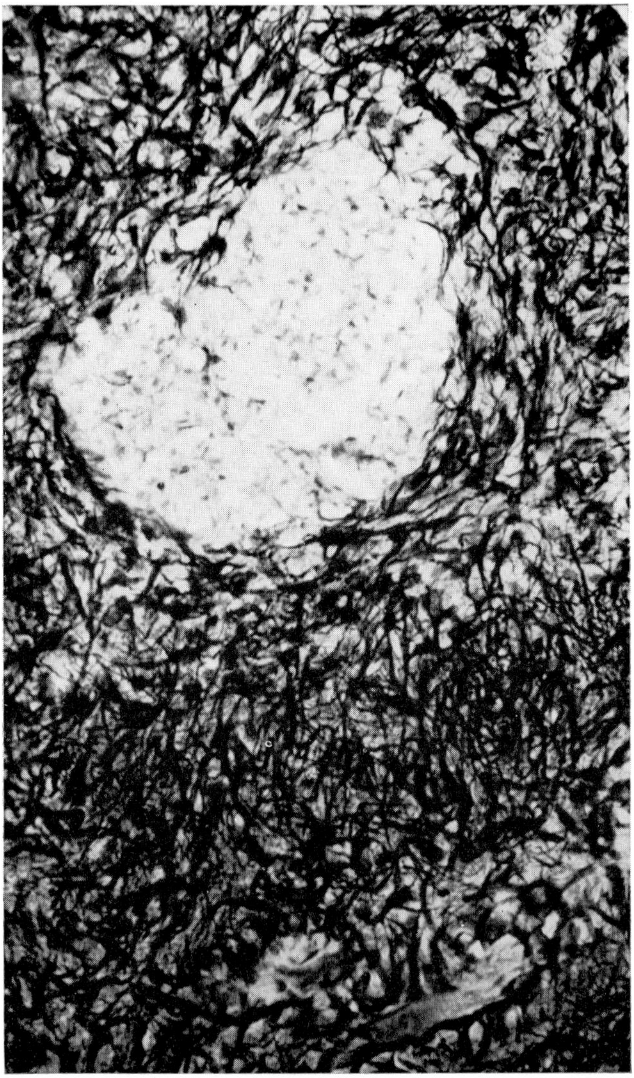

Fig. 4. Severe astrocytic changes in the hippocampus of a five-day-old hamster inoculated six weeks previously with the attenuated Langat virus. (Note the astrocytic tangles.) Cajal × 330.

weeks after infection. The hippocampal shrinkage reduced it to about one-third of its original size, while the severe microglial astrocytic reaction destroyed all the normal architectonics (Figs 3 and 4). At this stage some of the egg-shaped cell nests began to undergo calcification and occasionally these changes were present also in the cerebral cortex in the vicinity of the anterior horns of the lateral ventricles and in the corpora quadrigemina.

Hamsters inoculated at the age of 15 days, remained clinically unaffected although 30% had minimal inflammatory brain lesions during the first two weeks. While no lesions were found in the brain of hamsters inoculated intradermally beginning from three weeks after infection, a small proportion of the i.p. inoculated developed subacute lesions, without hippocampal involvement. However, in two hamsters destroyed 10 weeks after infection very severe and widespread changes were found in the cerebellum. These consisted of dense microglial and astrocytic proliferation, destruction of Purkinje cells, calcification and disruption of normal architectonics.

Attenuated Langat virus. Only newborn hamsters inoculated with the attenuated virus died during the first 4-6 days. Four-day-old hamsters survived the infection, but their growth was arrested and they remained stunted, while those five days old and older did not show any overt signs of disease. In spite of that all four- and five-day-old hamsters, inoculated by the intraperitoneal route had lesions in the brain similar to those in the 10-day-old hamsters infected with the virulent (TP 21) virus. However only 30% of hamsters inoculated by the intradermal route, irrespective of the dose of virus developed acute inflammatory lesions one week later. Subacute and chronic changes with severe involvement of the hippocampus were seen frequently in the i.p. inoculated animals (35%) and only occasionally in the i.d. infected (10%). In some cases the brain lesions were very severe and widespread and were common in addition to the hippocampus also in the olfactory lobe, paraterminal body, cerebral cortex, thalamus and midbrain. Only very occasionally were very mild inflammatory lesions found in the brain of hamsters inoculated with the attenuated strain of Langat virus at the age of 10 days or over.

Discussion

The experimental infections of mice showed only limited evidence of transplacental infection with the attenuated Langat virus. However, inoculations of newborn and suckling hamsters proved beyond a doubt that the developing brain is much more susceptible to virus infection than the adult brain and that permanent or long lasting lesions may result in immature animals from such infections. It should be borne in mind that in spite of the fact that adult hamsters are not susceptible to peripheral inoculations with either virulent or attenuated Langat virus, suckling and newborn were highly susceptible in the early life, while later during the suckling period they had the tendency to produce chronic and permanent brain lesions. The attenuated virus of WEE proved to be lethal for hamsters until the age of 12 days, however 15-day-old hamsters survived, but developed very severe and long lasting necrotic brain lesions. In contrast, adult hamsters inoculated with the attenuated virus developed an inapparent infection with inflammatory changes and little or no tendency for degenerative or necrotic changes (Zlotnik, unpublished).

Summary

Long term necrotising effects were produced in the brain of 15-day-old hamsters by peripheral inoculations of attenuated WEE virus. Younger animals died as a result of the infection.

Both the virulent and attenuated strains of Langat virus proved lethal to newborn hamsters. In suckling animals they proved to be capable of giving rise to progressive and proliferative lesions in the brain and to permanent deformity mainly of the hippocampus.

REFERENCES

Adams, J. M. (1968). *Neurology* **18,** 52.
Berman, P. H., Giles, J. P. and Krugman, S. (1968). *Neurology* **18,** 91.
Byers, R. K. and Meyer, E. (1952). *Amer. J. Dis. Child.* **84,** 543.
Coffey, V. P. and Jessop, W. J. E. (1959). *Lancet* **2,** 935.
Crome, L. and France, N. E. (1959). *J. Clin. Path.* **12,** 427.
Crome, L. and Stern, J. (1967). 'The Pathology of Mental Retardation', pp. 35 and 64. London: Churchill.
Davis, J. H. (1940). *J. Pediat.* **16,** 591.
Dayan, A. D., Gostling, J. V. T., Greaves, J. L., Stevens, D. W. and Woodhouse, M A. (1967). *Lancet* **1,** 980.
Diezel, P. B. (1954). *Virchows Arch.* **325,** 109.
Doherty, P. C. (1969). *J. comp. Path.* **79,** 413.
Doll, R., Hill, A. B. and Sakula, J. (1960). *Brit. J. Prev. and Social Med.* **14,** 167
Greenberg, M., Pellitteri, O. and Barton, J. (1957). *J.A.M.A.* **165,** 675.
Gregg, N. M. (1941). *Tr. Ophth. Soc. Australia* **3,** 35.
Haymaker, W., Girdamy, B. R., Stephens, J., Lillie, R. D. and Fetterman, G. H (1954). *J. Neuropath. exp. Neurol.* **13,** 562.
Ingalls, T. H. (1960). In 'Ciba Foundation Symposium on Congenital Malformations' (eds Wolstenholme and O'Connor), vol. 51. London Churchill.
Johnson, H. N. (1963). *Amer. J. Trop. Med. and Hyg.* **12,** 604.

Kass, A. (1951). *Acta Pediat.* **40,** 239.
Kibrick, S. and Benirschke, K. (1958). *Pediatrics* **22,** 857.
Knobloch, H. and Pasamanick, B. (1962). *New Eng. J. Med.* **266,** 1045.
Lennette, E. H., Megoffin, R. L. and Freeman, J. M. (1968). *Neurology* **18,** 21.
Lewis, L., Taylor, H. G., Sorem, M. B., Norcross, J. W. and Kindsratter, V. H. (1947). *Arch. Neurol. and Psychiat.* **57,** 430.
Lock, F. R., Gatling, H. B., Manzy, C. H. and Wells, H. B. (1961). *Am. J. Obst. and Gynec.* **81,** 451.
Michaelis, R. H. and Mellin, G. W. (1960). *Pediatrics* **26,** 200.
Nisenbaum, C. and Wallis, K. (1965). *Helv. paediat. Acta* **20,** 392.
Noran, H. H. (1944). *Am. J. Path.* **20,** 259.
Noran, H. H. and Baker, A. B. (1943). *Arch. Neurol. and Psychiat.* **49,** 398. (1945). *J. Neuropath. and exper. Neurol.* **4,** 269.
Pasamanick, B. and Knobloch, H. (1960). *Am. J. Pub. Health* **50,** 1737.
Platou, R. V. (1940). *Am. J. Dis. Child.* **60,** 1155.
Price, W. H., O'Leary, W., Lee, R., Parks, J. and Ganaway, J. (1963). *Am. J. Trop. Med. Hyg.* **12,** 782.
Shaeffer, M., Fox, M. J. and Li, C. P. (1954). *J.A.M.A.* **155,** 248.
Shinefield, H. R. and Townsend, T. E. (1953). *J. Pediat.* **43,** 21.
Smith, M. G. (1956). *Proc. Soc. exp. Biol. (N.Y.)* **92,** 424.
Swan, C., Tostevin, A. L. and Barham Black, G. H. (1946). *Med. J. Austral.* **2,** 889.
Swarts, C. L. and Kercher, E. F. (1954). *Pediat.* **14,** 735.
Wolf, A. and Cowen, D. (1959). *J. Neuropath. exp. Neurol.* **18,** 191.
Zeman, W. and Kolar, O. (1968). *Neurology* **18,** 1.
Zlotnik, I. (1968). *Br. J. exp. Path.* **49,** 555.
Zlotnik, I., Carter, G. B. and Grant, D. P. (1971). *Br. J. exp. Path.* **52** (in press).

DISCUSSION

Crome: This is a most important contribution. The question whether some of the encephalopathies of unclassified mental retardation might not be due to a virus is always in the minds of neuropathologists. But the only proved intrauterine infections have been from rubella and from cytomegalovirus. Influenza is doubtful. We do see changes like Dr. Zlotnik's in some cases without any history of encephalitis, but whether it was encephalitis is unknown. The only infection known nowadays not to have an overt period of clinical disease is post-encephalitic Parkinsonism. These are occasionally found, usually with involvement of the substantia nigra and with periventricular infiltration, but with no history of encephalitis. We need immunological tests in order to study this further.

Harris: I was interested in this paper because temporal lobe epilepsy is said often to follow a febrile illness with seizures. This was thought to be due to the anoxic effects of the seizures. Recently, however, it has been shown that many of these children have high titres of antibodies to adenoviruses. Certainly the E.E.G. picture in the acute stage is much akin to that in a virus encephalitis, with focal abnormalities that later disappear.

Zlotnik: I may add that these two viruses are not exceptions. Even with an entirely non-pathogenic virus, such as isolated from birds to which children have been found to have antibodies, and which is avirulent for the adult animal, when inoculated by the peripheral route will cause lethal encephalitis in the newborn mouse, even with the smallest dose. In the absence of maternal immunity, the baby, not getting antibodies from the colostrum, is open to infection.

Wigglesworth: Most of the human antibody protection is transplacental, surely, and the colostrum plays a relatively small part. Most viral antibodies are gamma G, aren't they?

Zlotnik: There are difficulties in relating human infections with animal experiments. In animals we know that the antibody level is not a measure of protection, for high levels of antibody to louping-ill virus in the monkey do not protect against intracerebral challenge.

Wigglesworth: But if the antibody transmission in the animal is different from that in humans, the animal may well be far more susceptible than the human neonate.

Zlotnik: In herpes the protection is not transmitted and whether protection is transmitted depends very much on the virus. For instance, you can get measles very early in life.

Wigglesworth: You can in fact get infants with herpes at birth, but whether through the placenta or the membranes is irrelevant. I've had instances of babies at 48 hours with necrotising encephalitis and calcification, so that it certainly can be pre-natal in man.

Kirman: There have been some suggestions that herpes infections in early life could be associated with disturbed behaviour.

Jellinger: Can poliovirus be caused by intrauterine infection? I've had one case of death from poliovirus at two days.

Zlotnik: Polio can be transmitted at any time during pregnancy. You can't predict which virus will penetrate. It might be that there is some defect in the placenta or something.

Wigglesworth: There must be an active protection rather than a passive one. The idea of the placenta as a membrane with a certain pore size is incorrect, since you may get anything from whole cells passing through it to small molecules being excluded.

Zlotnik: But the virus does not penetrate it!

Jellinger: Have you an idea of the pathogenesis of those calcified lesions? How do they develop?

Zlotnik: Hamsters calcify their lesions much more easily than do mice. After the acute phase the perivascular mononuclear cuffs are replaced by microglial cells. The virus is not present at this stage, but there must be some sort of antibody reaction, and the astrocytic reaction is more severe around these calcified lesions than in any other parts of the CNS. Early on the whole brain shows lesions, but later it is confined to certain areas; 20% of the animals after Langat virus have complete hippocampal destruction.

Kleihues: Your last group of animals that showed shrinkage of the hippocampus, do they show seizures?

Zlotnik: No symptoms whatsoever. It is most frightening! They appeared quite normal. This kind of hippocampal lesion has never been found in any other kind of disease, but the animals don't show any evident behavioural disorder.

Balázs: I'm fishing for models, animals with certain well-defined lesions in certain parts of the brain. Could you suggest some virus infections?

Zlotnik: Infections of guinea pigs with louping-ill virus, which is avirulent for adults, but after immunosuppresion an infection occurs and the virus persists. In those guinea pigs there is a selective destruction of Purkinje cells.

Hanefeld: Do you think it possible, Dr. Jellinger, that you as a neuropathologist may find no signs in the brain, although there was a previous history of encephalitis? In your cases of unclassified mental retardation, do you think you cannot exclude the previous occurrence of encephalitis?

Crome: There are a lot of cases in which encephalitis will have been a possible cause.

Hanefeld: Even with a history of encephalitis you may find nothing?

Crome and Zlotnik: Yes—

Jellinger:—both nothing and also scarring similar to non-inflammatory causes.

Zlotnik: And the same occurs in experimental animals. From six weeks after infection it may be difficult to find anything.

Jellinger: I would like to warn against identifying a febrile state with encephalitis. Experience shows that this is more often otitis media, or some other inflammatory lesion.

Davison: Does Dr. Crome see similar kinds of lesions in mentally normal children?

Crome: It's a question of degree. You find all sorts of lesions in the brains of children blind from various causes, and you can find an occasional granuloma.

Alkylating Agents and their Effects on the Adult Mammalian Brain

P. KLEIHUES

Introduction

Investigations have been carried out on an increasing number of alkylating agents which under physiological conditions may react with cell constituents. A wide range of biological actions have been attributed to this class of compounds including mutagenic, teratogenic, carcinogenic and cytostatic effects. Until recently, little attention has been paid to the interaction of alkylating agents with the nervous system. In 1965, Druckrey and his associates first reported the selective induction of brain tumours by systemic application of methylnitrosourea to rats. Subsequently, other nitrosamides have been found to be similarly effective and today these compounds seem to represent the most encouraging approach in experimental neuro-oncology. Some alkylating agents are potent carcinogens and also exert teratogenic effects on the nervous system when administered pre-natally, e.g., methylnitrosourea (von Kreybig, 1965; Koyama *et al.,* 1970) and methylazoxymethanol, the aglycone of the naturally occurring glycoside cycasin (Spatz *et al.,* 1967). The scope of this contribution is to give a comprehensive review of the carcinogenic action of alkylating agents on the nervous system in adult animals and to report on some experiments dealing with their acute effects on the brain and other tissues.

Carcinogenic Effects of Alkylating Agents on the Nervous System in Adult Animals

Before the discovery of neurotropic alkylating agents experimental tumour induction in the nervous system was restricted to the local application of carcinogens (mostly hydrocarbons) which themselves exerted no preferential effect on the brain. Consequently, the initial step in the production of such tumours included traumatic brain lesions and brain oedema. Malignant mesenchymal tumours frequently occurred and important features of human pathology such as te preferential location of tumours in different areas of the brain could not be investigated. Carcinogenic alkylating agents do not need to be applied at the site of tumour induction but may be administered systemically by different routes.

Type of Chemicals

Several compounds which may act as alkylating agents *in vivo* are capable of tumour induction in the nervous system. In Table 1 those agents are listed which by repeated administration to adult animals induce malignant tumours of the nervous system with an incidence of more than 50%. Like methylnitrosourea, most of these are acyl-alkyl-nitrosamides with the general structure

$$\text{ON-N}\begin{matrix}\nearrow \text{R1} \\ \searrow \text{R2}\end{matrix}$$

where R_1 is an alkyl residue (mostly a methyl group) and R_2 is an acyl residue. The neuro-oncogenic effect of phenyl-dimethyltriazene has recently been reported (Druckrey *et al.*, 1967). After subcutaneous injection, local sarcomas were only occasionally observed, indicating that the metabolism of this carcinogen may not take place at the site of injection. *In vitro* studies with microsomal fractions from various organs seem to suggest that the liver is the major site of its breakdown *in vivo* (Preussmann *et al.*, 1969b). Other triazenes (1-(pyridyl-3),3-dimethyl-triazene and 3-(dimethyltriazene)-pyridine-N-oxide) seem to be similarly effective in adult animals but detailed results have not yet been published (Preussmann *et al.*, 1969a).

In Table 2 alkylating agents are listed which may also induce tumours of the nervous system in adult animals but with an incidence of generally less than 20%. Their chemical structures are diverse and most of them affect the nervous system as well as various other organs. Methyl methane-sulphonate seems to be a rather weak carcinogen but after high intravenous doses several tumours were found in the surviving animals, all of them in the nervous system (Swann and Magee, 1969).

It should be mentioned that some of the compounds listed in Table 2, although not very effective in adult animals, have been shown to be potent neuro-oncogenic agents when administered pre-natally,

TABLE 1

Alkylating Agents which after repeated doses to Adult Animals induced Malignant Tumours predominantly of the Nervous System

Compound	*Animal*	*Route of application*	*Average total dose (g/kg)*	*No. of animals*	*Animals with tumours*		*Average survival time (days)*	*Reference*
					CNS	*PNS*		
N-Methyl-N-nitrosourea	rat	iv.	0.18	32	31	–	340	Druckrey *et al.*, 1967a
	rat	oral	0.435	26	16	4	163-238	Strobandt and Brucher, 1968
	rat	ip.	0.23	17	11	2	220	Mende and Kleihues, 1971
	rabbit	iv.	0.20*	27	19	–	300	Schreiber *et al.*, 1969
	rabbit	iv.	0.19*	28	21	–	268	Stavrou, 1969
	rabbit	iv.	0.15	25	14	–	349	Kleihues *et al.*, 1970
	dog	iv.	0.35*	10	4	–	390*	Warzok *et al.*, 1970
N,N′-Dimethyl-N-nitrosourea	rat	iv.	0.90	40	24	5	333	Druckrey *et al.*, 1967a
	rat	oral	1.30	17	9	5	396	Druckrey *et al.*, 1967a
N,N′,N′-Trimethyl-N-nitrosourea	rat	iv.	1.95	7	4	2	333	Druckrey *et al.*, 1967a
	rat	oral	1.30	14	9	7	450	Ivankovic *et al.*, 1965
N-Methyl-N-nitrosobiuret	rat	oral	2.70	16	7	3	400*	Druckrey *et al.*, 1971
1-Phenyl-3,3-dimethyltriazene	rat	sc.	1.25 (1.45)	21	11	3	410 (250)	Druckrey *et al.*, 1967b
	rat	oral	1.90	12	8	1	330	

* Approximation, calculated from data in the reference.

TABLE 2

Alkylating Agents which after repeated doses to Adult Animals produced a low incidence of Tumours of the Nervous System

Compound	*Route of application*	*Incidence of nervous system tumours*	*Reference*
Ethylnitrosourea	intravenous	< 30%	Druckrey *et al.*, 1967a
Diethylhydrazine	subcutaneous	< 20%	Druckrey *et al.*, 1966
Azoethane	subcutaneous	< 20&	Druckrey *et al.*, 1965b
Methylazoxymethanol	stomach tube	< 20%	Laqueur *et al.*, 1967
Methyl methanesulfonate	intravenous	< 15%	Swann and Magee, 1969
Dimethyl sulfate	inhalation	< 10%	Druckrey *et al.*, 1970a
Propansultone	intravenous	< 20%	Druckrey *et al.*, 1970b

e.g., ethylnitrosourea (Ivankovic and Druckrey, 1968; Kleihues *et al.*, 1968; Wechsler *et al.*, 1969), diethylhydrazine and azoethane (Druckrey *et al.*, 1968).

Route and Mode of Application

So far, it has only been possible to induce tumours of the nervous system in a high incidence in adult animals when the carcinogen was administered discontinuously over several months. When methyl-nitrosourea is given as a single dose of about 70-100 mg/kg most of the surviving animals die from malignant tumours in various organs. Brain tumours may also be observed but at a low incidence. After a single intravenous dose, the sites of tumour induction seemed to be randomly distributed between both parenchymatous and mesenchymal tissues (Druckrey *et al.*, 1967) whereas after a single oral dose a preferential occurrence at the site of application becomes apparent (Leaver *et al.*, 1969). The same compound, when administered discontinuously at low doses, induces malignant tumours almost selectively of the nervous system (Table 1). The route of application seems to be of minor importance since an equally high incidence of nervous system tumours could be obtained by either intravenous, intraperitoneal, or oral administration (Table 1). In the case of methylnitrosourea, however, it is necessary to ensure that no spontaneous hydrolysis occurs before the carcinogen is actually injected. Thomas *et al.* (1968) prepared a neutral solution of methylnitrosourea which after repeated intraperitoneal injections produced only local abdominal tumours, histologically classified as neurinomas. Mende and Kleihues (Table 1) used similar doses but prepared the carcinogen in a pH 6 buffer solution. Again, abdominal tumours (both neurinomas and sarcomas) were found but additionally 11 out of 17 animals died with malignant tumours of the central nervous system.

Dose, Tumour Incidence and Induction Time

Both the incidence of tumours and the induction time depend on the dose administered. The term induction time (or latent period) is generally used for the average survival time of animals from the beginning of the experiment and therefore does not truly reflect the beginning of tumour growth. Nevertheless, when calculated for a sufficiently large number of animals, it has revealed important quantitative aspects in experimental chemical carcinogenesis. On the basis of experimental data obtained with different types of carcinogen,

Druckrey (1967) has proposed the following relationship

$$d \times t^n = \text{constant}$$

where d is the amount of the carcinogen (administered either as single or repeated dose) and t stands for the induction time as defined above. n is a positive figure greater than one and characteristic not only for the carcinogen but also for the age and species of animals used in the experiment.

Similar dose-response relationships have been found for the induction of brain tumours both by pre-natal and post-natal application of various nitrosamides (Druckrey *et al.*, 1967; 1969).

Species of Animals

Comparative studies have been carried out on the neuro-oncogenic action of methylnitrosourea. As may be seen from Table 1, a high yield of nervous system tumours has been obtained in rats, rabbits and dogs. This compound, therefore, seems to be suitable for the investigation of the possible hazards of nitrosamides to higher animals. Attempts have also been made to use methylnitrosourea for the induction of brain tumours in primates, but so far without success.

Histopathological Classification of Tumours and Their Possible Site of Origin in the Nervous System

Generally, the morphological variety of tumours induced by alkylating agents seems to be smaller than that observed in human pathology (Zülch, 1969). It is beyond the scope of this paper to give a detailed description of the morphology of experimentally induced tumours of the nervous system (for review see Jänisch and Schreiber, 1969; Wechsler *et al.*, 1969) but the most relevant features may be summarised as follows:

1. The majority of CNS tumours induced by alkylating agents consists of malignant gliomas. Primary brain sarcomas have only occasionally been found and tumours of neuronal origin seem to be extremely rare, if present at all (Stroobandt and Brucher, 1968; Kleihues *et al.*, 1970). Further, we have never observed a tumour that could be classified as biologically benign. Infiltrating growth was always present and in several cases of methylnitrosourea induced tumours metastases via the cerebro-spinal fluid have been observed (Kleihues *et al.*, 1970).
2. Histopathologically, most tumours have been classified as

oligodendrogliomas, mixed gliomas (composed of both neoplastic oligodendrocytes and astrocytes), and ependymomas.

3. The histological appearance may depend on both the species and age of animals but the chemical structure of the alkylating agent seems to have little effect (Kersting and Thomas, 1968).
4. Tumours of the peripheral nervous system induced by various nitrosamides have mainly been classified as malignant neurinomas. There is some evidence that neoplastic Schwann cells do participate in their growth although mesenchymal cells may also be involved to a various degree (Kleihues *et al.*, 1968; Georgsson *et al.*, 1969; Jänisch *et al.*, 1970).
5. Tumours induced by alkylating agents are not randomly located within the nervous system. The majority of tumours seem to develop from a rather few circumscribed areas. In the peripheral nervous system these are the roots of the lumbosacral plexus and the proximal part of the trigeminal nerve (Wechsler *et al.*, 1969; Ivankovic and Druckrey, 1968). Within the central nervous system tumours preferentially occurred in the periventricular white matter of the cerebral hemispheres (Stavrou, 1969; Wechsler *et al.*, 1969; Kleihues *et al.*, 1970). In the adult mammalian brain glial cell proliferation persists in the subependymal layer (Lewis, 1968) and the possibility exists that such postembryonic germinal zones represent the site of origin of experimentally induced brain tumours.

Some Acute Effects of Neuro-oncogenic Alkylating Agents on the Brain and Other Tissues

Experiments have been carried out to investigate the acute effects of alkylating agents on the brain. The initial scope of these studies was to see whether potent neuro-oncogenic compounds such as methylnitrosourea would also predominantly affect the nervous system in the acute experiments. Therefore, in most experiments the brain and other organs were examined comparatively. For similar reasons in some experiments methyl methanesulphonate was used as well as methylnitrosourea, since methyl methanesulphonate seems to induce tumours predominantly of the nervous system, but at a much lower incidence than methylnitrosourea (see Tables 1 and 2).

Distribution and Metabolism *In Vivo*

There is evidence that the biological actions of N-nitroso compounds are caused by metabolically active (alkylating) breakdown products rather than by these compounds themselves (see Magee and

Barnes, 1967; Druckrey *et al.,* 1967; Magee, 1969). Acyl-alkyl nitrosamides such as methylnitrosourea and ethylnitrosourea are unstable in aqueous solutions (Garrett *et al.,* 1965) and their breakdown *in vivo* does not seem to require enzymic activity (Druckrey *et al.,* 1967). One would therefore expect that the primary distribution of these compounds (and of simple alkylating agents such as methyl methanesulphonate) in the body may influence the extent of their reactions with cell constituents. Quantitative studies on the penetration of different organs are difficult to carry out as these compounds undergo very rapid breakdown *in vivo.* The biological half-life in rat serum has been determined to be less than 5 min for methylnitrosourea and about 30 min for methyl methanesulphonate (Swann, 1968).

We have studied the distribution of [^{14}C] radioactivity in the rat 2 min after intravenous injection of N-[^{14}C] methyl-N-nitrosourea by means of total body autoradiography (Kleihues and Patzschke, 1971). At this very short time interval a rather uniform distribution of radioactively was observed throughout the body including the CNS and the mucous membranes of the gastro-intestinal tract. No significant regional differences were found within the CNS except that the concentration of radioactivity in the white matter was generally somewhat lower than in the grey matter. It was, therefore, concluded that the preferential location of experimental tumours in some areas of the CNS (as discussed in the preceding section) does not result from localised concentration of the carcinogen within the nervous system.

Acute Toxic Effects

A general feature of alkylating agents is their cytotoxic effect on proliferating cell populations. Bifunctional and polyfunctional alkylating agents are most effective in this respect and, therefore, have frequently been tested as anti-cancer drugs, including several nitrosamides (Skipper *et al.,* 1961; Schabel *et al.,* 1963; Rosso *et al.,* 1967; Wheeler and Bowdon, 1968).

Within 3-6 hours after a single dose of methylnitrosourea (50-100 mg/kg) severe cell lesions are found in rat organs with a high rate of cell turnover such as bone marrow, spleen and intestines (Leaver *et al.,* 1969; Kleihues, 1969). Cells in the late G_1 or early DNA synthesising phase of the cell cycle seem to be most sensitive (Roberts *et al.,* 1968). Similar observations have been made when methyl methanesulphonate was injected at sublethal doses. This effect on proliferating cells seems to be among the major factors determining the acute LD_{50}. No acute histopathological effects are seen in organs with a low cell turnover such as liver and kidney. In the adult mammalian brain there is a very low turnover of glial cells in some restricted subependymal areas (Lewis, 1968). Consequently, no gross pathological changes were observed in the CNS following the application of sublethal doses of methylnitrosourea or methyl methanesulphonate.

There is, however, some evidence of an acute neurotoxic effect of methylnitrosourea. Schein (1969) recently reported on episodes of tonic seizure activity in mice after a single dose of 100 mg/kg and similar episodes may be observed in rats when lethal doses are applied. From the work of Schein (1969) it appears that this effect on the brain results from a rapid decrease of brain NAD levels induced by methylnitrosourea.

We have recently studied the acute effect of methylnitrosourea on electrocortical activity in the cat brain (Hossmann and Kleihues). After infusion of 60 mg methylnitrosourea (corresponding to about 20 mg/kg) within 12 min into the carotid artery the EEG was recorded for 3-5 hours. Immediately after the infusion EEG changes were observed ranging from transient suppression of spontaneous barbiturate spindles to a complete suppression of EEG activity over the whole observation period. In some animals periodic episodes of complete EEG suppression were observed which lasted up to 20 min. Between such episodes the EEG recovered almost completely. Blood pressure and cerebral impedance were simultaneousnly recorded but remained unaffected, indicating that the EEG changes were a direct effect of methylnitrosourea on the brain and not due to reduced cerebral blood flow or to brain oedema. A systemic effect of methylnitrosourea is also unlikely to be responsible since intravenous injections of similar doses had no effect. Animals were killed within six hours after the infusion but no histopathological changes were observed by conventional light microscopy. One of the animals which survived for several days, however, showed extensive necroses in the brain on the side of the infusion.

Alkylation of Nucleic Acids

Alkylation of nucleic acids by carcinogenic N-nitroso compounds was first reported by Magee and Farber (1962) using radioactively labeled dimethylnitrosamine. After acid hydrolysis the major product of alkylation was shown to be 7-methylguanine in both DNA and RNA of rat liver. Comparative quantitative studies were performed by Swann and Magee (1968) on the extent of methylation of nucleic acids in several organs of the rat by different alkylating agents, including methylnitrosourea and methyl methanesulphonate. Methylnitrosourea methylated DNA to a similar degree in all organs investigated including the brain. Methyl methanesulphonate reacted with DNA to about the same extent as methylnitrosourea, the highest level of 7-methylguanine being present in the brain. Dimethylsulphate which, like methyl methanesulphonate, induced nervous system tumours at a low incidence (see Table 2), also reacted most extensively with brain DNA. The levels of alkylation produced by methylnitrosourea were generally higher in RNA whereas both dimethyl sulphate and methyl methanesulphonate caused higher levels of methylation in DNA. Wunderlich and Tetzlaff (1970) after intraperitoneal injection of [^{14}C] labeled methylnitrosourea found the highest levels of alkylation of nuclear DNA in organs with a high rate of cell turnover (bone marrow, spleen, foetuses, intestine) but the results for liver, kidneys and the brain are comparable to those reported by Swann and Magee (1968).

From the experimental data obtained so far, one may conclude that there is no quantitative correlation between the initial extent of alkylation at the (N)7 position of guanine and the carcinogenic response of the same organ. It should, however, be stressed that several problems related to the alkylation of nucleic acids are still unresolved. There is evidence that different fractions of RNA and DNA (Wunderlich *et al.*, 1970) may not react to a similar degree and that sites of alkylation other than the (N)7 position of guanine may influence the biological effects of alkylating agents (Loveless, 1969). Dr. H. D. Mennel and I have investigated the alkylation by methylnitrosourea and methyl methanesulphonate of HeLa cell nucleic acids. Methylnitrosourea methylated both DNA and RNA to a similar degree while in methyl methanesulphonate treated HeLa cells the level of 7-methylguanine was twice as high in DNA as in RNA, which basically corresponds to the observation *in vivo* of Swann and Magee (1968). In RNA from [^{14}C] methyl methanesulphonate treated cells there was, in additon to 7-methylguanine, a second peak of radioactivity which corresponded to the position of 1-methyladenine. Similar differences in the pattern of alkylation were found in rat brain RNA fractions after giving [^{14}C] labeled methylnitrosourea and methyl methanesulphonate *in vivo* (Fig. 1, work in progress with P. N. Magee).

Effects on Nucleic Acid Synthesis

The effect of methylnitrosourea and methyl methanesulphonate on the incorporation of thymidine (methyl[^{3}H]) into DNA of several organs of the rat was investigated at different time intervals up to 48 hours. A single intraperitoneal dose of methylnitrosourea (100 mg/kg) led to an almost complete inhibition of DNA synthesis within 6 hours

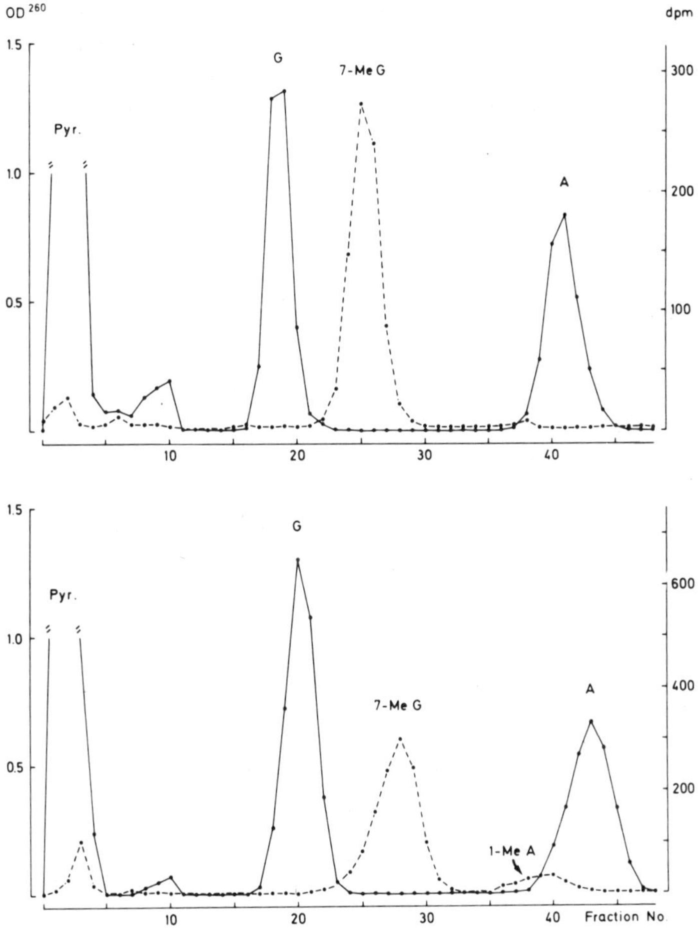

Fig. 1. Alkylation of rat brain ribosomal RNA by methylnitrosourea and methyl methanesulphonate. Adult rats received an intravenous injection (1 mM/kg) of N-[^{14}C]methyl-N-nitrosourea (135 μCi/mM) or [^{14}C]methyl methanesulphonate (311 μCi/mM) and were killed two hours later. Ribosomal RNA was extracted from the microsomal fraction and hydrolysed in N HCl (60 min, 100° Cels.). The purine bases were separated on a Dowex 50 (H^+ form) column using an exponential gradient solution (1-3 N HCl). The radioactive peaks eluted between guanine (G) and adenine (A) were identified as 7-methylguanine (7-MeG) and 1-methyladenine (1-MeA). *Upper:* methylnitrosourea; *lower:* methyl methanesulphonate.

(Kleihues, 1969). This effect was present in all organs investigated but somewhat more marked in those with a high cell turnover (e.g., spleen, intestine, bone marrow). Both organ-dependent and dose-dependent differences were mainly reflected by the duration of the recovery phase rather than by the degree of maximal inhibition. Similar observations were made when methyl methanesulphonate (100 mg/kg) was used but the maximal effect was already present after 3 hours (Mende and Kleihues).

It was further investigated whether or not the inhibition of DNA synthesis was quantitatively related to the acute LD_{50}. It was found that equimolar doses of methylnitrosourea (100 mg/kg) and ethylnitrosourea (120 mg/kg) affected DNA synthesis in rat intestines to a similar degree. This dose (about 1 mM/kg) corresponds to the LD_{50} for methylnitrosourea while that for ethylnitrosourea is twice as high (240 mg/kg). One may, therefore, conclude that factors other than the inhibition of DNA synthesis participate in the acute toxic effect of methylnitrosourea. This seems to be important as the difference in the toxicity between methyl- and ethylnitrosourea is still larger when equimolar doses are applied transplacentally to rat foetuses (see Wechsler, p. 179).

Investigations of the effect of methylnitrosourea on RNA synthesis *in vivo* were first performed using orotic acid-6-[^{14}C] as precursor. There was a significant decrease in the specific activity of kidney RNA after 2-3 hours, but a similar drop in the total amount of [^{14}C] radioactivity in the acid soluble precursor pool indicated that this effect was related to the uptake of orotic acid from the blood (or rapid secretion via the urine) rather than to macromolecular synthesis itself. When uridine [^{14}C] was used as a precursor a significant decrease in the specific activity of RNA was neither present in the kidney nor any other organ of the rat including the brain. Similar results were obtained with methyl methanesulphonate.

Inhibition of Protein Synthesis

The intraperitoneal injection of methylnitrosourea (100 mg/kg) causes a marked inhibition of the incorporation of [^{14}C]-1-leucine into proteins of several organs of the rat. The specific activity of proteins was already significantly reduced after 1.5 hours, the maximal effect being present at 2-3 hours after the application of methylnitrosourea. At this time the incorporation of L-leucine-1-[^{14}C] into proteins was reduced by 30-45% in various organs including the brain. In the liver methylnitrosourea caused a disaggregation of polyribosomes as revealed by sucrose density analysis of the postmitochondrial supernatant. The relative increase of monosomes paralleled the inhibition of protein synthesis which approached control values within 9 hours. Although protein synthesis was inhibited to a similar degree in the brain, changes in the cerebral polysome profiles were considerably less marked than those observed in the liver. When weanling rats were treated with a similar dose of methylnitrosourea, no inhibition of the incorporation of labelled L-leucine into brain proteins was observed but the polysome profile showed a significant increase of monosomes. At the same time the specific activity of total amino acids in the acid soluble pool of treated animals was more than 50% higher when compared with control animals.

When the MG^{++} concentration was lowered from 5 to 2 mM and the KCl concentration raised to 0.25 M the methylnitrosourea induced

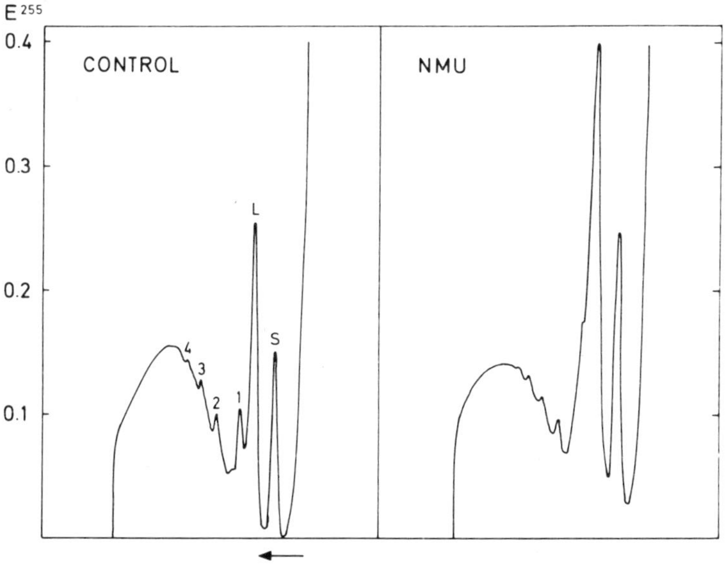

Fig. 2. Effect of methylnitrosourea on the polyribosomal profile from rat brain. Weanling rats (10 days old) received an intraperitoneal injection of methylnitrosourea (100 mg/kg) or a similar volume of citrate buffer (controls) and were killed three hours later. The post-mitochondrial supernatant (2 mM $MgCl_2$; 0.25 M KCl) was treated with Na-deoxycholate and analysed on an exponential sucrose gradient (Spinco SW 40 rotor; 40,000 rpm; 195 min). The direction of sedimentation is indicated by an arrow. In the control animals the position of the small (S) and large (L) ribosomal subunits and that of monosomes (1) and oligoribosomes (2-4) is indicated.

disaggregation of polysomes was paralleled by a substantial increase in the relative amount of ribosomal subunits (Fig. 2). Again, this effect was more marked in the liver than in the brain.

Disaggregation of rat liver polyribosomes has also been observed (Mizrahi and Emmelot, 1964; Villa-Trevino, 1967) during the inhibition of protein synthesis by dimethylnitrosamine which was first reported by Magee (1958) and Magee and Hultin (1962). Villa-Trevino suggested that the breakdown of polysomes might result from a defect in messenger RNA and that methylation of messenger RNA could be the underlying cause for both the instability of polysomes and the inhibition of protein synthesis. The acute effects of methylnitrosourea are not, as in the case of dimethylnitrosamine, mainly restricted to the liver and, therefore, protein synthesis is inhibited in other organs as well. The increase of ribosomal subunits rather than of monomeric ribosomes, as observed in polysome profiles from liver and brain of methylnitrosourea-treated animals may be tentatively interpreted as reflecting an inhibition predominantly of steps involved in the initiation of peptide chains.

Summary

There are several acyl-alkyl nitrosamides and aryl-dialkyl triazenes which after repeated administration to adult animals induce malignant tumours predominantly of the nervous system. The neuro-oncogenic effect of these and other biological alkylating agents has been reviewed. Information has accumulated on the morphology and classification of experimentally induced tumours, but little is yet known about their sequential development and their site of origin in the nervous system.

Experiments have been carried out on the acute effects of methylnitrosourea and related alkylating agents on the brain and other organs. Early effects of methylnitrosourea include a suppression of electrocortical activity, a decrease in brain NAD concentrations, alkylation of nucleic acids, and an inhibition of DNA and protein synthesis. There was no reaction in the acute experiment which could be positively related to the carcinogenic effect of this class of compounds.

REFERENCES

Druckrey, H. (1967). *UICC Monograph Series* 7, 60.

Druckrey, H., Ivankovic, S. and Preussmann, R. (1965a). *Z. Krebsforsch.* **66**, 389.

Druckrey, H., Preussmann, R., Ivankovic, S., Schmidt, C. H. and So, B. T. (1965b). *Z. Krebsforsch.* **67**, 31.

Druckrey, H., Preussmann, R., Matzkies, F. and Ivankovic, S. (1966). *Naturwissenschaften* **53**, 557.
Druckrey, H., Preussmann, R., Ivankovic, S. and Schmahl, D. (1967a). *Z. Krebsforsch.* **69**, 103.
Druckrey, H., Ivankovic, S. and Preussmann, R. (1967b). *Naturwissenschaften* **54**, 171.
Druckrey, H., Ivankovic, S., Preussmann, R., Landschutz, C., Stekar, H., Brunner, U. and Schagen, B. (1968). *Experientia* (Basel) **24**, 561.
Druckrey, H., Kruse, H., Preussmann, R., Ivankovic, S. and Landschutz, C. (1970a). *Z. Krebsforsch.* **74**, 241.
Druckrey, H., Kruse, H., Preussmann, R., Ivankovic, S., Landschutz, C. and Gimmy, J. (1970b). *Z. Krebsforsch.* **75**, 69.
Druckrey, H., Landschutz, C., Preussmann, R. and Ivankovic, S. (1971). *Z. Krebsforsch.* **75**, 229.
Garrett, E. R., Goto, S. and Stubbins, J. F. (1965). *J. pharmac. Sci.* **54**, 119.
Georgsson, G., Wessel, W. and Thomas, C. (1969). *Z. Krebsforsch.* **72**, 12.
Hossmann, K. A. and Kleihues, P. Unpublished results.
Ivankovic, S. and Druckrey, H. (1968). *Z. Krebsforsch.* **71**, 320.
Ivankovic, S., Druckrey, H. and Preussmann, R. (1964). *Z. Krebsforsch.* **66**, 541.
Jänisch, W., L geman, A., Dietz, W. and Schreiber, D. (1970). *Exp. Path.* **4**, 317.
Jänisch, W. and Schreiber, D. (1969). *Experimentelle Geschwulste des Zentralnervensystems.*
Kersting, G. and Thomas, C. (1968). *Verh. Dtsch. Ges. Pathol.* **52**, 384.
Kleihues, P. (1969). *Arzneim.-Forsch.* **19**, 1041.
Kleihues, P., Matsumoto, S., Wechsler, W. and Zülch, K. J. (1968). *Verh. Dtsch. Ges. Pathol.* **52**, 371.
Kleihues, P., Zülch, K. J., Matsumoto, S. and Radke, U. (1970). *Z. Neurol.* **198**, 65.
Kleihues, P. and Patzschke, K. (1971). *Z. Krebsforsch.* **75**, 193.
Koyama, T., Handa, J., Handa, H. and Matsumoto, S. (1970). *Arch. Neurol.* **22**, 342.
Von Kreybig, T. (1965). *Z. Krebsforsch.* **67**, 46.
Leaver, D. D., Swann, P. F. and Magee, P. N. (1969). *Brit. J. Cancer* **23**, 177.
Lewis, P. D. (1968). *Nature* **217**, 974.
Loveless, A. (1969). *Nature* **223**, 206.
Magee, P. N. (1958). *Biochem. J.* **70**, 606.
Magee, P. N. (1969). *Ann. N.Y. Acad. Sci.* **163**, 717.
Magee, P. N. and Barnes, J. M. (1967). *Adv. Cancer Res.* **10**, 163.
Magee, P. N. and Farber, E. (1962). *Biochem. J.* **83**, 114.
Magee, P. N. and Hultin, T. (1962). *Biochem. J.* **83**, 106.
Mende, C. and Kleihues, P. Unpublished results.
Mizrahi, I. J. and Emmelot, P. (1964). *Biochim. Biophys. Acta* **91**, 362.
Preussmann, R., Druckrey, H., Ivankovic, S. and von Hodenberg, A. (1969b). *Ann. N.Y. Acad. Sci.* **163**, 697.
Preussmann, R., von Hodenberg, A. and Hengy, H. (1969). *Biochem. Pharmacol.* **18**, 1.
Roberts, J. J., Brent, T. P. and Crathorn, A. R. (1968). In 'The Interaction of Drugs and Subcellular Components in Animal Cells' (ed. P. N. Campbell). London: J. & A. Churchill.
Rosso, R., Donelli, M. G., Reyers-Degli Innocenti and Garrattini, S. (1967). *Europ. J. Cancer* **3**, 125.

Schabel, F. M., Johnston, T. P., McCaleb, G. S. and Montgomery, G. A. (1963). *Cancer Res.* **23**, 725.

Schein, P. S. (1969). *Proc. Soc. exp. Biol. Med.* **131**, 517.

Schreiber, D., Jänisch, W., Warzok, R. and Tausch, H. (1969). *Z. ges. exp. Med.* **150**, 76.

Skipper, H. E., Schabel, F. M., Trader, M. W. and Thomson, J. R. (1961). *Cancer Res.* **21**, 1154.

Spatz, M., Dougherty, W. and Smith, D. W. E. (1967). *Proc. Soc. exp. Biol. Med.* **124**, 476.

Stavrou, D. (1969). *Z. Krebsforsch.* **73**, 98.

Stroobandt, G. and Brucher, J. M. (1968). *Neuro-Chirugie.* **14**, 515.

Swann, P. F. (1968). *Biochem. J.* **110**, 49.

Swann, P. F. and Magee, P. N. (1968). *Biochem. J.* **110**, 39.

Swann, P. F. and Magee, P. N. (1969). *Nature* **223**, 947.

Thomas, C., Sierra, J. L. and Kersting, G. (1968). *Naturwissenschaften* **55**, 183.

Villa-Trevino, S. (1967). *Biochem. J.* **105**, 625.

Warzok, R., Schneider, J., Schreiber, D. and Jänisch, W. (1970). *Experientia* **26**, 303.

Wechsler, W., Kleihues, P., Matsumoto, S., Zülch, K. J., Ivankovic, S., Preussmann, R. and Druckrey, H. (1969). *Ann. N.Y. Acad. Sci.* **159**, 360.

Wheeler, G. P. and Bowdon, B. J. (1968). *Cancer Res.* **28**, 52.

Wunderlich, V., Schutt, M., Bottger, M. and Graffi, A. (1970). *Biochem. J.* **118**, 99.

Wunderlich, V. and Tetzlaff, I. (1970). *Arch. Geschwulstforsch.* **35**, 251.

Zülch, K. J. (1969). *Arzneim. Forsch.* **19**, 1503.

Teratogenic and Oncogenic Effects of Ethylnitrosourea on the Developing Nervous System of Rats

W. WECHSLER*

Introduction

The discovery of the oncogenic action of the alkylating agent ethylnitrosourea (ENU) by Druckrey and co-workers (Druckrey *et al.*, 1966; Ivankovic *et al.*, 1966; Druckrey *et al.*, 1967; Ivankovic and Druckrey, 1968) marked the beginning of a new era of experimental neuro-oncology. Chemical carcinogens thus became available, which after systemic administration selectively produced tumours of the central and peripheral nervous system in rats under particular experimental conditions. ENU is an alkyl-nitrosamide and has the formula:

$$O=N-N\begin{matrix} \diagup C_2H_5 \\ \diagdown CONH_2 \end{matrix}$$

The degradation of ENU occurs spontaneously and rapidly, and the metabolites, which are considered as proximate and ultimate carcinogens are diazoethane and the carbonium ion. These metabolites act in various organs with a variety of cell constituents. The mode of action of ENU appears to be ethylation of nucleic acids and proteins at the molecular level (Swann and Magee, 1970, 1971). Because of its instability ENU must act locally but preferentially after resorption by the blood stream. Therefore, the route of administration is not as important as in the case of the topical carcinogens, e.g. the polycyclic hydrocarbons.

This group of carcinogens therefore can be administered intravenously, subcutaneously, intraperitoneally or by feeding and

* Presented by P. Kleihuis.

inhalation. Obviously oral administration and inhalation could closely simulate the natural conditions of man and animals.

It is the aim of this report to discuss the oncogenic effects of ENU and also to demonstrate its teratogenicity with particular reference to the lesions produced in the nervous system of rats after administration during pregnancy and during the first four weeks of post-natal life.

Teratogenic Effects of Ethylnitrosourea

The first reports of teratogenic effects exerted by ENU administered intravenously to pregnant rats were published by Druckrey *et al.* (1966), von Kreybig and Schmidt (1967), Ivankovic and Druckrey (1968) and von Kreybig (1968). ENU passes the placental barrier and is able to damage the developing embryo and foetus, particularly between the 12th and 15th day of gestation, provided that the dosage is higher than 40 mg/kg of body weight. Malformations observed were described as ectro-, oligo- and syndactylia of the fore- and hindlegs (Druckrey *et al.*, 1966; von Kreybig and Schmidt, 1967, Ivankovic and Druckrey, 1968; von Kreybig, 1968).

ENU is also able to affect the development of the brain. After giving a single dose of 60-80 mg/kg ENU at the 13th, 14th and 15th day of gestation, malformations of the brain, particularly in the hemispheres were observed (von Kreybig and Schmidt, 1967; von Kreybig, 1968).

To study quantitatively and qualitatively the cytotoxic and teratogenic effects of ENU, 93 pregnant Sprague-Dawley rats (CD-rats, Charles River Breeding Laboratories, Wilmington, Mass., 01887, U.S.A.) have been subjected to single i.v. injections of ENU at different times during pregnancy, namely 5, 7, 9, 12, 15, 20 and 22 days. A total number of more than 900 embryos, foetuses and offspring have been used to evaluate both, the lethal dose and the teratogenicity for the different stages of development. The dose-levels varied from 10 to 400 mg/kg.

ENU is toxic at all periods of ante-natal development, although the dose required to give a specified toxic response varies. The most sensitive period is from five to nine days of gestation; later periods are less sensitive. After birth the sensitivity decreases gradually, and there is no great difference between two- to four-week-old and adult animals. The vulnerability of embryos and foetuses to teratogenic effects is greatest between the 9th and 15th day of pregnancy. Earlier periods of gestation and later periods of foetal development are less vulnerable for teratogenic lesions, but for different reasons. The biological toxicity expressed as LD 50 or LD 100 is different for the various periods of gestation, and for foetal animals is 2-10 times greater than that for

a b c d

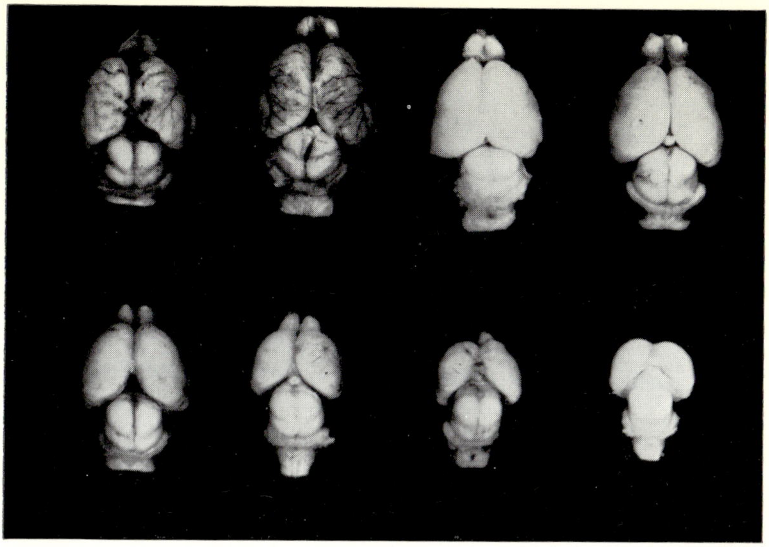

e f g h

Fig. 1. Malformations of the brain in Sprague-Dawley rats, produced with different dose levels of ENU on the 12th day of gestation.
(*a*) normal brain on the 22nd dies post coitum (dpc).
(*b*) brain of a newborn rat.
(*c–h*) newborn rats the pregnant mother of which received 10, 40, 60, 80, 100, and 120 mg/kg ENU of body weight i.v.

a b c d

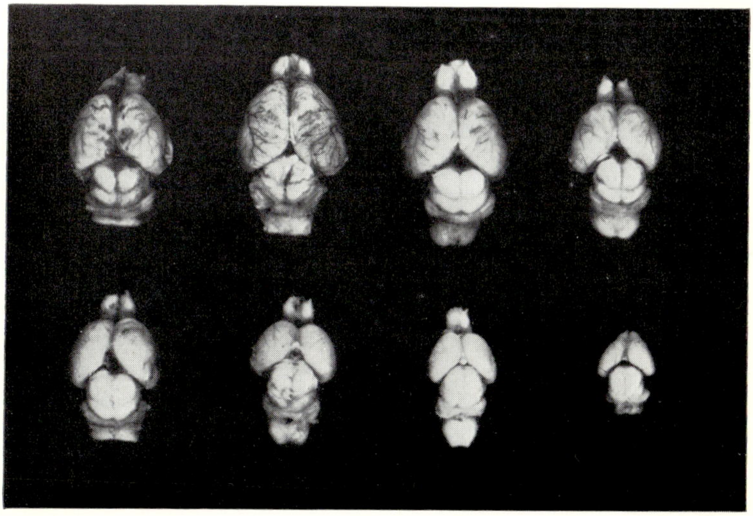

e f g h

Fig. 2. Malformations of the brain in Sprague-Dawley rats, produced with different dose levels of ENU on the 15th day of gestation.
(*a*) normal brain on 22nd dpc.
(*b*) brain of newborn rat.
(*c–h*) newborn rats, the pregnant mother of which received 30, 40, 60, 80, 100, and 150 mg/kg ENU on the 15th dpc i.v.

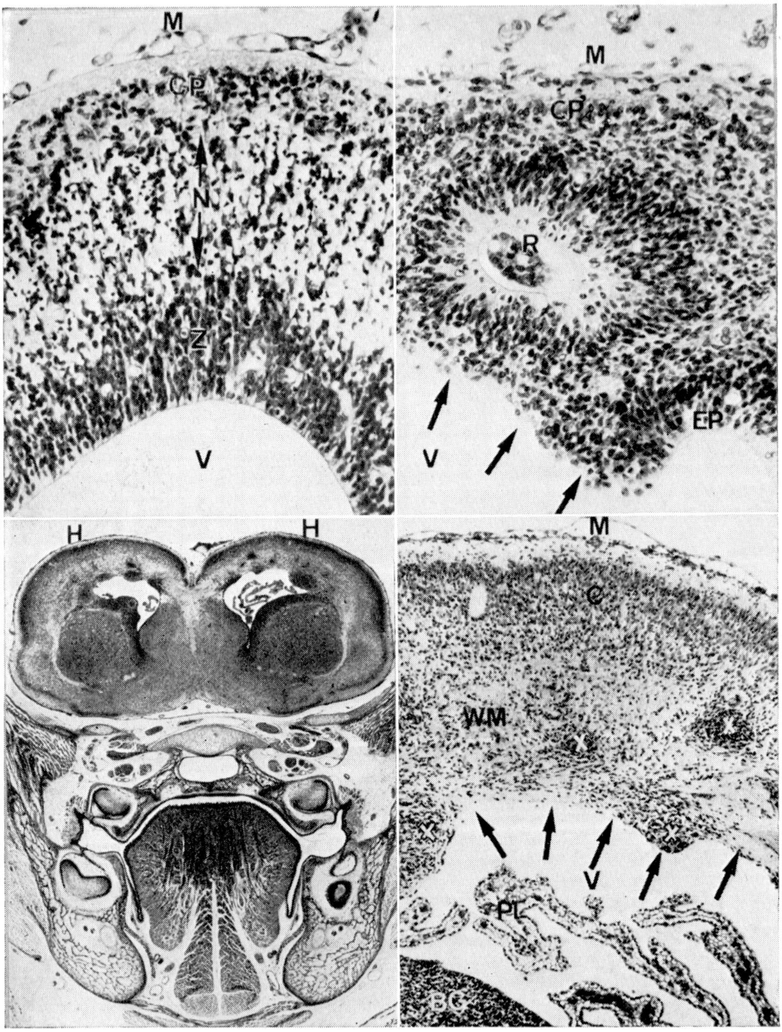

Fig. 3. Acute toxic lesions as determinants for the teratogenic effects in the brain hemispheres. Pregnant Sprague-Dawley rats received a single i.v. injection of 80 mg/kg ENU on 15th dpc. The resulting lesions are showing after different periods of survival.

(*a*) survival time, 24 h. Parietal region of the foetal hemisphere with necrosis (N) between the ventricular/subventricular cell zone (Z) and the neurons of the primitive cortical plate (CP). M = meninx primitiva, V = ventricle.

(*b*) survival time 3 days. Frontal region of the hemisphere exhibiting severe lesions with disruption (arrows) of the ventricular ependyma (EP), rosette formation (R), and disturbed patterns of the ventricular, subventricular and intermediate zones. CP = unaffected immature neurons of the primitive cortical intermediate zones.

(*c–d*) survival time 8 days. Frontal section of the head of a newborn rat. Note the microcephalic appearance of the hemispheres (H), demonstrating a variety of lesions, e.g. a reduced cortex (C), a damaged ventricular surface (arrows) and several heterotropic cellular aggregates (x), located close to the lateral ventricle (V) and in the white matter (WM). M—meninges, PL—choroid plexus. H & E (*a*) and (*b*) × 240, (*c*) × 6, (*d*) × 95.

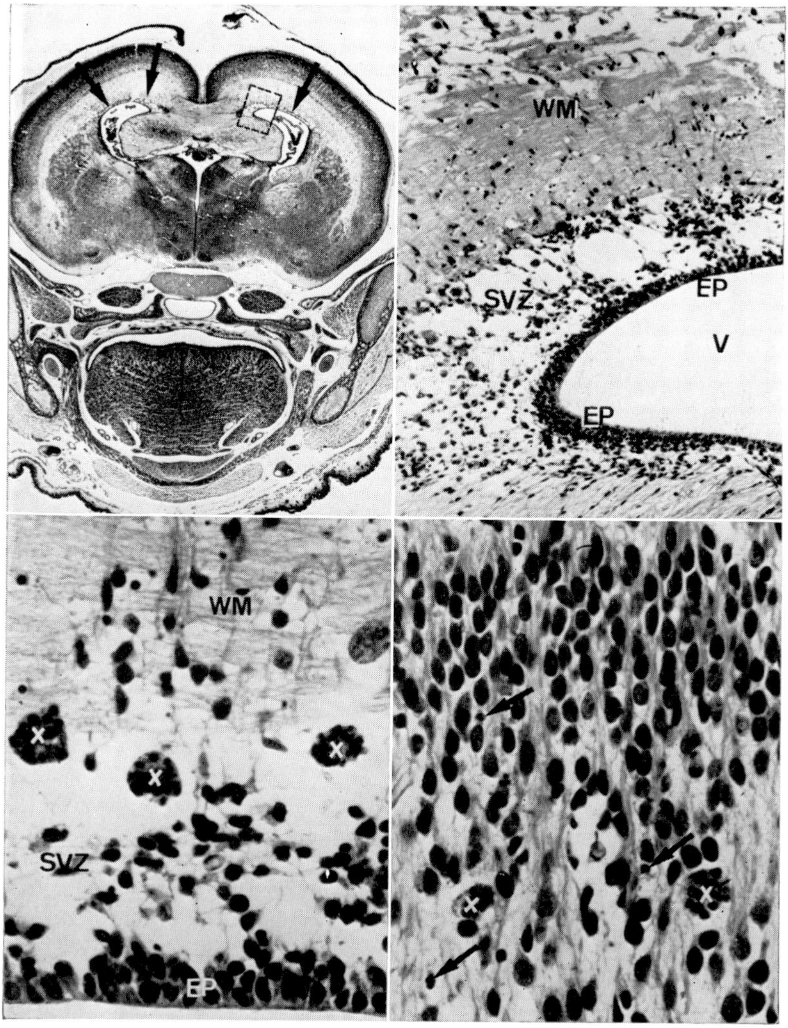

Fig. 4. Selective vulnerability of the foetal rat brain shortly before birth, after treatment with ethylnitrosourea. Pregnant Sprague-Dawley rats received a single i.v. injection of 120 mg/kg ENU on the 22nd dpc. The brain of the newborn rats was examined after 24 h. Cytotoxic lesions developed with preference in the subependymal zones of the lateral ventricles.

(*a*) Frontal section of the head and parietal brain. The paraventricular zones of the lateral ventricles (V) demonstrate microcystic destructions (arrows). All other parts of the brain are unaffected. H & E × 6.

(*b*) Magnification of the marked region with the damaged area of the brain hemispheres. Note the extensive cytotoxic lesions in the subventricular zone (SVZ) and the moderate lesions in the white matter (WM). The ependyma (EP) of the lateral ventricle (V) seems to be unaffected. H & E × 125.

(*c*) Formation of cytotoxic giant cells (x) in the disruptured subventricular zone (SVZ). H & E × 500.

(*d*) Cortex of the hemispheres with normal appearance of the nerve cells. Some very few glial cells are pyknotic (arrows) and some cytotoxic giant cells (x) can be observed. H & E × 600.

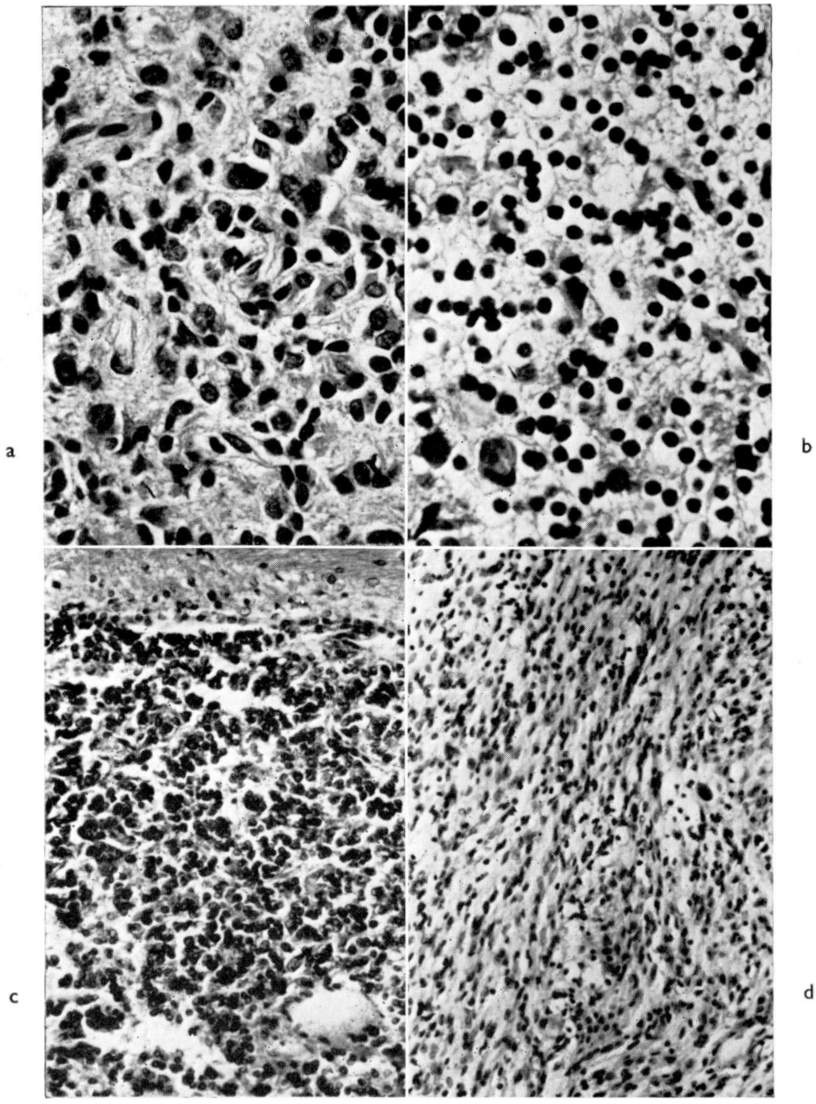

Fig. 5. Histopathology of transplacentally induced tumours with ENU in the offspring of treated mother rats.
(*a*) Astrocytoma. H & E ×500.
(*b*) Oligodendroglioma. H & E ×500.
(*c*) Anaplastic ependymoma. H & E ×240.
(*d*) Anaplastic neurinoma. H & E ×240.

adult animals (LD 0 for adult Sprague-Dawley rats = 300 mg/kg ENU, LD 50 approximately = 375 mg/kg ENU, LD 100 = 450 mg/kg ENU).

Teratogenic effects of the nervous system are dependent on the dosage and the time of application of ENU. As a general rule the brain is more vulnerable than the spinal cord, and the spinal cord more vulnerable than the peripheral nervous system. With respect to the topic of this conference emphasis will be placed on brain damage only. Within the brain the hemispheres are the preferred sites for lesions. A dose of 80 mg/kg ENU injected i.v. to pregnant Sprague-Dawley rats on the 12th day of gestation produces agenesis of the olfactory bulbs and severe hypoplasia of the hemispheres, while other parts of the brain, including the cerebellum, appear normal or less disturbed (Fig. 1). The same dose applied to pregnant rats on the 15th day of gestation leads only to a marked impairment of the development of the brain hemispheres (Fig. 2). The brain can also be damaged on the 20th and the 22nd day of pregnancy; however, the persisting lesions in the hemispheres and the cerebellum are moderate (Fig. 3). It is also possible to damage the brain after birth with increased dose-levels. Newborn rats and young animals up to the age of two weeks will suffer permanently from structural changes, particularly within the hemispheres and the cerebellum.

The malformations produced in the brain are caused by cytotoxic effects, which develop as early as three and six hours after the injection (Fig. 4). It is of interest that the lesions are predominantly found in those parts of the brain lying between the ventricular ependyma and the cells of the primitive cortex. This regional increase in vulnerability may be explained by the fact that cells located in the subependymal zones are largely in the S-phase of the mitotic cycle (Fujita, 1966). This would mean that proliferating cells are more susceptible than cells in interphase. Repair mechanisms in other organs are well documented after cytotoxic lesions; to what extent repair occurs in the central nervous system remains to be determined.

Oncogenic Effects of Ethylnitrosourea

ENU is a powerful resorptive carcinogen. After single or multiple injections into adult rats, a large number of tumours develop in different organs, including the haematopoietic system, the stomach, intestine, uterus, breast, the brain and the spinal cord (Druckrey *et al.*, 1967; Ivankovic and Druckrey, 1968). Studying newborn, 10- and 30-day-old BD IX rats, Druckrey *et al.* (1970) observed an increasing susceptibility with a shortening of the latency period for tumour growth, and a shift of the tumour spectrum to those developing within the nervous system and the kidney. A selective neuro-oncogenic effect is observed, when the compound is administered during pregnancy. The susceptibility of the foetus to neoplastic growth later in life is greatest in the third period of gestation. No tumours could be induced before the 12th day of gestation in rats (Ivankovic and Druckrey, 1968). This is the reason why ENU is particularly suited to produce a high incidence of tumours of the central and peripheral nervous system in offspring of mother rats, which received the compound even as a single dose between the 15th and the 22nd day of gestation (Druckrey *et al.*, 1966; Ivankovic *et al.*, 1966; Druckrey *et al.*, 1967; Ivankovic and Druckrey, 1968; Kleihues *et al.*, 1968; Wechsler *et al.*, 1969; Zülch and Mennel, 1970; Napalkov, 1971; Koestner *et al.*, 1971).

The susceptibility to tumour induction at the 15th day of gestation is approximately 50 times higher than the susceptibility of adult BD rats (Ivankovic and Druckrey, 1968). Our own experiments suggested an approximately 70-fold increase at the 20th day of gestation in Sprague-Dawley rats (Swenberg *et al.*, 1971). Tumour growth is dependent on the age of application during ante- and post-natal periods of life, the dosage, the route of application, but also dependent on genetic factors inherent in different strains of rats (Druckrey *et al.*, 1970).

Transplacentally induced tumours develop at preferred sites within the brain, the spinal cord, the cranial nerves, the spinal roots, and particularly in the large nerves of the lumbosacral and the brachial plexus. The tumours of the nervous system fall into the following main groups: gliomas, ependymomas and neurinomas. The neurogenic neoplasms demonstrate a varied spectrum of differentiation and anaplasia, and most of them have to be considered as malignant (Fig. 5). The morphology of the tumours, including ultrastructural details essential for classification, have been described particularly by Ivankovic and Druckrey (1968), Kleihues *et al.* (1968), Wechsler *et al.* (1969), Zülch and Mennel (1970), and Koestner *et al.* (1971).

Discussion

The alkylating agent ethylnitrosourea is potentially teratogenic and oncogenic in experimental rats. The biological effects are dose-dependent and vary greatly in different periods of ante- and post-natal life. Among the factors involved in teratogenesis and/or oncogenesis are dosage, age of application, and strain-dependent genetic differences.

It is legitimate to compare the biological effects of ethyl- and methylnitrosourea (MNU), since it is known that MNU is also a potent resorptive carcinogen and teratogen (for *oncogenesis* see Druckrey *et al.,* 1967; Jänisch and Schreiber, 1969; Stroobandt and Brucher, 1969; Leaver *et al.,* 1969; Stavrou, 1969; Kleihues *et al.,* 1970; Warzock *et al.,* 1970; Swenberg *et al.,* 1971; and for *teratogenesis* see Napalkow and Alexandrow, 1968; Napalkow, 1971; von Kreybig, 1968; Koyama *et al.,* 1970 and Wechsler, 1970, 1971). When calculated on a comparable quantitative basis, MNU is more toxic than ENU. Because of its relatively low toxicity, ENU is an ideal candidate for transplacental tumour induction. ENU induces transplacentally selectively tumours of the nervous system. A comparable neuro-oncogenic effect can be obtained when adult rats receive repeated small doses of MNU over a period of weeks and months, while ENU in similar experiments is oncogenic in a variety of organs. This suggests the hypothesis that at the molecular level differences in methylation versus ethylation of cellular constituents may determine the different response.

It may be possible that compounds like ENU affect the nervous system also in hitherto unknown ways. Alkylating compounds may interfere especially during development with cellular constituents of various organs and induce permanent changes which are expressed, e.g. as mutagenic effects in later generations, or e.g. as diseases of the nervous system, which are as yet not fully understood. The biological effects of alkylating N-nitroso-compounds were well recognised in recent years. It should be mentioned that agents of this type are produced by chemical and pharmaceutical industries. They are constituents of natural products (Haskell *et al.,* 1954; Matsumoto and Strong, 1963; Arison and Fendale, 1967) and formed by inert precursors in the gastric juice of animals and man (Sander, 1967; Lyinski and Epstein, 1970). Others are used as chemotherapeutic agents in cancer treatment, for instance 1,3-Bis(2-chloroethyl)-1-nitrosourea (Wheeler and Bowdon, 1965, 1968; Schabel *et al.,* 1963) and 1-(2-chloroethyl)-3-cyclohexyl-1-nitrosourea (Bray *et al.,* 1970; Oliverio *et al.,* 1968, 1970). Whether alkylating agents might be hazardous to human health, is widely discussed (Magee, 1971) and should be clarified in the near future.

Summary

The alkylating agent ethylnitrosourea (ENU) has to be considered as oncogenic, teratogenic, and mutagenic. Experimental results are summarised in this report, concerning the oncogenic and teratogenic actions of ENU in different rat strains. ENU acts as a resorptive carcinogen systemically after introduction by various routes. The increased susceptibility of rat foetuses, newborn and 10-day-old rats demonstrates that the peri-natal period of development is particularly suited for tumour production. A single contact with the metabolites of the carcinogen is sufficient to produce tumours in the offspring of the treated mother rats. The selectivity to tumours of the central and peripheral nervous system is surprising and is restricted to the pre-natal period of life and newborn rats. Since the effects are dose-dependent, a number of essential and modifying factors in oncogenesis could be evaluated.

ENU is also teratogenic in rats. The type of malformation depends on the dosage and the stage of development. The central nervous system has the longest determining period extending from the ninth day of gestation until birth and the second week of post-natal life. Malformations of the brain show a predilection for different parts of the central nervous system, and the lesions are seen in the cerebral hemispheres, the olfactory bulbs and the cerebellum. No causal relationship is detectable between the teratogenic and oncogenic effects in transplacental ENU experiments.

Whether ENU may cause other persisting molecular lesions in the nervous system, particularly in the brain, is of potential interest with respect to the pathogeneis of a number of aetiologically undetermined neurological and psychiatric diseases.

ACKNOWLEDGEMENTS

Supported in part by Grant CA 11224 from the National Institutes of Health, Bethesda, Maryland, U.S.A., and a visiting and consulting professorship of the Ohio State University, Columbus, Ohio, U.S.A.

In addition I would like to thank Miss U. Beckmann and Mr. H. Göldner for the skilled technical and photographic assistance and Mrs. U. Wiesner for the excellent editorial help with this article. I am grateful to Prof. Dr. H. Druckrey, Freiburg, Germany, the initiator and stimulator of our research in this field.

REFERENCES

Arison, R. N. and Fendale, E. L. (1967). *Nature, London* **214,** 1254.

Bray, D., Oliveiro, V., Adamson, R., Devita, V. (1970). *Proc. Amer. Assoc. Cancer Res.* **11,** 12.

Druckrey, H., Ivankovic, S., Preussmann, R. (1966). *Nature* **210,** 1378.

Druckrey, H., Preussmann, R., Ivankovic, S., Schmähl, D. (1967). *Z. Krebsforsch.* **69,** 103.

Druckrey, H., Schagen, B., Ivankovic, S. (1970). *Z. Krebsforsch.* **74,** 141.
Druckrey, H., Landschütz, Ch., Ivankovic, S. (1970). *Z. Krebsforsch.* **73,** 371.
Fujita, S. (1966). In 'Evolution of the Forebrain' (eds R. Hassler and H. Stephan), p. 180. Stuttgart: Georg Thieme Verlag.
Haskell, T. H., Ryder, A., Bartz, Q. R. (1954). *Chemother., N.Y.* **4,** 141.
Ivankovic, S., Druckrey, H., Preussmann, R. (1966). *Naturwissenschaften* **53,** 410.
Ivankovic, S. and Druckrey, H. (1968). *Z. Krebsforsch.* **71,** 320.
Jänisch, W. and Schreiber, D. (1969). 'Experimentelle Geschwülste des Zentralnervensystems'. Jena: Gustav Fischer Verlag.
Kleihues, P., Matsumoto, S., Wechsler, W., Zülch, K. J. (1968). *Verh. Dtsch. Ges. Path.* **52,** Togung, 372. Stuttgart: Fischer.
Kleihues, P., Zülch, K. J., Matsumoto, S., Radke, U. (1970). *Z. Neurol.* **198,** 65.
Koestner, A., Swenberg, J. A., Wechsler, W. (1971). *American J. Pathol.* **63,** 37.
Kreybig von, T. (1968). *Arzneimittelforsch.* suppl. **17,** 1, Editio Cantor KG, Aulendorf/Württ.
Kreybig von, T. and Schmidt, W. (1967). *Arzneimittelforsch.* **9,** 1093.
Leaver, D. D., Swann, P. F., Magee, P. N. (1969). *Brit. J. Cancer* **23,** 177.
Lijinsky, W. and Epstein, S. S. (1970). *Nature, Lond.* **225,** 21.
Magee, P. N. (1971). *Fd. Cosmet. Toxicol.* **9,** 207.
Matsumoto, H. and Strong, F. M. (1963). *Arch. Biochem. Biophys.* **101,** 299.
Napalkov, N. P. and Alexandrov, V. A. (1968). *Z. Krebsforsch.* **71,** 32.
Napalkov, N. P. (1971). In 'Problems of Oncology' (Russian) **17,** 1.
Oliverio, V. T., Vietzke, W. M., Williams, M. K., Adamson, R. H. (1968). *Proc. Amer. Assoc. Cancer Res.* **9,** 56.
Oliverio, V. T., Walker, M. D., Hayes, S. L., De Vita, V. T. (1970). *Proc. Amer. Assoc. Cancer Res.* **11,** 61.
Schabel, F. M., Jr. (1963). *Cancer Res.* **23,** 8725.
Sander, J. (1967). *Arch. Hyg.* **151,** 22.
Sander, J. (1970). *Arzneimittelforsch.* **20,** 418.
Stavrou, D. (1970). *Acta neuropath. (Berlin)* **15,** 220.
Stroobandt, G. and Brucher, J. M. (1968). *Neuro-chirurgie* **14,** 515.
Swann, P. F. and Magee, P. N. (1970). 10th Intern. Cancer Congress, Houston, Texas, p. 3.
Swann, P. F. and Magee, P. N. (1971). *Biochem. J.* in press.
Swenberg, J. A., Koestner, A., Wechsler, W. (1971). *J. Neuropath and Exper. Neurol.* **30,** 122.
Swenberg, J. A., Koestner, A., Wechsler, W. (1971). *Amer. J. Path.* **62,** 11a.
Warzock, R., Schneider, J., Schreiber, D., Jänisch, W. (1970). *Experientia* **26,** 303.
Wechsler, W. (1970). 6th Intern. Congr. Neuropathology, p. 128. Paris: Masson.
Wechsler, W. (1971). *J. Neuropath. and Exper. Neurol.* **30,** 120.
Wechsler, W., Kleihues, P., Matsumoto, S., Zülch, K. J., Ivankovic, S., Druckrey, H. (1969). *Ann. N.Y. Acad. Sci.* **159,** 360.
Wheeler, G. P., Alexander, J. A. (1965). *Cancer Res.* **25,** 1770.
Zülch, K. J. and Mennel, H. D. (1970). 6th Intern. Congr. of Neuropathology, p. 60. Paris: Masson.

DISCUSSION

Balázs: I was very interested in your finding that RNA synthesis didn't seem to be affected, but protein synthesis was reduced, because this means that there is a dissociation between the two processes, and that there was basically a translational defect. The polysome profile did not give much of a lead, but to prepare polysomes from brain is rather more tricky than from other organs. You require a much higher magnesium and potassium concentration than when using liver. You need to go up to about 12 mM of magnesium to get a good polysome profile from the brain. Yours were very nice, but probably if you go higher with Mg^{++} and K^{+} you may find that in your controls the monomeric peak may be smaller. In that case there may be a possibility that even in the polysome profile there may be evidence of a translational defect.

Kleihues: Using a Mg^{++} concentration of 5 mM we found a relative increase of monomeric units in both the liver and brain of rats treated with methylnitrosourea. When the Mg^{++} concentration was lowered to 2 mM (0.25 M KCl) the breakdown of polyribosomal units was paralleled by an increase of ribosomal subunits rather than of monomeric ribosomes (Fig. 2). Evidence has accumulated in recent years that a ribosome cycle exists in mammalian cells similar to that in bacterial protein synthesis. After chain termination ribosomes dissociate and exchange their subunits before a new messenger or cistron is read. The accumulation of subunits, as observed in rats treated with methylnitrosourea may therefore be tentatively interpreted as reflecting an inhibition predominantly of steps involved in chain initiation.

Magee: I would like to ask Dr. Kleihues, and Dr. Balázs too, whether it seems unlikely that the actual mechanism of the inhibition by the same agent will be fundamentally different in the brain and in the liver.

Kleihues: I do not expect this to be different, and I am still not convinced that it is different, but the response of the polysome profile was indeed very different in the brain and in the liver, although the inhibition of protein synthesis was of similar degree in both. I do not conclude, therefore, that there is a different mechanism of action. At present it seems not to be unlikely that there are relative differences in the different organs of chain elongation or chain initiation, although this is not proven by these studies.

Balázs: May I suggest that it is known that the lability of the brain polysomes increases with age? This very important dependence on Mg^{++} and K^{+} ions also increases with age. Now, the toxic effect probably is no different in the very young animal from the older one. Could this difficulty be overcome by studying the polysome profile in young animals where you do not have the difficulty of the lability? In that case you may get a lead as to whether there is an increase or not of monomeric units.

Kleihues: We did it in 130 g rats and in 10-day-old rats. We could look at newborn rats and see whether the pattern differs. Personally I do not think this very likely, but I will be happy to take up this suggestion.

Davison: Could you explain why it is that the specific activity of the amino acids in the brain is higher in treated than in control animals? Is it also true of liver? What about plasma?

Kleihues: In adult rats there was a decrease of specific activity (S.A.) of proteins and an increase of the S.A. of amino acids in the free pool. Now, on calculation you get an inhibition of protein synthesis of about 50%. In weanling rats, on the other hand, there was no significant difference in specific activity of proteins, but the specific activity of the amino acids in the acid soluble pool was twice as high. Taking the differences in the pool sizes into account you get the same 50% figure.

Davison: Why are the S.A. higher?

Kleihues: In adult animals there was an accumulation in the acid soluble pool caused by inhibition of protein synthesis. This seems to be a general phenomenon.

Davison: It is a widespread effect?

Kleihues: Yes, in all organs, including the serum.

Balázs: There is biochemical and A.R.G. evidence that in the brain the rate of protein synthesis in neurones is higher than in glial cells. The animals were killed in your experiments 30 min after the injection of the labelled amino acid; this may be too long since at that time the rise in the labelling of proteins is already slowing down as a result of the exponential decrease in the concentration of the precursor in the blood. If the treatment affected preferentially the rate of protein synthesis in the nerve cells one would expect a substantial increase in the content of radioactivity in the amino acid pool in the tissue. The treatment apparently also affected the time course of the removal of the labelled amino acid from the blood, and as a consequence the incorporation rate in unaffected cells, let us say in the glia, may remain linear for a longer time than in controls, which may have masked the reduction in the rate of neural protein synthesis since the time-lapse between injection and sacrifice was relatively long. However, to clarify the question whether or not the rate of protein synthesis is affected when the difference compared with controls is observed in the content of radioactivity in the free amino acids rather than in the labelling of proteins, one ought to determine the flus of the labelled amino acid from blood into the tissue and from the tissue amino acid pool into protein.

Kleihues: We made a preliminary study of the specific activity of brain and liver proteins at different intervals and we chose a maximal period of 30 min. Even up to 60 min there was no decline of specific activity of L-leucine-1-(^{14}C) within the brain or in the liver. We homogenise the brains, so we do not know what happens to neurones and glia. I know

the work on separating neurones and glia, and that there are changes in the kinetics of labelling between these cell types. We are trying to do this, too. This could give an explanation, especially in the weanling rats.
Balázs: Yesterday I talked about compartmentation. With (U-^{14}C) leucine you get C^{14} incorporated into the amino acids of the Krebs cycle. Now, leucine is one of the precursors which shows signs of metabolic compartmentation, and if you estimate glutamine and glutamate respectively relative to that of leucine (Patel, A. J. and Balázs, R. (1971). *Biochem. J.* **121**, 469) you may get an indication whether you have affected the free pool in the neurones or not.
Kleihues: This is a very good suggestion.
Cremer: You had rats surviving after E.N.U. with very small brain weights. Could you tell us more about these?
Kleihues: As far as I know, Dr. Wechsler has not done special studies on behaviour of these animals. But Laqueur and Spatz have obtained similar effects with methane-azoxy methanol derived from cycasine. They found microcephaly in these animals; they also did behavioural studies, finding considerable differences (Hadad *et al.* (1969) *Science* **163**, 88).
Cavanagh: I get the impression that the dose to produce this effect is rather higher than that to produce tumours.
Kleihues: Yes. This is important.
Cavanagh: This is probably due to massive depopulation of the subependymal layer?
Kleihues: I think so. There is a close dose relationship to brain weight reduction. The carcinogenic effect, however, does not follow a close dose relationship. There is the same incidence of tumours whether you use a high or a much lower dose.
Jellinger: Was there a relationship between loss of brain weight and real malformations?
Kleihues: No, I don't think so. With a very high dose there was an incaeasing number of ectopias, but with a lower dose there was a general loss in weight of the organ.

Recently it has been shown that the virus of panleukaemia in cats produces cerebellar malformations, previously thought to be 'spontaneous'. During the last third of gestation in cats, we have used ethylnitrosourea (i.v. 50 mg/kg) and all kittens showed after birth marked cerebellar malformations, which were symmetrical and principally affected the medial parts. Not only was there a general loss of granule cells but also microgyria and a great distortion of the whole architecture. Purkinje cells lay at all levels, including ectopic islands outside the cortex. This effect is dose-dependent but may also be species-dependent too, but we have never seen these changes in mice.

Jellinger: Were the microgyria changes associated with porencephalic defects?

Kleihues: No.

Wigglesworth: The fact that carcinogenic doses are very much lower than in the adult is of considerable interest. Are there any compounds, that the human foetus might come in contact with, that could produce such an effect.

Kirman: What about 'sweeteners'–cyclamates–in food?

Kleihues: All these effects are restricted to this group of alkylating agents, but there is no positive evidence for their being in any way causal to human brain tumours.

Magee: Although cyclamates are not alkylating agents, nonetheless they are reported to be a carcinogenic, producing tumours in rat bladder. A carcinogenic agent does not have to be an alkylating agent, so that it cannot be excuded.

Stern: Dr. Schoental at Carshalton has lately been working on alkaloids which, when eaten in small amounts by the mother, produce brain tumours in the offspring.

Cavanagh: I have seen these tumours and they are very like those produced by nitrosourea.

General Discussion

OPENED BY P. N. MAGEE

The two papers of Dr. Wechsler and Dr. Kleihues have been on nitroso compounds, and here we do meet the problem, namely to what extent is this work, interesting though it may be to oncogenesis, relevant to the problem of mental retardation in man? We really do not know what the effects of low doses on the mentality and behaviour of animals might be. There is quite good evidence that these compounds can occur in the environment, and I would like to talk about this. In Tabe 1 the nitrosamide compounds are those that produce brain tumours, but more research has been done on the allied nitrosamines,

TABLE 1

DIMETHYLNITROSAMINE	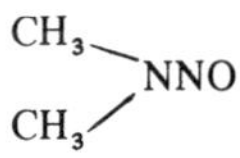
N-NITROSOMETHYLUREA	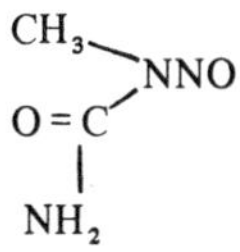

which so far as I know, do not produce brain tumours, but they do produce tumours of just about every other organ. One would imagine that results obtained with one compound could be extrapolated to the other type of compound. The alkylating agent produced by these compounds is a carbonium ion, and there is evidence as we have already heard that this produces alkylation of nucleic acids and other cell components.

Whether or not nitroso compounds act by alkylation, methylmethanesulphonate, an alkylating agent which is not a nitroso compound, has been found by us to produce brain tumours 19 months later when given to a young adult rat. Moreover, in answer to an earlier question from Dr. Clayton, a number of these alkylating agents do find their way into various aspects of industry. Ethylmethanesulphonate, a related compound, produces tumours in the kidney, but not in the brain, so that the reverse of the nitrosourea situation occurs here, the methyl agent affecting the brain and the ethyl agent affecting other organs. All I want to stress is that the effects of the nitroso compounds could be due to their alkylating action, although not necessarily so.

A more practical question is whether man is going to be susceptible to the action of these compounds. One can approach this by looking at a whole range of species, which can be done with the nitrosamines with which most work has been done (Table 2). No insusceptible species

TABLE 2

Species Reported to be Susceptible to Carcinogenesis by Nitrosamines

Rat	Rabbit
Mouse	Dog
Hamster	Monkey
Guinea pig	Rainbow trout

TABLE 3

Metabolism of [^{14}C] dimethylnitrosamine by tissue slices *in vitro*

Tissie	O_2 *Uptake* (μl O_2/g wet wt./hour)	$^{14}CO_2$ *Production* (percent ^{14}C added)
Rat liver	760	5.2
Human liver	240	3.0
Rat kidney	2,560	0.5

Montesano, R. and Magee, P. N., *Nature, Lond.* **228**, 173-174 (1970).

appear to have been found, so that on this basis it is unlikely that man would not be susceptible to the carcinogenic action of this group of compounds. They are also very powerful mutagenic agents as well as carcinogenic agents. But if it was felt that further evidence of the susceptibility of man was wanted, as my colleagues and I did, the only way to approach this problem would be to study the metabolism of one of these compounds by human tissues. In Table 3 the results of some experiments by Dr. Montesano (Montesano, R. and Magee, P. N. (1970) *Nature, Lond.* **228**, 173) of the metabolism of dimethyl nitrosamine by tissue slices *in vitro,* including rat liver, human liver and rat kidney. The metabolism of the compound labelled with C^{14} is measured by the production of $C^{14}O_2$ *in vitro* in a Warburg apparatus. The human liver compares favourably with rat liver, and similarly looking at alkylation of nucleic acids as an index of another parameter of metabolism, again the human liver activity is of the same order as the rat liver. Perhaps we can conclude, therefore, that man would be susceptible to these compounds, if exposed to them.

The final question is whether man is going to be exposed to this class of compounds. The answer appears to be yes. In Table 4 is a list of non-industrial sources of nitrosamines, particularly the trace amounts in tobacco smoke, in various foods, in plants, e.g. cycasin, and a number of micro-organisms which can produce nitrosamines, notably streptocytosin which was developed as an antibiotic. This latter

TABLE 4

Some Reported Non-industrial Sources of Nitrosamines and Related Compounds

Food	*Tobacco smoke*
Fish	
Meat	*Plants*
Mushrooms	Solanum incanum
Wheatflour	Cycas circinalis
Cheese	
Milk	*Microorganisms*
African spirits	Streptomyces

material is closely related to nitrosomethylurea, except that it has a sugar attached to a nitrogen. It is a remarkably potent diabetogenic agent in a number of species, and produces kidney tumours in rats.

The situation may be rather more sinister even than this, in that these simple molecules are formed by the reaction between nitrites and secondary amines, particularly in a slightly acid medium. In the mammalian stomach the medium is slightly acid and the reaction occurs between nitrites and secondary amines here with the formation of nitrosamines. Nitrates can also give this reaction if micro-organisms are present. Nitrites are, of course, used in food as preservatives, particularly bacon, and moreover nitrites, derived from nitrates in water, can readily occur, and the average daily intake is known. Secondary amines, of course, occur in the diet and also endogenously, e.g. proline, pyrrolidine in the urine, pressor amines and so forth. Deliberate feeding of animals with secondary amines and nitrites can produce tumours (Magee, P. N. (1971) *Food Cosmetic. Toxicol.* **9**, 207) and brain tumours have been also produced by feeding ethylurea with sodium nitrite (Ivankovic, S. and Preussmann, R. (1970) *Naturwissenschaften* **57**, 460).

What we do not know with regard to our present problem is how much of this kind of damage is needed in the brain at a sensitive stage of development. I am doubtful about this. Certainly, with regard to carcinogenesis this is very relevant since very small changes are adequate which are irreversible, but how much brain damage is necessary to have an effect leading to mental retardation is unknown. These agents could perhaps occur in the environment of pregnant women.

Davison: Cigarettes contain a large amount of nitrates, I believe. Is there a relationship between smoking in pregnancy and birth weight and brain weight?

Magee: The amounts may be too small to have an effect.

Cavanagh: So far we have been concerned with single large doses to produce an effect, but we must also consider the effects of smaller doses over a longer period of time at a critical period.

Jellinger: Is there any cumulative effect?

Magee: It is possible in carcinogenesis, but whether this could have an effect on mental retardation is difficult to say.

Crome: Smoking has certainly been shown to be harmful and reduces learning ability in the children of smoking mothers in social class V, suggesting that several factors are accumulating, which is a fairly common situation in mental retardation.

These herbicides that are teratogenic, do they have an alkylating action?

Magee: In general, not, but whether alkylation is the important point is not certain, of course.

Kirman: Margarine made from mouldy peanuts produced acute liver atrophy, is this relevant to the elaiomycin story?

Magee: You are referring to aflatoxin, and this is a good example. This is not, so far as we know, an alkylating agent, although it is highly carcinogenic.

Wigglesworth: With Dr. Butler, I found that with the administration of aflatoxin to pregnant rats we got foetal growth retardation, but this has since been shown to be due to reduction of maternal food intake. We didn't produce tumours in the offspring, nor has anyone else; but malformations have been produced in the hamster (Elis, J. and Di Paolo, S. A. (1967) *Amer. J. Path.* **83**, 53).

Crome: Tumours are of course not an important cause of mental retardation, except for tuberous sclerosis and neurofibromatosis.

Jellinger: There is a small percentage of large infantile cerebral tumours which are associated with neurological deficit and mental defects, most of those tumours arise from the deeper parts of the cerebrum.

Dobbing: Dr. Marsh Edwards of Sydney University noticed that in one hot season there were a number of abnormalities occurring in his guinea pig colony. This led him to expose pregnant guinea pigs for about one hour to raised temperatures. He produced a number of gross anomalies when exposed at 20-25 days of gestation and at 45-50 days and he produced true microcephaly. The incidence was remarkably high considering the mild change in temperature.

Giroud: You speak about the nitrosamine content in the food. Are there variations with the preservation methods?

Magee: Yes. Foods preserved with sodium nitrite have nitrosamines in them. In 1960 in Norway a number of sheep went down with 'hepatitis' which was traced to the consumption of fish meal preserved in sodium nitrite. Fish when slightly rotten contains a lot of amines and in the presence of sodium nitrite, you can easily get nitrosamines formed. In the case of the sheep the amount present was enough to kill the animals.

Giroud: Tobacco remains the most dangerous item. It is well known that the growth of the foetus in heavily smoking women is slower, and many people think that the weight of the newborn is reduced and the intelligence may also be affected. Indeed, even in normal homozygotic twins differences have been found in intelligence according to the weight of the newborn. We know from underdeveloped countries that the early stages of post-natal feeding is very important for brain development.

Zlotnik: About two years ago a large colony of mice infected with Langat virus was tested by behavioural methods which had been shown to be sensitive to the effects of many drugs. Even though these animals had gross brain changes, little behavioural abnormality could be detected (Seamer, J. and Peto, S. (1969) *Lab. Anim.* **3**, 129): It shows that severe encephalitis might have a lesser effect than some drugs.

Jellinger: The same is true with large tumours.

Balázs: Although the neurobiological techniques of morphology and biochemistry have improved a lot in recent years, what hope is there for behavioural tests showing the functional results of the different treatments?

Jellinger: There is still a big gap between human pathology and experimental situations, and often too, gross pathological changes may sometimes be found which were almost completely asymptomatic.

Laurence: This is of course a problem only of detection, and in situations of stress these animals would surely fail. The same holds true for mildly damaged hydrocephalics, that only show inadequacy by failing to make a good go of their lives.

Dobbing: This is one point surely. We X-irradiated heads of six-day-old rats and when adults they had cerebella that were distorted and only half the normal size. Body weight and growth were unchanged. The usual behavioural methods could not distinguish them, but when stressed by an agility test for a food reward they were immediately detected.

There is a further point, which is that there is a world of difference between the effects of a lesion in the developing plastic brain and one in the adult formed brain. We tend not to take this into account.

Laurence: Similarly apparently undetectable damage in premature children subsequently grow up to be behavioural problems. Some damage must have led to this, although this was not detectable.

O'Connor: You can devise a certain number of tests which might be appropriate for less important animals, for instance measurement of short term memory, but this might not be possible for the hamster. Individual tests must be developed, such as rhythm discrimination. Hippocampal destruction when bilateral in humans leads to short term memory loss, but whether this is relevant to small mammals is unknown.

The question is, whether there is a one-to-one correspondence between destruction and behaviour and it is often difficult in the subnormal to make such a correlation. For instance, in microcephaly there are many examples of considerable intelligence levels but with very slowed responses.

Kleihues: By choice of the animal your chances may be increased. This was shown with our studies on cerebellar damage in cats, whereas no effects occurred in rats. In tumour production we use rats, but perhaps this is bad as there are no spontaneous tumours in rats. In the dog, however, spontaneous tumours often occur and perhaps this would be a better species, particularly in the occurrence of preferential location of tumours and so forth.

Drillien: Referring back to real life and stress, I studied the behaviour at seven of children at all birth weights who had, or had not been exposed to complications of pregnancy and delivery, and I found that as birth weights decreased children who were subjected during the first five years of life to stressful situations in the home showed behaviour disturbances when faced with stress. When the home situation was stable, they did not show these disturbances. Children with normal birth weights etc. with very stressful situations, did not show much

disturbance. It was those who had suffered from possible perinatal damage who were more vulnerable.
Laurence: The same occurs in the mildy hydrocephalic child.
Woollam: I've kept a number of rabbits with hydrocephalus by Vitamin A deficiency for years. They have had practically no cerebral cortex, but they have been quite indistinguishable from normal rabbits.
Zlotnik: To devise a test you must choose your condition or your species. Thus hamsters are very shy and it is virtually impossible to test them, but certain strains of mice are very good for certain behavioural tests and may even be trained to do tests.
O'Connor: In relation to Dr. Drillien's point with regard to behaviour, learning is obviously important, but so also is excitability, which is, I suppose, also affected by lesions or chemicals. A considerable variability is found in this in subnormality. This is an important variable, but because of its effects on learning not often mentioned.
Dobbing: I think we should not be too keen to find an absolutely comparable model of mental retardation, but all these features mentioned by Dr. O'Connor are capable of being found in a rat, and the goal should be in testing to find differences rather than direct analogies with the human qualities.
Kirman: To reinforce Dr. O'Connor's experience, when one is dealing with the mildly retarded and considers employability, one continuum is intelligence, but others are drive and persistence, and willingness to learn and to adapt socially. These factors seem to be to a large extent independent. The problem is the extent to which this set of categories is influenced by the lesions or influence by upbringing and other inherent temperamental properties. These distinctions are very difficult.
Laurence: I know of two identical twin girls, one with I.Q. 135, the other a hydrocephalic with I.Q. 125; the latter should have performed well in life, but her behaviour was out of all proportion to the differences in I.Q. She had no self-reliance, no drive, no persistence, and so on.
Sylvester: Dr. Zlotnik, does inbreeding play an important part in your strains of animals and do genetic influences come to influence the results?
Zlotnik: They were outbred hamsters, but we are continuing this work now on inbred strains of mice.
O'Connor: There is a very simple reaction that could be used in esting, and that is speed of reaction to stimulus. This is characteristically retarded in all subnormals, but it is a very crude method, and general in its relevance.

Dobbing: Rats previously undernourished tend to respond to a sharp bang by 'freezing' which then confuses their responses over the next few minutes. Also they are hyperactive, and hyperkinetic. This, too, confuses their performance on testing.

O'Connor: You have to avoid that presumably by some kind of conditioning.

4
Aetiology and Epidemiology of Unclassified Mental Retardation

Perinatal Factors Affecting Mental Development of Low Birthweight Infants

C. M. DRILLIEN

Introduction

Over many years my main research interest has been what happens to low birth weight infants and why. Although infants of low birth weight have a greatly increased risk of mental and neurologic defects, the converse (that children with these handicaps have a greatly increased risk of low birth weight) does not hold. Thus, my interest in and knowledge of brain dysfunction or damage which is presumably associated with mental retardation, is peripheral. Nevertheless, low birth weight may provide a useful model for study because of the wide variation in later mental status of infants of similar birth weight, ranging from obvious mental deficiency withoor without cerebral palsy and epilepsy through minor degrees of mental retardation, often associated with minor degrees of neurological impairment, to the good or superior intelligence of children who appear to have emerged from the hazards associated with low birth weight completely unscathed.

Consideration of differences in the perinatal histories of low birth weight infants who subsequently present with major handicaps, minor impairments or are completely normal, may throw some light on the aetiology of unclassified mental retardation in general.

Past and Present Studies

In my previous studies (Drillien, 1964) I was more concerned with outcome than aetiology at a time when there was little agreement about what happened to low birth weight infants. Although the incidence of residual handicap reported from different centres varies, it is now generally agreed that major handicaps (which are predominantly mental and neurological) are significantly increased at birth weights of 2000 g and under; that low birth weight children without major handicaps in normal school tend to score less well on tests of intelligence and scholastic achievement than do larger-born children and also that low birth weight children perform less well scholastically than would be expected from their intelligence level, possibly due to an increase in behavioural difficulties and specific educational problems.

In 1966 I started collecting for study another group of infants of 2000 g and under in an endeavour to elicit what were the differences in genetic endowment, familial and maternal characteristics, intra- and extra-uterine environment and immediate post-natal care which might account for the wide variation in outcome. Many of these children are still very young and their mental status at school age may be quite different from that found at the time of their last examination; thus, for the purpose of this preliminary analysis, I have had to make predictions. In the main, what is presented here is hypothesis rather than proven fact. The data are co-relational and require submission to some such statistical techniques as multiple regression or multivariate analysis. This will be done when the children are older and their later status more clearly defined.

One of the interesting aspects of this study has been the identification of a syndrome of transient abnormal neurologic signs in the first year which we have called 'transient dystonia associated with low birth weight'. In this aspect of the study I have received valuable assistance and advice from colleagues in paediatric neurology, Dr. T. T. S. Ingram and Dr. J. K. Brown. Children who exhibited transient dystonia tend to be somewhat retarded in all fields of development at later ages and to have more problems of behaviour (particularly hyperkinetic behaviour) in the second and third years of life. We believe that some of these children will have difficulties at school age because of a mild degree of mental retardation associated with behaviour problems and specific educational difficulties and that this syndrome may be prognostic of minimal brain dysfunction.

In the following analyses children have been classified as entirely normal if they have never shown any abnormal neurological signs and on tests of mental development at the time of their last examination were performing well up to what would be expected for a child from that particular family. Children classified as suspect exhibited transient dystonia in the first year and in mental development were definitely not performing up to expectation though not obviously retarded. Children classified as handicapped for the most part had obvious mental retardation or neurological defects; a few were handicapped mainly by physical defects. Children who were not performing up to expectation *or* had exhibited transient dystonia, were classified as 'status unpredictable' and omitted from most analyses.

Aetiologic Factors and Later Status

The aetiology of low birth weight is multiple and since aetiology is likely to be related to outcome; the basic causes of handicap associated with low birth weight may be obscured by follow-up studies which do not take aetiology into consideration. An advance was made with the recognition that the small-for-date infant presented a different problem from the prematurely delivered appropriate weight infant. Recent prospective studies have taken gestational age into account and to some extent this has clarified the problem of relating outcome to aetiology. However, my current study indicates that among all small-for-date infants there is still a multiple aetiology: in particular that those who are exceptionally small-for-date stand out as a separate group.

I have been using the Denver intrauterine growth charts (Lubchenco *et al.*, 1963) as illustrated in Fig. 1 and have superimposed on this an additional line which represents 60% of the Denver 50th centile, 60% of the mean being a level originally suggested by Warkany (1961) as indicating gross intrauterine growth retardation. At the time this chart was constructed U.K. standards were not available. The dotted line indicates 60% of U.K. means of weight for gestational age, made available recently from the British Perinatal Mortality Survey data (Butler and Alberman, 1969). Infants whose weight-for-gestational-age came on or below this line have been called very small-for-date (VSFD).

Of all surviving infants of 2000 g or less at birth born in the Simpson Memorial Maternity Pavilion, Edinburgh, in recent years, 35% were SFD and of these one-third (12% of the total) could be considered VSFD. The distribution in my survey sample is different as I have been selecting cases to give more nearly equal numbers in different birth weight/intrauterine growth groups.

Table 1 examines some factors which may have a bearing on both aetiology and outcome.

Maternal Characteristics

HEIGHT AND SOCIAL CLASS

Nearly one-half of mothers of VSFD infants were short and one in five was very short, being less than 5 ft; this was not associated with an excess of poor-type mothers. One-third of mothers of SFD infants were

TABLE 1

Some adverse factors in the perinatal history of infants of 200 g or less at birth by intrauterine growth (I.U.G.) and later status of the child

				MOTHER			PREGNANT	INFANT	
I.U.G.	*Later status*	*No. Cases*	*%*	*Short*	*Poor Social grade*	*Infertile*	*Late comp.*	*Cong. anomalies*	*Wt. loss > 10%*
					percentage				
VSFD	Normal	18	35	59	12	24	17	24	6
	Suspect	13	25	53	8	46	46	46	23
	Handicapped	9	18	25	13	63	33	75	–
	*All	51	100	46	14	36	27	44	10
SFD	Normal	31	43	45	14	24	45	31	6
	Suspect	13	18	23	15	33	62	38	16
	Handicapped	11	15	40	20	20	73	70	20
	* All	72	100	34	19	25	48	44	11
> 25 Centile	Normal	49	52	18	22	22	41	14	37
	Suspect	13	14	23	8	46	15	54	53
	Handicapped	15	16	13	33	40	23	67	60
	* All	93	100	19	23	27	33	34	44

* Including 'status unpredictable'.
Some standards from control populations:
Short maternal stature 22% (1);
Poor social grade 9% (2);
Maternal infertility 22% (3).
(1) Butler and Bonham (1963); (2) Drillien (1964); (3) Drillien (1968).

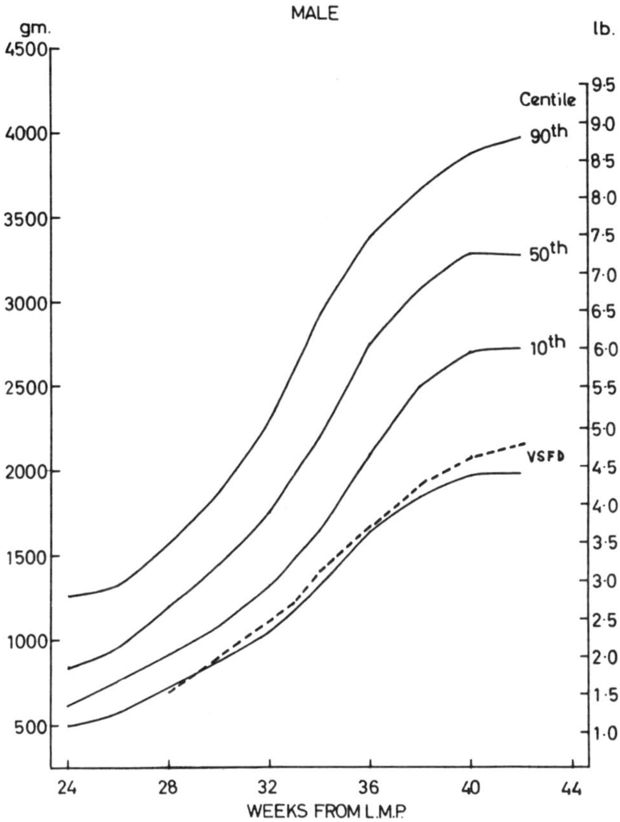

Fig. 1. Denver intrauterine growth chart (Lubchenco *et al.*, 1963).

short and more of these were of poor social class. Women having adequately grown infants were no more likely to be short than the general population of mothers, although the highest incidence of poor-type mothers and of unmarried mothers was found in the well-grown group, possibly associated with the maximum incidence of known attempted abortion in this intrauterine growth group.

INFERTILITY

Relative infertility (defined as difficulty in conceiving, and/or frequent abnormal outcome in conceptions) has been demonstrated as a significant association with a number of congenitally determined

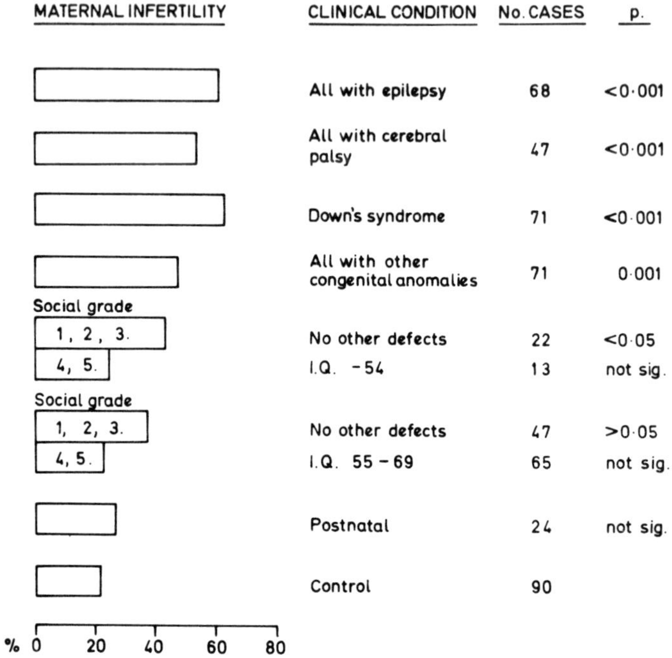

Fig. 2. Maternal infertility by clinical condition of mentally handicapped children.

disabilities (Ingram and Russell, 1961; Drillien *et al.*, 1962, 1966) since Murphy (1947) reported a significant excess in the reproductive histories of all mothers of infants with congenital anomalies who died during a five year period in Philadelphia.

In a retrospective study of 400 mentally handicapped children in Edinburgh (Drillien, 1968) maternal infertility was not increased in cases of mental handicap of post-natal origin or in mothers of poor social class whose children had no defects other than mental retardation. In all other clinical categories there was a signficant increase in maternal infertility as shown in Fig. 2.

In this current group of low birth weight infants, infertility was increased in the VSFD group.

Pregnancy Factors

Threatened abortion was increased in most intrauterine growth groups. Third trimester complications were least common in the VSFDs and most common in the SFDs, with moderate or severe toxaemia being the predominant late complication in both groups. Antepartum haemorrhage was the predominant late complication in the pregnancy histories of well-grown infants.

Characteristics of the Infant

CONGENITAL ANOMALIES

The incidence of congenital anomalies in all groups was increased above the 9% minor anomalies and less than 2% major anomalies found in some control groups (Drillien, 1964; Drillien, 1968).

In the study of mentally handicapped Edinburgh children already mentioned, one-quarter of survey subjects presented with well-recognised clinical syndromes (including Down's). Of the remainder, 29% of those classified as suffering from mental retardation only had minor congenital anomalies. Of those suffering from physical or neurological defects in addition to mental retardation, more serious and/or less common congenital anomalies were present in 56%.

POST-NATAL WEIGHT LOSS

As would be expected, significant weight loss of more than 10% of birth weight was common in the well-grown more prematurely delivered infants and uncommon in SFD and VSFD infants.

This then is the total picture related to intrauterine growth. Division of survey subjects into normal, suspect and handicapped reveals more obvious differences in these factors and permits of some interesting speculations.

Very Small-for-Date Infants

When later status was normal there was a high proportion of short mothers (59%) and a low incidence of all other possibly significant factors.

When the child had obvious handicap the mother was no more likely to be short than would occur by chance, but there was a very high incidence of infertility of mother and of associated congenital anomalies in the infant; two situations which I believe to be indicators of developmental abnormality, with subsequent mental and neurological defect being more likely to have originated in early gestation rather than being caused by damage to a potentially normal central nervous system at a later stage of gestation. These handicapped children experienced few post-natal complications, had little weight loss and caused little anxiety in the newborn nursery.

In the suspect group the figures for infertility and congenital anomalies were mid-way between the extreme groups of complete normality and obvious abnormality. Here was the highest incidence of late pregnancy complications and of infants who caused anxiety in the post-natal period from a variety of complications such as biochemical disturbances and respiratory disorders. Thus, it appears that among VSFD infants we have two main situations: (1) very small infants born to very small mothers who are genetically small and not stunted women who have failed to fulfil their growth potential because of poor environment of upbringing. The children are likely to be normal except that they remain of very small stature; (2) developmentally abnormal infants who have failed to grow *in utero* because of some early disturbance during the period of organogenesis and who are likely to show later mental and neurologic defects. A third group may have suffered from adverse factors in late pregnancy and in the early neonatal period and have sustained minor impairments rather than major handicaps.

Small-for-Date Infants

Among the rest of the small-for-dates late pregnancy complications, significant post-natal weight loss and other post-natal complications were increased in the histories of suspect children and more so in the handicapped group. There was also a high incidence of associated congenital anomalies in the handicapped. Perhaps here we have the situation in the handicapped of additional damage being caused in later pregnancy and post-natally to an already developmentally abnormal central nervous system while in the suspect group minor impairment is produced primarily by adverse perinatal factors (such as pre-natal malnutrition and pre- and post-natal hypoxia) associated with severe toxaemia and placental insufficiency.

The suggestion that placental insufficiency predisposes to minor impairment rather than major handicap is strengthened by examining the later status of 26 VSFD and SFD infants whose mothers were found to have abnormally low oestriol excretions in later pregnancy. The proportion of suspect children was doubled (35% as compared with 18%) and the proportion of handicapped children halved (8% as compared with 19%) as compared with the VSFD or SFD offspring of 97 mothers who had normal oestriol levels or whose oestriol excretions were not measured. Although the numbers are small the difference in trend is on the borderline of significance at the 0.05 level ($X^2 = 5.131$ for 2 df). Three-quarters of the mothers with low oestriol excretions had toxaemia or chronic disease.

Well Grown Infants

Among the well grown late pregnancy complications (predominantly antepartum haemorrhage) appeared to bear no relation to outcome, being most often reported for the entirely normals.

In most intrauterine growth groups threatened abortion was increased, particularly when later status was suspect or definitely abnormal. The highest incidence (39%) of threatened abortion associated with later abnormality was in the well grown group. I do not think that first trimester bleeding *per se* is primarily associated with later status; rather that this bleeding is an indicator of two possible situations: (1) a developmentally abnormal foetus, or (2) a normal foetus with somewhat insecure implantation; this normal foetus is more likely to be delivered prematurely with or without third trimester bleeding.

This hypothesis is strengthened by examining the association of threatened abortion both with later status and congenital anomaly. Of 47 children with a history of threatened abortion, 21 were normal of whom only three had associated congenital anomalies compared with 8 of 15 suspect children and 10 of 11 handicapped children.

As in other intrauterine growth groups, so among the well grown, associated congenital anomalies were increased in the suspect and more so in handicapped children. Maternal infertility was increased in both suspect and handicapped groups.

There is also a suggestion here that malnutrition in the neonatal period may be as important in determining later status in this group as pre-natal nutrition in the SFD group.

Post-natal Nutrition

If we are considering the possibility of malnutrition at a critical period of brain development it may in fact be inappropriate to select weight for gestational age at birth as a measure of adequacy of nutrition. Because of differences in feeding behaviour and post-natal weight gain by maturity, the prematurely delivered infant whose weight for gestational age is adequate or good at birth may weigh no more than the small-for-date infant when both reach a post-conceptional age of 40 weeks. This is illustrated by Fig. 3 which shows post-natal weight curves for two male infants, the one 1250 g at 29 weeks (just below the 50th

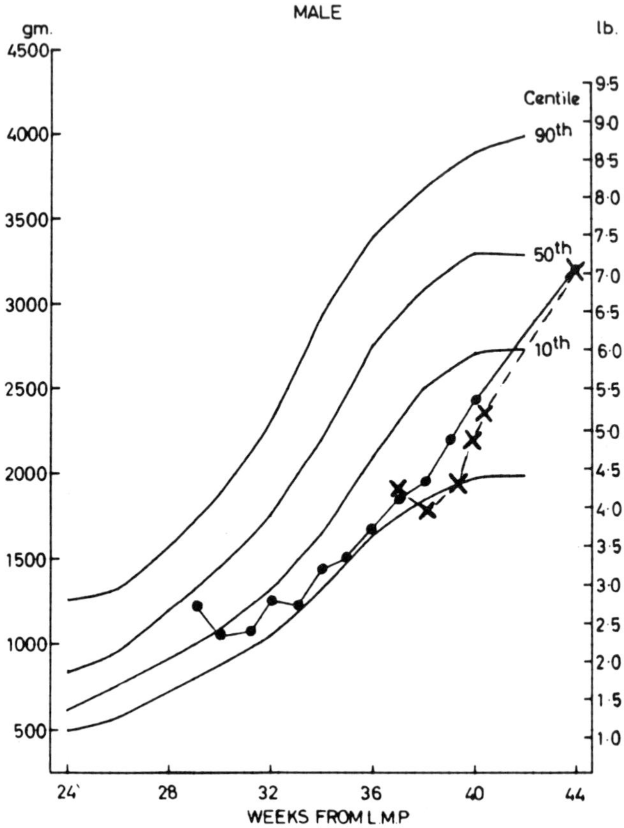

Fig. 3. Post-natal weight curves for two infants; the one appropriate weight prematurely delivered, the other small-for-date.

centile) and the other 1900 g at 37 weeks (far below the 10th). If the period from 29 to 33 weeks is critical for brain development, it could be that the appropriate weight prematurely delivered infant was at greater risk from malnutrition. If 36 to 40 weeks is critical then the SFD infant might be at greater risk. Both boys appear to be mentally retarded in the I.Q. range 65-75.

The possible importance of post-natal nutrition is highlighted in Table 2 which gives mean values of some measures of post-natal nutrition of infants of 3 lb (1360 g) and under born 1948-60 and their status at school age. It seemed likely that poor prognosis for infants born 1953-54 was associated with the extreme delayed feeding

TABLE 2

Some measures of post-natal nutrition and status at school age for infants of 3 lb. (1360 g) or less at birth by date of birth (1948-70)

	Year of birth			
	1948-52	*1953-54*	*1955-60*	*1966-70*
	Mean values			
Per cent birth weight lost	15	21	16	9
Day lowest weight recorded	9	15	11	8
Day birth weight regained	24	33	26	16
Status at school age	Percentage			
Normal school. Class for age	35	6	31	(50)
Normal school. Retarded	35	18	22	(34)
Special school ± Cerebral palsy, Epilepsy	30	76	47	(16)

( ) = Prediction.

practised at that time. Certainly highly significant correlations were obtained at ages 3-11 years between the results of intelligence tests and measurements of weight loss and gain in the post-natal period. I have added to this table mean values for like weight infants born 1966-70. It appears that in Edinburgh we are doing something (though I would guess not enough) in maintaining nutrition in the immediate post-natal period nearer to what it would be *in utero,* which may account for the improved prognosis of low birth weight infants in recent years.

Transient Dystonia Associated with Low Birth Weight

As mentioned earlier, a number of low weight infants in this study group who were neurologically normal at the time of their discharge from maternity hospital presented in the first six months of life (conceptional age) with abnormal neurological signs. Essentially these consist of a syndrome of abnormal extensor muscle tone which is identical to the dystonic stage of diplegia described by Ingram (1964) but in most cases is transient and does not lead to diplegia.

Incidence

The incidence of transient dystonia increased with decreasing birth weight (Table 3). More obvious signs were detected in 13% of those weighing 1751-2000 g with a gradual increase to 43% of those of birth weight 1250 g and under. The incidence was rather higher in males of all birth weights.

TABLE 3

Incidence of abnormal neurological signs in the first year by birth weight excluding all children with definite cerebral palsy at one year

Abnormal neurological signs	*Birth weight (g)* -1250	1251-1500	1501-1750	1751-2000
		Percentage		
Nil	43	64	56	74
Minor	14	11	28	13
More obvious	43	25	16	13
Total	100	100	100	100
No. cases	21	28	68	81

Later Status

At a conceptional age of one year all children were assessed developmentally using the Gesell (1941) schedule with the results shown in Table 4. Mean D.Q. was reduced in all fields of development in those who had exhibited transient dystonia with retardation more marked in gross locomotion than in adaptive and personal-social

TABLE 4

Mean development quotient (D.Q.) at one year by birth weight and neurological signs, excluding all children with physical handicaps and definite cerebral palsy

Birth weight (g)	*Abnormal neurological signs*	*D.Q. Locomotor*	*Other*	*No. cases*
1500 and under	1. Nil	96	91	26
	2. Minor	91	93	6
	3. More obvious	79	82	15
	1-3	17	9	
1501-2000	1. Nil	99	95	93
	2. Minor	89	88	27
	3. More obvious	82	85	20
	1-3	17	10	

behaviour and language. The degree of retardation appeared to increase with increasing severity of the early abnormal signs. It was not possible to make a similar comparative assessment at age two years as many children who had exhibited transient dystonia in the first year were difficult or impossible to test at two years because of over-activity and poor concentration.

Relation to Intrauterine Growth Status and Congenital Anomalies

There was a significant excess of transient dystonia in the poorly grown (birth weight for gestational age at or below the 10th centile) as compared with the well grown (birth weight above the 25th centile). There was also a significant increase in transient dystonia among infants with congenital anomalies.

Since congenital anomalies are known to be increased in VSFD and SFD infants it could be that the excess of transient dystonia was due simply to this association. Table 5 examines this possibility and demonstrates that (1) whatever the intrauterine growth status transient dystonia was nearly twice as common in infants with associated congenital anomalies and (2) whether or not the infant had congenital anomalies transient dystonia was nearly twice as common in those who

TABLE 5

Incidence of transient abnormal neurological signs in the first year in infants with and without congenital anomalies, by intrauterine growth status

	Abnormal neurological signs	*Intrauterine growth per centile (Denver)*			
		10th and under		*> 25th*	
		No.	*%*	*No.*	*%*
No congenital anomalies	Nil or minimal	37	82	51	91
	Obvious	8	18(A)	5	9(C)
	Total	45	100	56	100
Congenital anomalies present	Nil or minimal	26	67	19	83
	Obvious	13	33(B)	4	17(D)
	Total	39	100	23	100

[(1) B/A = 1.8, D/C = 1.9; (2) A/C = 2.0, B/D = 1.9]

were SFD. Thus, whatever is the brain dysfunction or damage that produces this abnormal neurological picture, it seems that in some cases it may be due to disturbance in early gestation and in some others to disturbance in late gestation.

Relation to Post-natal Complications

I could find no association between the incidence of transient dystonia and any adverse perinatal state in isolation (such as hypoxia, respiratory distress syndrome, hypoglycaemia, hyperbilirubinaemia). The only single factor which appeared to be important was the amount of weight loss. However, as many adverse post-natal states are interrelated further analysis is needed here.

Summary

This present study suggests that low birth weight infants can be divided into three main categories with different purposes: (1) those who are prematurely delivered and/or of low birth weight primarily because of developmental abnormality of the foetus. There is a high incidence of associated congenital anomalies and of mental and neurological handicaps. Infants may be small-for-date or appropriate weight with an excess of very small-for-date infants. (2) Growth-retarded infants (all SFD) who have suffered from hypoxia and malnutrition in the third trimester and appropriate weight but post-natally malnourished infants. These are less likely to have major handicaps but may show mild degrees of mental retardation and minor neurologic abnormalities at later ages. (3) Appropriate weight prematurely delivered infants precipitated into the world too soon because of complicating factors such as antepartum haemorrhage, attempted abortion and cervical incompetence. These are potentially normal infants and we may expect a marked improvement in their prognosis with modern methods of premature baby care.

REFERENCES

Butler, N. R. and Bonham, D. G. (1963). 'Perinatal Mortality. The First Report of the 1958 British Perinatal Mortality Survey'. Edinburgh: Livingstone.

Butler, N. R. and Alberman, E. D. (1969). 'Perinatal Problems. The Second Report of the 1958 British Perinatal Mortality Survey'. Edinburgh: Livingstone.

Drillien, C. M. (1964). 'The Growth and Development of the Prematurely Born Infant'. Edinburgh: Livingstone.

Drillien, C. M. (1968). *Arch. Dis. Childh.* **43**, 283.

Drillien, C. M., Ingram, T. T. S. and Russell, E. M. (1962). *Arch. Dis. Childh.* **37**, 282.
Drillien, C. M., Ingram, T. T. S. and Wilkinson, E. M. (1966). 'The Causes and Natural History of Cleft Lip and Palate'. Edinburgh: Livingstone.
Gesell, A. and Amatruda, C. S. (1941). 'Developmental Diagnosis'. New York: Hoeber.
Ingram, T. T. S. (1964). 'Paediatric Aspects of Cerebral Palsy'. Edinburgh: Livingstone.
Ingram, T. T. S. and Russell, E. M. (1961). *Arch. Dis. Childh.* **36**, 34.
Lubchenco, I. O., Hansman, C., Dressler, M. and Boyd, E. (1963). *Pediatrics* **32**, 793.
Murphy, D. P. (1947). 'Congenital Malformations. A Study of Parental Characteristics with Special Reference to the Reproductive Process'. 2nd ed. Philadelphia: Lippincott.
Warkany, J., Monroe, B. B. and Sutherland, B. S. (1961). *Amer. J. Dis. Child.* **102**, 2, 127.

DISCUSSION

Crome: As a pathologist I derived a good deal of comfort from Dr. Drillien in being shown how difficult factor analysis is in these situations and that you often have to accept multiplicity of causes. When I began to examine brains of mentally retarded individuals usually in the clinical history there was a yearly statement of *in statu quo,* and scarcely more than that. Nowadays the history not untypically runs something like this: Rather elderly mother of Social Class V, illegitimate child, some infection in the first trimester of pregnancy, pre-eclamptic toxaemia, breach presentation, delayed second stage, forceps delivery, difficulty of resuscitation, neonatal jaundice, the only item being missing is shortness of the mother! It is extremely difficult to determine in such cases what was the decisive factor, and we often have to accept that we shall not be able to determine this.

Drillien: This sort of data obviously needs to be submitted to sophisticated statistical treatment. What I'm trying to do with each baby at the time of birth is to decide on the evidence whether this baby is likely to have suffered in early gestation and be developmentally abnormal, whether it suffered some adverse factor in later pregnancy from toxaemia, etc., or whether it was potentially normal at the moment of birth, but then suffered—or had various combinations of these. I am trying to decide this at the beginning and trying to see how this correlates with later status. So far, it looks fairly successful in that the ones that seem potentially normal infants at birth seem normal later. It seems extraordinary what the normal human infant can put up with post-natally. I have five very small infants (1000 g or less), prematurely delivered, with the usual post-natal complications of such infants, but all five are quite normal.

Wigglesworth: It is possible to be depressed by the high incidence of mental handicap in the follow-up of low birth weight babies, but we should remember how rapidly changing this situation seems to be. At Hammersmith in two series from 1961-64 and 1965-68 there were 123 babies less than 1500 g equally divided between those four-year periods. In the first period there was recognisable neurological deficit in 12%, in the second period it was only 5%. Whatever the reasons there seems to be a considerable change in prognosis for these very low birth weight babies.

Drillien: There is also a big improvement in this group in the Edinburgh figures. It contains the largest number of accidental premature deliveries. But the 1500-2000 g group of babies does not seem to be improving in the same way. This group contains more small-for-dates babies, or ones who have suffered some insult before birth.

Dobbing: I think this vulnerable period in the human being, which is four-fifths post-natal, is also a period of opportunity, that is to say it is potentially recoverable in crude terms if one can stimulate a good growth rate. Dr. Wigglesworth didn't mention that between his two periods the greatest development that has taken place in the management of the newborn has been the practice of early feeding and of keeping them warm, so that their calories are used for growth.

Wigglesworth: It does seem possible by proper feeding of normal weights-for-birth babies to keep their head circumference growth to within the normal range, whereas in babies small-for-dates it does not seem possible.

Giroud: I was very interested in two facts. It is interesting to note the frequency of infertility and also the frequency of abnormal function in the placenta. This is certainly as you say and that it is most important for our interpretation of the facts.

I want to put two questions. The first, what is the fate of the newborn with other abnormalities? Is it better than the others or is there little difference? Secondly, what is the fate of the oversized child from a diabetic mother?

Drillien: The risk to the diabetic baby is in the immediate post-natal period. If it survives, there is very little difference in their later status, apart from the fact that they are more likely to get juvenile diabetes. I have not noted any increase in congenital malformations in infants of diabetic mothers. If they survive, they do very well.

Wigglesworth: It would be interesting to know where the information on abnormalities comes from. In fact, the most important thing of babies from diabetics is that they should be normal at birth if the diabetes is properly controlled. The really big babies coming to me at post-mortem have come from undiagnosed maternal diabetes. The brain is not particularly large and may if anything be slightly small, even in real macrosomia where the liver may be as large as that of a one-year-old infant.

Kirman: I am struck by the rarity of diabetic mothers amongst those with retarded children, but we haven't made a special study of this.

Dobbing: There is also a rarity of diabetic mothers amongst the largest babies in the population, isn't there? Dr. Neligan at Newcastle selected a group of very large babies, none of whom came from diabetic mothers, and although he has only followed them for six or seven years they, I understand, tend to be rather better of in performance than normal.

Wigglesworth: The big non-diabetic babies dying for other reasons do seem to have rather larger brains, while big diabetic babies do not.

Drillien: I was hoping that Dr. Holt would tell me what is the brain damage or dysfunction that produces this abnormal neurological picture in the first year.

Holt: I was meaning to ask you, but perhaps you answered this in your paper, whether you could distinguish between those that go onto the established picture of cerebral palsy and those with the transient picture, but when young they all look the same. Presumably on this basis you think the pathology is dissimilar, or not?

Drillien: We are getting more and more confused because a number of our dystonic cases are entirely normal at one year, but come back with abnormal signs about three months after gaining independent locomotion rather late. Some of these at two years have mild diplegia, but I don't know the end of the story. I have not met anyone else who has recognised this picture. In the States they said they certainly saw this picture at 4-5 months, but they all went onto true diplegia. They did not recognise this degree of abnormality as completely resolving.

Holt: I know seven or eight babies whom I would say were indeed cerebral palsied but who then recovered. I counted this as a spontaneous recovery of cerebral palsy. I suspect that in those places where they see a lot of young babies they are aware of those with apparent cerebral palsy who spontaneously clear up.

Drillien: Did you see this 15 to 20 years ago? I didn't see it in the '50s. There is no relation to neonatal jaundice.

Kirman: The Isle of Wight study shows a continuum of clumsiness, but I don't know what the background is. Presumably it is relevant to this problem.

O'Connor: Does anyone know what picture Prechtel's children showed who became dyscalculic and were hyperactive at a later age?

Drillien: Prechtel only really studied 'normal' babies, and they didn't show this sort of picture.

Somatic Growth in Severe Mental Retardation

A. T. RUNDLE

Introduction

In some ways, the inclusion of somatic growth in a study of unclassified mental retardation is somewhat misleading, as it may suggest that this group is sufficiently homogeneous to constitute an entity amenable to the growth study approach. As Marshall (1968) has pointed out, not only is the condition a heterogeneous one, but the attempt by some authors to subdivide it into different categories (which bear little or no relationship to the basic pathology) can be dangerous. Furthermore, any attempt to consider somatic growth as an abstract idea, divorcing it from the social and psychological environment to say nothing of its interaction with sexual development can lead to sterile conclusions.

It would be impossible to undertake a comprehensive survey of somatic growth as applied to the mentally retarded child in the time allowed, this has, by necessity, limited this communication to a brief description of the severity of the problem, and how some of the investigations in the last decade have, if nothing else, reinforced my opening remarks on the heterogeneous nature of the sample.

The history of the attempts to apply the study of growth as a diagnostic tool in mental retardation is not new, dating as it does to the initial studies of Tarbell (1883). Improved mathematical methods and the introduction of computer techniques has, in the last decade, provided the stimulus for renewed interest, which, together with our increasing knowledge on the aetiological mechanisms involved, is at last producing meaningful information.

Frequency of Growth Abnormalities

Over the last 10 years we have been fortunate in being able to study the somatic growth of 236 females aged 5-18 years and 194 males, all of whom could be classified as undifferentiated as defined in the 'Statistical Manual for the use of Institutions' (1946), and we are currently taking 11 linear measurements, weight, five subjective estimates of sexual maturation and several biochemical estimates at least once each year. By necessity, this communication will have to be limited mainly to our findings on stature, and that, principally in the form of a cross-sectional approach.

The distribution of the sample is shown in Fig. 1, in which the height of each subject has been rated in terms of the percentile of the normal height for age from the data of Scott (1961). From these data

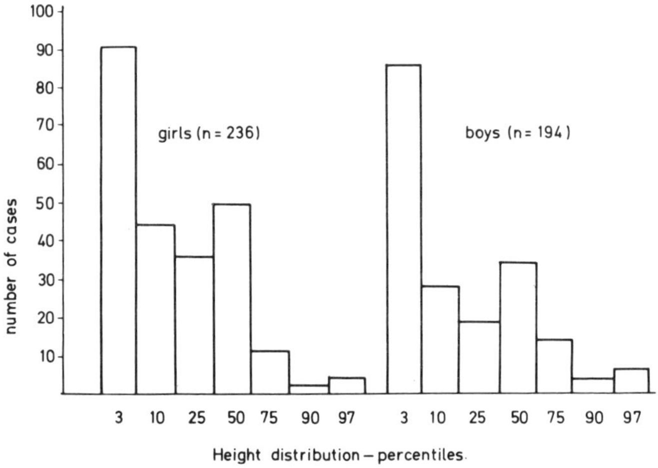

Fig. 1. Height distribution of 236 mentally retarded girls and 194 mentally retarded boys age 5-18 years rated in terms of the percentile of normal height for age.

two things are self-evident, first that a large proportion of the sample can be considered as having retarded stature (i.e. less than the 25th percentile of their normal peers), and secondly the presence of a bimodal distribution, which we were first able to detect in a study on the sexual development of mentally retarded girls (Rundle and Sylvester, 1965). An explanation of this bimodality is, at first sight, fairly simple. Mead (1914) observed that the more severe the mental retardation, the greater the retardation of height (more recently supported by the studies of Kugel and Mohr, 1963; Roberts and

Clayton, 1969). The latter authors were able to confirm that this bimodality was not simply a product of our population, and were able to detect in the abnormal mode evidence for physiological immaturity and a tendency to lower birth weights. This evidence together with others (e.g. Dutton, 1958; 1959) suggests that the two modes consist of one where growth conforms to a normal population and a second where some pathological process is operative.

Although the general trend of the data suggests a high frequency of growth failure, it is surprising how often the growth mechanism can be considered normal. Considering the bias in the selection of subjects, one would expect to find extremes in the range of correlations between different parameters of growth, but as has been demonstrated elsewhere, a considerable number of the correlation coefficients fall between 0.5 and 0.75, with quite a few in the 0.75-0.95 range (Rundle, 1970).

Cross-sectional investigations as outlined above, can be criticised as having severe limitations, being sufficient to describe the frequency of abnormalities but yielding little or no information on the mechanisms involved. An investigation of these will require a large number of longitudinal studies covering the whole period from early childhood to the attainment of adult status (one is tempted to suggest this should be further expanded to include both uterine growth and possible geriatric changes) and to analyse the data not only as simple growth curves, but also the first and second derivatives of it (i.e. the velocity and acceleration curves). To this end, we have been following a series of cases for several years, and although it would be premature to report on the results of this investigation, I would like to give two examples of the use to which this type of data can be put.

Figure 2 compares the cumulative frequencies of a series of pre- and post-pubertal boys aged 5-18 years, in which the height increment for one year has been rated in terms of the percentile expected of the normal for age (the criterion for puberty being genital stage 3 on the ratings of Tanner, 1961). The height velocities of the pre-pubertal boys is significantly lower than either the post-pubertal or the expected normal, but after puberty the height velocity of the mentally retarded boys approaches norality.

Figure 3 shows a weight growth curve and its first and second derivative. Also marked are three maturational landmarks, menarche, and the attainment of breast and pubic hair stage 3 (Tanner, 1961). Although weight is notoriously difficult to interpret (being sensitive to exogenous and endogenous factors) several interesting factors emerge. On the simple growth curve, menarche seems to exert little effect, but on the velocity curve this milestone coincides with the period of

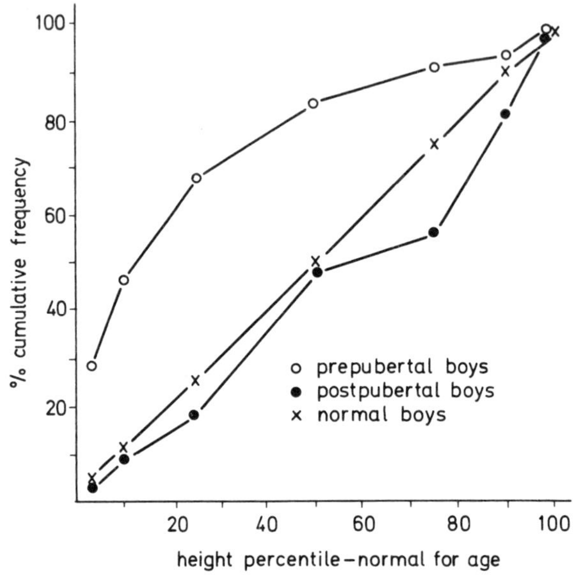

Fig. 2. Percentage cumulative frequencies of 68 pre-pubertal mentally retarded boys aged 5-16 years and 49 pubertal mentally retarded boys (genital development stage 3 or more) rated in terms of the height percentile, normal for age.

maximum velocity, whereas the attainment of breast stage 3 is accompanied by a transient decrease in velocity. The accleration curve shows no effect of menarche, but the appearance of the two maturational indices is marked by a reversal of a period of deceleration. One further interesting point in the acceleration curve is the physiological significance of the age nine years which appears to be the point of transition from acceleration to deceleration, there is nothing in either the growth data or the patient's clinical notes to explain any physiological change at this age.

Causation of Growth Defects

Any attempt to summarise the multitude of factors influencing growth would necessitate the covering of factors as dissimilar as environment (social and psychological), physiological mechanisms (state of the endocrine organs, response to infections) genetics, nutrition etc. To demonstrate the complexity of the subject I shall outline only three studies that we have made, the first on the effect of

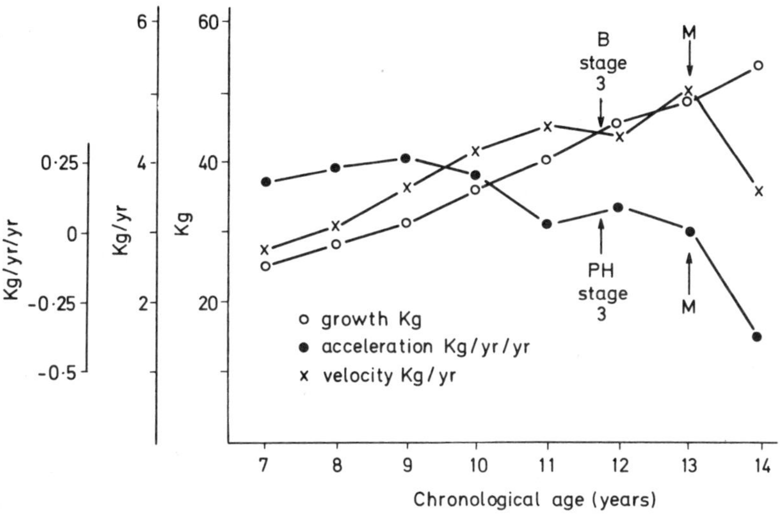

Fig. 3. Weight growth, velocity and acceleration curves of a mentally retarded girl. M, the recorded age of menarche, B and P.H. are the ages at which the breast and pubic hair was first noted to have attained stage 3 (Tanner, 1962).

the bias of socio-economic origins on the stature of the sample, the second on the possible degree of involvement of the thyroid gland, and thirdly on the possible relationship between the growth anomalies and retarded sexual maturation.

Socio-economic Bias

The relationship between stature and sibship size and the socio-economic status of the father is well-documented (Scottish Council for Research in Education, 1953; Douglas and Blomfield, 1958; Miller *et al.*, 1960; Thomson, 1959). In view of the considerable bias towards the lower social groups (IV and V) shown by mentally retarded persons (Registrar-General's Statistical Review 1952-53) it was decided to test if this bias played any significant part in the reduction of mean height in our sample, and this analysis has been reported in detail elsewhere (Rundle and Sylvester, 1967). Briefly, we were able to show that the bias did exist and it would account for some of the reduction in height of the sample as a whole. We were able to approximate this reduction in mean height for 11-year-old children as 2 cm which although significant suggests that some much more important factors exist. In this study we were surprised that we were unable to detect any change in size due to sibship size.

Effect of Thyroid Dysfunction

Investigations into the thyroid state (as measured by the levels of serum thyroxine-iodine) suggest that this may be one of the major causative factors in growth retardation (Rundle, 1971). Of the 127 cases investigated, 15 subjects (eight female and seven males) were found to have a thyroxine-iodine level less than 3.0 μg/ml and of these 15 cases, 11 were severely subnormal for height (i.e. on or below the 25th percentile of the normal). Details of this investigation are set out in Table 1. In an attempt to assess whether this hypothyroidism was a

TABLE 1

The distribution of 54 girls and 73 boys aged 4 to 18 years with respect to their height (in percentiles of the normal for age from the normal data of Scott (1961))

	Boys		*Girls*		*Both sexes*	
Height percentile	*Hypo-thyroid*	*Euthyroid*	*Hypo-thyroid*	*Euthyroid*	*Hypo-thyroid*	*Euthyroid*
3rd	3	33	6	23	9	56
10th	1	8	1	4	2	12
25th	2	7	0	6	2	13
50th	0	10	1	8	1	18
75th	0	4	0	2	0	6
90th	1	4	0	3	1	7
97th	0	0	0	0	0	0

transient feature of childhood, 330 adult mentally retarded subjects were investigated, and 6.7% of the sample was found to be hypothyriotic. It appears that the thyroid is more involved in the somatic growth failure than may have previously been suspected, although Wilkins (1966) has shown that in a series of cases in which short stature was the presenting feature more than 10% showed signs of hypothyroidism, a proportion remarkably similar to that in the mentally retarded population.

Retarded Sexual Maturation and Growth Anomalies

In the section on growth velocity, I touched on the observation of differences between the pre- and post-pubertal boys, with the latter more closely approximating the normal. As our survey has now covered more than 10 years, including several years prior to and several years after the onset of the pubertal spurt we are now able to make some estimate on the relationships between the age of onset of puberty and its relationship to somatic growth. But first, a brief comment on the way in which the data will be presented (Rundle and Sylvester, 1970). One of the most informative ways of analysing growth data, is to present the growth curve or the velocity curve, not in chronological sequence, but in terms of years before and after maximum velocity (Israelsohn, 1960), similarly it is possible to present the growth data in terms of years before and after a given landmark in sexual maturation (menarche, breast, development of pubic hair stage for girls; appearance of moustache, voice breaking, genital development stage in boys). Probably the simplest maturation criterion is menarche in girls, since this is non-subjective, and appears to be a dramatic event. However, much caution must be applied as menarche is not just a single dramatic event but one of a gradual process, and of course menarche does not necessarily imply ovulation. Using menarche as the maturational index, and if the normal age for menarche is assumed to be 13.05 years (Scott, 1961) it is possible to carry out a cross-sectional survey of, say, stature in terms of years from menarche and further to rate these as the normal expected percentiles. Figure 4 shows the comparison of two histograms, A shows the data on 87 girls rated in respect to their chronological age, and B the same series rated in terms of years from menarche. The transposition of the data causes a noticeable shift of the data towards the normal expected frequencies (unshaded) but there still remains a considerable number of cases lying below the 25th percentile. One serious difficulty in this type of exercise is that the use of a single maturational criterion in this way eliminates those cases (probably the most abnormal) who will never achieve full adult status. If, however, we keep the inherent dangers of this technique in mind, it is safe to suggest that late maturation of the mentally retarded (Rundle and Sylvester, 1963, 1965) is either one of the major causative factors in the growth retardation, or, of course, they are both symptoms of underlying physiological or pathological mechanisms. Before leaving this topic, mention must be made to the findings of Wilkins (1966) that the largest single cause of stunted growth was due to what he has termed constitutional retarded growth and adolescent development, of which he found no less than 30.9% of the cases he investigated. This group had been slow in both growth and osseous development throughout childhood, the onset of puberty was delayed but they eventually matured sexually and achieved reasonably normal stature. It is interesting to speculate what proportion of the severely mentally retarded patients are of this type and if the mechanisms involved are abnormal in some way.

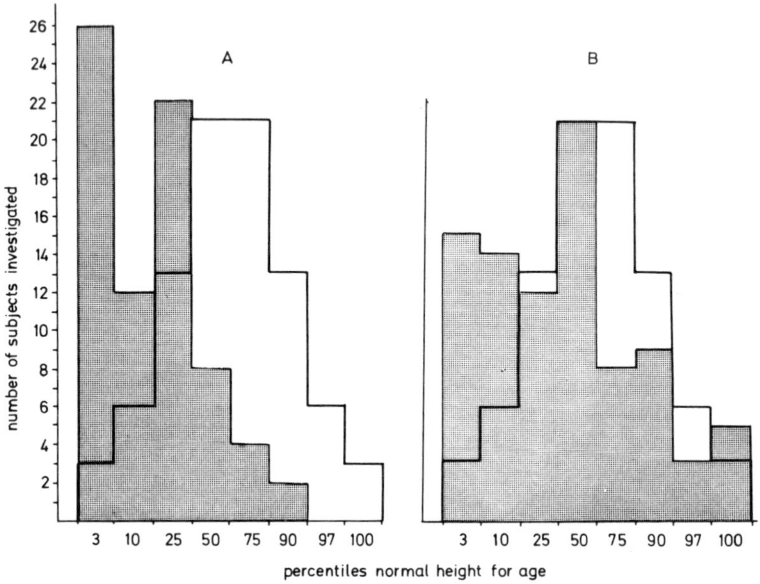

Fig. 4. Height distribution of 87 mentally retarded girls (shaded areas). A, rated in terms of the normal percentiles for age, B, similarly rated but in terms of years from menarche. Unshaded areas show the normal expected frequencies.

The Large Child

A survey on the literature of the growth of the mentally retarded subject would suggest, at least superficially, that the only anomalies one would expect to find are those involving reduction in size. For some reason the occasional child who is significantly taller than his normal peers has been studiously neglected, probably due to the aetiological point of view that the tall child usually belongs to Albright's category of what 'endocrinology is not' (1951).

In any mentally retarded population the tall child is occasionally encountered for example in our sample of 550 cases, 10 have been found to exceed the 97th percentile of their normal peers. Perhaps in a normal population these would have little or no significance, but in the mentally subnormal population where the reverse is usually the case they become of disproportionate interest. We became interested in this group following the observation by my clinical colleague, Dr. P. Sylvester, that the mentally retarded children who exhibited severe behaviour disorders often seemed to be taller than their institutionalised peers. In spite of the claims of Dutton (1964) that there was a failure of growth in psychotic boys we have investigated a series of 16 boys and 17 girls with acute behavioural problems, and these data are set out in Table 2. The first striking observation on this group is that

TABLE 2

The distribution of 16 males and 17 females aged 12-18 years with the stature and trunk length rated as S.D. from the mean of normal for age. All cases exhibiting severe behaviour disorders

Deviation from normal mean for age	*Stature*		*Trunk length*	
	Males	*Females*	*Males*	*Females*
−2 S.D.	0	2	1	1
−1 S.D.	2	4	2	0
Mean	4	0	4	4
+1 S.D.	5	7	7	6
+2 S.D.	5	4	2	3
+3 S.D.	0	0	0	3
Total	16	17	16	17

there are only two girls and no boys with a stature approaching −2 S.D. from the normal. Even taking into account sampling errors in such a small group, this is in marked contrast to the group as a whole (180 cases out of 530). The second observation is an apparent sex-difference, although the males have a stature predominantly above the normal mean (84% of the sample) the contribution of trunk length to stature more closely resembles the normal with only 66% of the sample above the normal, whereas it is the trunk length which is increased at the expense of the leg length in the females.

Although there are considerable dangers in drawing too many hard conclusions from such a small heterogeneous sample, this group shows at least that analysis of growth data may enable the investigator to subdivide a large mass of apparently unrelated conditions and provide the starting point for further investigation.

Intelligence and Growth Defects

Finally, a few comments on the possible relationship between intelligence and the degree of physical impairment.

There is considerable contemporary interest in the possible correlation between poor physique and retarded intellect in consequence of inadequate nutrition (Cabak and Majdanvic, 1965; Cravioto *et al.*, 1966; Pollitt and Granoff, 1967; Stock and Smythe,

1963), congenital disease (Campbell and Reynolds, 1949; Chazan *et al.*, 1951; Linde *et al.*, 1966) and particularly the association between mental retardation and congenital heart disease (Ross, 1939). All the studies subsequent to that of Tarbell (1883) support, in substance, his findings that mental defect correlates with impaired physical growth and sexual maturation. Mosier *et al.* (1965) in a study of 2472 mentally retarded children showed positive correlations between I.Q. and several anthropometric estimates, but as these authors point out, the errors introduced by variations in techniques may differ considerably between different I.Q. groups. The patients with lowest I.Q. are the least co-operative and tend to be measured least accurately. Such measurements (at least in our experience) would be too low, rather than too high, thus contributing towards a spurious correlation.

The opening remarks of this communication doubted the suitability of a heterogeneous mixture of low-grade mentally retarded subjects as an exercise in the study of growth. This is even more questioned in any discussion on the interrelationship between growth and intellect. Drash and Money (1968) have shown that where such relationship does exist, it does so in those cases which do not deviate too far from the measure of the central tendency, i.e. to be near the average for one thing is to be near the average for all things. They also point out the need to investigate homogeneous groups, clinically identified, since only by so doing will the common factors regulating both physique and intelligence be recognised.

REFERENCES

Albright, F. (1951). Introduction. In 'Textbook of Medicine'. Philadelphia: Cecil and Loeb.

Cabak, V. and Majdanvic, R. (1965). *Arch. Dis. Childh.* **40**, 532.

Campbell, M. and Reynolds, G. (1949). *Arch. Dis. Childh.* **24**, 294.

Chazan, M., Harris, T., O'Neill, D. and Campbell, M. (1951). *Guy's Hospital Reports* **100**, 331.

Cravioto, J., DeLicardie, E. R. and Birch, H. G. (1966). *Pediatrics* **38**, 319.

Douglas, S. W. B. and Blomfield, J. M. (1958). 'Children under Five'. London: Allen & Unwin.

Drash, P. W. and Money, J. (1968). In 'Human Growth, Body Composition, Cell Growth, Energy and Intelligence' (D. B. Cheek, ed.). Philadelphia: Lea and Febiger.

Dutton, G. (1958). The Physical Approach to Amentia. M.D. Thesis: London.

Dutton, G. (1959). *Arch. Dis. Childh.* **34**, 331.

Dutton, G. (1964). *Brit. J. Psychiat.* **110**, 101.

Israelsohn, Wilma, J. (1960). In 'Human Growth' (J. Tanner, ed.). London: Pergamon.

Kugel, R. B. and Mohr, S. (1963). *Amer. J. ment. Defic.* **68**, 41.

Linde, L. M., Rasof, B., Dunn, O. J. and Rabb, E. (1966). *Pediatrics* **38**, 92.

Marshall, W. A. (1968). *Develop. Med. and Child. Neurol.* **10,** 390.
Mead, C. D. (1914). *Pediat. Sem.* **21,** 394.
Miller, F. J. W., Court, S. D. M., Walton, W. S. and Knox, E. G. (1960). 'Growing up in Newcastle-upon-Tyne: a Continuing Study in Health and Illness in Young Children and their Families'. London: Oxford University Press.
Mosier, D. H., Grossman, H. J. and Dingman, H. F. (1965). *Pediatrics* **36,** No. 3, part 11, Suppl.
Pollitt, E. and Granoff, D. (1967). *Inter-Amer. J. Psychol.* **1,** 93.
Registrar-General (1952-53). 'Statistical Reviews of England and Wales'. Supplement on Mental Health.
Roberts, G. E. and Clayton, B. E. (1969). *Develop. Med. Child. Neurol.* **11,** 584.
Ross, M. (1939). *J. Pediat.* **14,** 21.
Rundl, A. T. (1970). In 'Mental Subnormality: Modern Trends in Research' (B. W. Richards, ed.). London: Pitman Medical and Scientific Publishing Co. Ltd.
Rundle, A. T. (1971). *J. Ment. defic. Res.* **15,** 51.
Rundle, A. T. and Sylvester, P. E. (1963). *J. Ment. defic. Res.* **7,** 10.
Rundle, A. T. and Sylvester, P. E. (1965). *Amer. J. Ment. defic.* **69,** 635.
Rundle, A. T. and Sylvester, P. E. (1967). Proceedings of the 1st Congress of the International Association for the Scientific Study of Mental Deficiency.
Rundle, A. T. and Sylvester, P. E. (1970). *J. Ment. defic. Res.* **14,** 196.
Scott, J. A. (1961). 'Report on the Heights and Weights of Schoolchildren in the County of London in 1959'. London County Council.
Scottish Council for Research in Education (1953). 'Social Implications of the 1947 Scottish Mental Survey'. London: London University Press.
'Statistical Manual for the use of Institutions for Mental Defectives'. New York State Hospital Press, Utica. American Association for Mental Deficiency (1946).
Stock, M. B. and Smythe, P. M. (1963). *Arch. Dis. Childh.* **38,** 546.
Tanner, J. M. (1962). 'Growth at Adolescence', 2nd ed. Oxford: Blackwell.
Tarbell, G. C. (1883). Proceedings of the Association of Medical Officers of the American Institute for Idiotic and Feebleminded Children.
Thomson, A. M. (1959). *Eugenics Review* **51,** 157.
Wilkins, L. (1966). 'The Diagnosis and Treatment of Endocrine Disorders in Childhood and Adolescence', 3rd ed. Springfield: Charles C. Thomas.

DISCUSSION

Balázs: Did you look at any other possible hormonal defects?

Rundle: Yes, but unfortunately not in so-called unclassified retardation as yet.

Balázs: One would like to know whether in those very small children there is a defect in growth hormone production. Some years ago Reiss (Reiss, M., Hillman, J. and Davis, R. H. (1963) *J. clin. endocr. Metab.* **23,** 11) did some work on mentally retarded patients of small stature who seemed to respond to chorionic gonadotrophin. There may be a subgroup in this population who may have a defect in other hormone production.

Rundle: I was associated with Reiss (Halkerston, I. D. K., Hillman, J., Palmer, D., Reiss, M. and Rundle, A. T. (1957) *J. Endocrinol.* **16**, 156) in this work and I think we found that choriogonadotrophic was selectively used on young boys with undescended testes to bring these down. There was physical improvement, but also behavioural deterioration. They certainly grew more rapidly, but this was a specialised group.

Kirman: How many of this series of Dr. Rundle's were unable to chew or had swallowing difficulties?

Morris: Supplementary to that I would like to know about the dietary intake on a long-term basis? We often find growth increments that we never expected when we take them into an ordinary paediatric ward.

Laurence: As a corollary, is there any information about subnormals who are not in institutions?

Rundle: One has to be very careful about the nutritional side. There is no doubt about their rate of growth increasing on change to another environment, but how much is due to nutritional changes, and how much to change of atmosphere, attention and so forth, is unknown. All these factors are known to have a marked effect and very quickly.

Holt: Did Dr. Kirman have anything else in mind?

Kirman: Simply that over the years we get a chronic recurrence of this problem with those that cannot feed themselves, especially those that cannot chew. As there is a shortage of nurse time for feeding them, they get fed with a kind of 'skilley' which has a limited nutritional value. Even homogenising a normal diet, because it is too stiff it tends to be diluted, and the protein and calorie value is reduced.

Rundle: I have always been careful in the use of body weight in these analyses. It is too easily measured and therefore it is inaccurate. Velocity of growth is a much more sensitive index.

Sylvester: This particular group do in fact have ordinary school dinners. Nursing time is very important, but I don't know whether this is deficient, but they certainly get vitamin supplements. Were you asking about special swallowing difficulties?

Kirman: If you cost our hospital diets we are well to the bottom of the table, as you well know, but at Queen Mary's we spend about three times as much per head as St. Laurence's does. What relation this bears to calorie intake, I'm not sure, but it must bear some relationship.

Sylvester: We are often scrutinised by various people and inadequate diets are certainly a great problem.

Rundle: If one deals with physiological mechanisms when using a longitudinal study on single cases and looking for differences in velocity curves, and so forth, one is possibly going to derive oblique information, but it would be more accurate to deal with fewer cases and ensure their adequate nutrition as well as the other factors. But to do this is practically impossible in the circumstances in which one has to work.

Holt: Would you like to answer Dr. Laurence's earlier question on the growth of mentally retarded children outside institutions, because behind this is a question as to the value of extensive studies on growth in places where there is a biased population, under a not very good nutritional state, perhaps selected from a particular social group?

Rundle: There is very little information in the literature on this, particularly on longitudinal studies of large enough series and with accurate measurements. This is always very difficult in such cases.

Crome: Does anyone know whether undernutrition and institutionalisation can depress thyroid function?

Clayton: It can certainly depress growth hormone secretion. Moreover, we have got very similar results to Dr. Rundle's in a survey with Roberts, and of course these patients came from a very different background, coming to Great Ormond Street for the investigation of mental retardation.

Laurence: This probably answers my question.

Crome: Is it possible, therefore, that the 15% depression of thyroid function can be explained by undernutrition in institutions?

Clayton: No, undernutrition as such has to be very severe before it affects pituitary function, and this has been well observed in adults during the war where all sorts of hormonal events occurred associated with malnutrition. Severe malnutrition as such in children will probably not lead to thyroid deficiency, but there is no doubt that deprivation of children can lead to a failure to secrete growth hormone, and this is well documented.

Holt: Is there any relation between growth hormone secretion and exercise, and would this have any bearing on this question?

Clayton: There is a relation between growth hormone secretion and exercise, but I am not sure of its relevance here. I was thinking of growth hormone secretion in response to specific tests. This can be grossly impaired or indeed absent in emotionally deprived children, as recorded by Blizzard's group (Powell, G. F., Brasel, S. A. and Blizzard, R. M. (1967) *New Engl. J. Med.* **276**, 1279).

Crome: Dr. Rundle said that one of the myths is lack of testicular function in mongolism, but how was this measured?

Rundle: Whether measured by size or by testosterone output, the myth can be shown to be false.

Kirman: To revert to the other matter, I was not suggesting that the reduced stature of these severely retarded patients was due to the institutional conditions. I was asking if institutional conditions could fog the results, because our own observations show that at the time of entering hospital the same can be recorded, but not so dramatically as Dr. Rundle's figures show.

Psychiatric Aspects of Unclassified Mental Retardation

B. H. KIRMAN

Role of the Psychiatrist

It is now a well established tradition that mental handicap is the concern of the psychiatrist. This was not always so and Ireland (1877) had difficulty in obtaining medical cover of any kind for the Larbert Institution. Until the introduction of the National Health Service the hospital medical officer caring for the mentally retarded tended to be a factotum and only recently has grudging concession been given his status as psychiatrist. Much of the attention of such workers has necessarily been directed to description of organic syndromes (Brushfield, 1924; Brushfield and Wyatt, 1926, 1927, 1928; Brushfield, 1928). Much of our own text (Hilliard and Kirman, 1965) is devoted to physical problems as is work by Richards (Richards, 1960, 1963, 1964; Richards *et al.*, 1965; Richards and Rundle, 1959) among many other psychiatric colleagues.

Psychiatrists are primarily concerned with aberrations of human behaviour and relationships, and with attempts to rectify these. One of the earlier attempts to influence behaviour in the severely retarded was that of Itard in 1798. His work was followed by that of Seguin (1846) on the psychological treatment of idiots. His positive views as to the role of psychological influences were supported by Pinel (1806) despite the latter's nativist philosophy, which foreshadowed the tendency at a later date to attribute the main role in mental handicap to genetic factors. This more pessimistic approach to the effect of psychological efforts to improve the mentally handicapped derives to a large extent from the work of Binet and Simon (1914), though they at times expressed a contrary view.

Among the more seriously mentally retarded, more than a half fail to be assigned to any definite clinical syndrome or aetiological group

(Tables 1 and 2). Limited research has been done on the mildly handicapped, but a higher proportion of them resist clinical classification and the importance of other factors than the degree of brain damage is better recognised. There are different psychological considerations in regard to the unclassified group of retarded children, in that their condition is recognised later, they are more often mildly

TABLE 1

Aetiological Factors in 200 Consecutive Admissions.
From Berg and Kirman (1959)

Group A: Due to known factor	19 (9.5%)
1. Environmental:	
Kernicterus due to rhesus incompatibility	6
Kernicterus of prematurity	1
Meningitis, tuberculous	4
Meningitis, influenzal	1
Pertussis immunisation	1
2. Genetic:	
Phenylketonuria	3
Cerebral lipidosis:	
Amaurotic family idiocy	1
Unclassified	1
Galactosaemia	1
Group B: Probably due to factor indicated	8 (4%)
1. Environmental:	
Maternal rubella	1
Therapeutic irradiation of mother	1
Thiouracil treatment of mother	1
Septicaemia, neonatal	1
Septicaemia, with sinus thrombosis	1
Gastro-enteritis with coma	1
Encephalitis	1
2. Genetic:	
Hypoglycaemia	1
Group C: Other factors implicated	111 (55.5%)
1. Environmental:	
Birth trauma: probable	27
Birth trauma: possible	9
2. Genetic?:	
Family history of mental retardation	18
Family history of mental disorder, epilepsy or other neurological abnormality	10
3. Unknown:	
Mongolism	46
Sturge-Weber syndrome	1
Group D: No factors suggested	62 (31%)

TABLE 2

Diagnosis of Mental Subnormality in N.E. Scotland. From Innes *et al.* (1968)

Clinical type	*Number*	*Percentage*
Down's syndrome	242	8.4
Birth injury	91	3.1
Encephalomeningitis	61	2.1
Cretinism	9	0.3
Klinefelter's syndrome	9	0.3
Tuberous sclerosis	6	0.2
Congenital syphilis	5	0.2
Phenylketonuria	5	0.2
Toxoplasmosis	2	0.07
Kernicterus	2	0.07
Gargoylism	1	0.03
Lead poisoning	1	0.03
Marfan's syndrome	1	0.03
Microcephaly	1	0.03
Autism	1	0.03
Achondroplasia	1	0.03
Craniostenosis	1	0.03
Encephalocoele	1	0.03
Meningocoele	1	0.03
Thalidomide dysgenesis	1	0.03
Retrolental dysplasia	1	0.03
Methaemoglobinaemia	1	0.03
Diabetes and talipes	1	0.03
Porphyria	1	0.03
Pierre Robin syndrome	1	0.03
Total classified	447	15.5
Total cases	2887	100

handicapped and attitudes to them are not conditioned by the effect of a recognisable syndrome.

Much of the credit for the newly awakened interest in the potential of the mentally handicapped and the possibility of improving their achievement and behaviour must go to the psychologists rather than to psychiatrists. Burt (1922) recognised the variation in incidence of retardation according to class and social milieu. O'Connor and Tizard (1956) showed that the simple expedient of placing high grade patients in open employment was successful in a high proportion of cases and provided, indeed, a better criterion of success than attempts at prediction. The Clarkes (1965) have exposed the previous under-estimation of the potential of the moderately and severely retarded patient (trainable imbecile). Psychotherapy has been open to the

TABLE 3

Classification of a series of 645 patients admitted to hospital with severe mental retardation (Angeli and Kirman, 1971).

Classification	*Patients*	*(%)*	*Sibs*	*Half-sibs*	*Affected sibs* *S.S.N.*	*E.S.N.*	*Miscarriages*	*Stillborn*
Unclassified	330	(51)	666	63	31	16	92	14
Environmental	155	(24)	280	30	2	3	30	8
Down's syndrome	104	(16)	237	37	3	2	22	4
Congenital hydrocephalus	24	(4)	45	6	0	0	4	3
Total	645	(100)	1305	137	43	22	157	29

TABLE 4

Empirical risk of affected siblings of 645 severely mentally handicapped propositi by aetiological classification (Angeli and Kirman, 1971).

Classification	*Sibs*	*S.S.N.*	*%*
1. Unclassified	666	31	$4.7^{n.s.}$
2. Environmental	280	2	0.7*
3. Down's syndrome	237	4	$1.7^{n.s.}$
4. Other genetic syndromes	77	7	9.1*
5. Congenital hydrocephalus	45	0	$0^{n.s.}$
Total	1305	44	3.4

* Significant at 5% level but not at 1%.
$^{n.s.}$ Not significant.

criticism that results have often been difficult to demonstrate objectively. In this respect, whilst not being unduly influenced by the pessimism of Binet, it is important to accept his plea for objective measurement, and this is a contribution which contemporary clinical psychologists are particularly qualified to make on the basis of a more rigorous training in the assessment of behaviour than is usually afforded to the practising psychiatrist. Work by Woodward (1962) based on Piaget's methods has enabled a more precise assessment of the very retarded or very disturbed child, whilst that of Gunzburg (1960) provides an objective record of social adjustment.

Many psychiatrists have ignored the mentally handicapped when considering psychotherapeutic provision on the assumption that co-operation in psychotherapy requires a good level of intelligence and verbal fluency. Thus, Healy and Bronner (1936) stated that 'counselling or psychotherapy do not seem applicable to mental defectives'. O'Connor is among those who have demonstrated that the contrary is true (O'Connor and Yonge, 1955). If, indeed, we look upon much of neurotic and maladaptive behaviour as being learned then there is no reason why the mentally retarded should not respond to attempts to replace this by more acceptable responses. We know that they condition and that they can learn, albeit more slowly than those of better intelligence. In fact there is some evidence to suggest that unsatisfactory behaviour is more easily modified in those of lower intelligence since in them it may result from lack of appropriate

TABLE 5

Analysis of aetiology = in 645 patients (Angeli and Kirman, 1971).

	Total Number	*Male*	*Female*	*Age on admission* 0-5	*5-10*	*Over 10*
1. Down's syndrome	104	66	38	82	16	6
2. Environmental	158	84	74	115	31	12
3. Unclassified	327	182	145	230	80	17
4. Congenital hydrocephalus	24	14	10	18	4	2
5. Genetic entity group	32	17	15	23	7	2
(a) Tuberous sclerosis	7	5	2	3	3	1
(b) Phenylketonuria	14	6	8	11	2	1
(c) Hurler's syndrome	4	4		2	2	
(d) Sturge-Weber syndrome	2		2	2		
(e) Hypercalcaemia	1		1	1		
(f) Familial muscular dystrophy	1	1		1		
(g) Familial hyperglycinaemia	1		1	1		
(h) Low's syndrome	1	1		1		
(i) 'Cri-du-Chat' syndrome	1		1	1		
Total	645	363	282	468	138	39

TABLE 6

Suggested environmental factors in 155 cases (Angeli and Kirman, 1971).

Environmental factor	*Number of cases*
Rubella, maternal	14
Prematurity (birth weight <4 lb)	20
Perinatal damage	64
Icterus neonatorum	9
Subdural haematoma	12
Postnatal infection	28
Lead	2
Cerebral thrombosis	4
Total	155

instruction, whereas in those of higher intelligence it may stem from temperamental difficulties which may be less tractable. Mary Sheridan's work with neglectful mothers is an example of this trend (Sheridan, 1956).

Parent Counselling

It would seem that the psychiatrist might well be fitted by his training in personal relationships to help families with handicapped children. Particularly in the case of severely handicapped children it appears that this form of expertise is more likely to be necessary for the parents than for the child directly. In this connection the family must be seen as a unit. Effective psychiatric support is likely to be best given when the psychiatrist is a member of a team with a psychologist and psychiatric social worker, with other possible members such as the speech therapist and with other specialists available (Kirman, 1966). There is no reason why such clinics should not be run by interested paediatricians or school medical officers (Hutchison, 1967), but it must be recognised that the function should not be limited to 'diagnosis' with the emphasis solely on the physical and biological aspect. It is essential that a psychotherapeutic role should be adopted at the outset, though this will need to be combined with practical advice. The survey by Tizard and Grad (1961) indicated that 14% of parents felt that their case had been poorly handled, and 41% found unsatisfactory features when they were told the facts about their child's backwardness. It is clear that all such difficulties will not be met by the provision of special psychiatric clinics, since the same survey revealed difficulties on the parents' part in regard to ordinary medical treatment for their child. Interested psychiatrists can help in the task of public, and more particularly professional, education in this respect.

In his preface to Eileen Brooke's (1967) presentation of the 1963 census of patients in psychiatric beds, the Chief Medical Officer suggests that increasing provision of community services for the subnormal is having an effect on the hospital population. Whilst this may be part of the matter, and whilst the shortage of hospital beds may also be relevant, there is doubtless also an element of change in public and professional opinion. Less parents reject their retarded child and this may be because of a change of attitude in the medical adviser. Certainly the services of a psychiatrist at the time when parents first appreciate their child's handicap can be most helpful in softening the blow, in helping them to face reality and in helping the parents not to feel isolated or rejected. Although this is a sensitive and difficult area it should be capable of objective exploration to find out to what extent this form of help is needed.

Parental Attitudes

Families with a seriously mentally handicapped child have to make considerable adjustments. Many manage this with considerable success. Others have a varying degree of difficulty. It is possible to think of a continuum in regard to distribution of affection and care, in the centre of which are those families which can accept the handicapped child realistically and devote to him a reasonable proportion of their material and emotional resources without unduly depriving themselves and other members of the family. At one extreme re those who completely reject the child, who may for example, 'put him away' and tell the other children and neighbours that the child has died. At the other extreme are those who over-protect. In the case of severely handicapped children this is sometimes associated both with parental failure to admit or recognise the abnormality and with relative deprivation of the other children. Sometimes such parents want to put the normal child in a residential nursery so that they can devote themselves entirely to the abnormal child. In the case of the mildly handicapped, over-protection can have a suffocating effect on the personality of the child and may be associated with gross parental underestimation of mental capacity. The attitude of professional advisers and, more particularly, of a psychiatric team can make a considerable impact on such pathological family attitudes and relationships.

It is easy to attribute parental depression to the fact of having a retarded child, but in the following case depression preceded the arrival of the first retarded child. K.A. was born when her mother was aged 22. Mother became depressed during the pregnancy and felt she should not have the baby. Talipes was noted at birth and at six weeks the mother noticed she (the baby) was not taking notice. She was taken to a number of eminent authorities although no cause for the severe retardation was found and she was placed in residential accommodation at the age of five. The parents were unable to continue to pay the fees there and she was moved to hospital. The second child was normal, but the third child born when the mother was 27 proved to be severely retarded like the first. When the third child was seen at the age of two years the mother appeared very depressed. She was pessimistic about the future of the child and wanted her in residential care; she complained that nobody understood her feelings of despair and her impatience at being confronted 'endlessly with mentally retarded children'. She underwent a hysterectomy after the birth of this child. Mother was particularly resentful because she had asked for genetic counselling after the birth of the first abnormal child and had been (reasonably) reassured. She felt that the medical profession had misled her in this respect. She tended to be continually critical of care and treatment provided for her children. Prior to placing her last child she abandoned her almost entirely to the care of a devoted nannie.

Circumstances placed a considerable burden on this mother who was already ill-prepared to tolerate it. The history illustrates the fact that even in familial and presumably genetically determined instances of severe retardation the condition may remain unclassified. At the time when genetic advice was sought there was no reason to quote a higher figure than 3% risk which is the estimate derived from our more recent survey (Angeli, in preparation; Angeli and Kirman, 1971; Kirman, 1971), and in line with Penrose's earlier findings (1938). There was no logical basis for resentment in this case but logic plays only a limited part in the response to this type of psychological trauma.

The following illustrates another depressive reaction. A.P. at 15 months was profoundly retarded. Her mother at age 23 had a premature baby weighing 2 lb which lived 8 hours. She married during that pregnancy and states she received tablets from her G.P. to 'bring on the period'. The second child lived three days and death followed operation for (?) duodenal atresia. The third child was A.P. who was noted to be abnormal immediately after birth. Even after this third child the parents say they were advised by their G.P. to have another but they were beginning to think of adoption. They were depressed and felt—'We are not like other people'. The mother felt she was being punished for ever because she took tablets during her first pregnancy and because it was sinful to become pregnant before marriage. The child was placed in hospital at the age of 10 months.

The following case illustrates over-protection: N.B. was referred at the age of 49 years, with a history of meningitis treated in hospital when she was a baby, by a 'Harley Street Specialist', who is said to have declared that she would never be fit for school and was always to have her own way. At 49 she was mildly retarded but had had no schooling and had never worked. She had been cared for by her mother until the latter's death six years earlier after which she had lived with her married sister and nearly wrecked the marriage because she 'got on the husband's nerves'. She was placed in a job in a laundry and, after four years of hostel life, arrangements are being made for her to have a flat of her own. Had she not been over-mothered she might have become independent in the normal way and had the 'Harley Street Specialist' not pronounced the fateful words (if indeed he did) she might have had the benefit of schooling. The judgements pronounced, or thought to be pronounced, by professional advisers may often have a much more profound effect than is realised by those who make them.

Imposed Behaviour Patterns

Until the operation of the Mental Health Act of 1959 almost all the mentally handicapped in hospital were formal patients. The views put forward by Russel Barton (1959) on 'the Institutional Neurosis' were perhaps as much applicable to the psychiatric unit for the mentally handicapped as that for the mentally ill. Overcrowding, understaffing, regimentation and deprivation of liberty with inadequacy of occupational outlet and incentive led to patterns of maladjustment. Attempts to escape were, perhaps, evidence of normality but were seen as proof of psychopathy and sometimes led to a vicious spiral of conflict ending in violence and removal to the special hospital (Rowan, 1958). The psychiatrist was identified with authority and lost his therapeutic role, or failed to gain it. If he is to be successful, the psychiatrist must be seen by the patient to be actively interested in rehabilitation and not as a custodian.

The relationship between mental retardation and delinquency has been critically reviewed by Woodward (1955) and by O'Connor and Tizard (1956), who showed the lack of specific correlation both in careful studies reported by others and in their own material. The proportion of those in locked wards seemed to depend more on hospital policy than on the type of patient. The findings of Castell and Mittler (1965) suggest that on the basis of a preliminary survey there are still in hospitals for the mentally retarded a considerable proportion of people within the dull normal or mildly retarded range who should be capable of rehabilitation. Presumably they account for many of that total of more than 4000 patients formally detained as subnormal or severely subnormal under the Act. Apart from those who are detained, or who are considered anti-social, there is an unknown number in hospital or elsewhere who are regarded as mentally handicapped, but whose prime problem is neurosis or psychosis. There is need for much more research to measure the size of these categories and to determine the adequacy of psychiatric and social support. On the evidence available this is clearly inadequate and the weight of the burden placed on the service makes this almost inevitable in present circumstances, the hospitals being for 'disposal' rather than for rehabilitation. Two valuable research projects could be to measure intelligence by age and length of stay of a sample of the institutional population; and to survey the manner in which the mentally handicapped, who appear before the courts, or against whom proceedings are contemplated, are dealt with. This second study might particularly review the use made of the probation service in this connection.

Child Psychosis and Autism

There is no clear distinction between these conditions and unclassified mental handicap despite much work by Creak (1961, 1964); Wing (1966) and others. The core cases in the rigorous study by Hermelin and O'Connor (1970) were selected on clinical and arbitrary grounds. The best guide to prognosis in autism is measured intelligence, perhaps because this also serves to some extent as a measure of social co-operation. On the other hand, the attempt to define autism or infantile psychosis implies the use of criteria other than intelligence. Although heterogeneous in origin, the treatment of autism demands attempts at education and behaviour shaping in which consistency of regime and persistence of effort may be the chief desiderata for all cases.

Similar therapeutic principles apply to that hard core of the mentally handicapped who exhibit unacceptable behaviour to such a degree as to cause them to be rejected by almost every agency. They may be destructive to others, to themselves, to objects, be noisy, smear faeces, be hyperactive, isolated or negativistic. To some extent these bad cases may be the result of bad conditions. Long-term physical and chemical restraint have been employed. Experience has shown that a proportion of these cases if subjected to continued effort over a period of months may be shaped into acceptable patterns of behaviour (Abbas and Donoghue, unpublished observations). Work by Gregg (unreported) at the Fountain Hospital showed that by persistent effort simple industrial tasks could be substituted for undesirable behaviour in a group of such patients; so far as could be judged, as well as easing management there was considerable work satisfaction in the group.

Classification and Epidemiology

Biological diagnosis is of limited value to the parents or psychiatrist. Knowledge of a clinical diagnosis may have a blinkering effect on attitudes. Intellectual capacity and behavioural responses are all important in practice. The Isle of Wight study (Rutter *et al.*, 1970a, b) gives a useful perspective to the need for practical help and guidance, showing the tendency for aggregation of psychological, neurological and psychiatric handicaps. The results of this study are a powerful argument in favour of an integrated multi-disciplinary service. If an argument for the co-ordination of different disciplines in research in this field is needed it can be found in the results of the Perinatal Survey (Butler and Bonham, 1963; Pringle *et al.*, 1966; Butler and Alberman, 1969).

REFERENCES

Abbas, A. and Donoghue, E. (Unpublished observations).

Angeli, E. (in preparation) M.D. Thesis.

Angeli, E. and Kirman, B. H. (1971) (in print). Proceedings of Second Congress of the International Association for the Scientific Study of Mental Deficiency. Warsaw, 1970.

Barton, R. (1959). 'The Institutional Neurosis'. Bristol: Wright.

Berg, J. M. and Kirman, B. H. (1959). *Proc. Roy. Soc. Med.* **52,** 787.

Binet, A. and Simon, T. (1914). 'Mentally Defective Children' (trans. Margaret Drummond). London: Edward Arnold.

Brooke, E. M. (1967). 'A Census of Patients in Psychiatric Beds'. London: H.M.S.O.

Brushfield, T. (1924). *Brit. J. Child. Dis.* **21,** 241.

Brushfield, T. and Wyatt, W. (1926). *Brit. J. Child. Dis.* **23,** 178, 254 and 265.

Brushfield, T. and Wyatt, W. (1927). *Ibid.* **24,** 98 and 209.

Brushfield, T. and Wyatt, W. (1928). *Ibid.* **25,** 96.

Brushfield, T. (1928). *Proc. Roy. Soc. Med.* **22,** 138.

Burt, C. (1922). 'Mental and Scholastic Tests'. London: P. S. King.

Butler, N. R. and Bonham, D. G. (1963). 'Perinatal Mortality'. Edinburgh: Livingstone.
Butler, N. R. and Alberman, E. D. (eds) (1969). 'Perinatal Problems. The Second Report of the 1958 British Perinatal Mortality Survey'. London: Livingstone.
Castell, J. H. F. and Mittler, P. J. (1965). *Brit. J. Psychiat.* **3,** 219.
Clarke, A. M. and Clarke, A. D. B. (1965). 'Mental Deficiency: The Changing Outlook', 2nd ed. London: Methuen.
Creake, M. (1961). Schizophrenia syndrome in childhood. Progess report of working party. *Cerebral Palsy Bull.* **3,** 501.
Creake, M. (1964). Schizophrenia syndrome in childhood. Further progress report of working party. *Develop. Med. Child. Neurol.* **4,** 530.
Gunzburg, H. C. (1960). 'Social Rehabilitation of the Subnormal'. London: Baillière, Tindall & Cox.
Healy, W. and Bronner, A. (1936). 'New Light on Delinquency and Its Treatment'. New Haven: Yale Univ. Press.
Hermelin, B. and O'Connor, N. (1970). 'Psychological Experiments with Autistic Children'. Oxford: Pergamon Press.
Hilliard, L. T. and Kirman, B. H. (1965). 'Mental Deficiency', 2nd ed. London: Churchill.
Hutchinson, A. (Chairman) (1967). 'Stress in Families with Handicapped Children'. London: National Society for Mentally Handicapped Children.
Innes, G., Kidd, C. and Ross, H. G. (1968). *Brit. J. Psychiat.* **114,** 35-41.
Ireland, W. W. (1877). 'On Idiocy and Imbecility'. London: Churchill.
Itard, J. M. G. (1798). 'The Wild Boy of Aveyron', translated by G. and M. Humphrey (1932). New York: The Century Co.
Kirman, B. H. (1966). *Brit. med. J.* **1,** 41.
Kirman, B. H. and Angeli, A. (1970). *Roy. Soc. Hlth. J.* **90,** 311-315.
Kirman, B. H. (1971). In 'Genetic Counselling in Relation to Mental Retardation (J. M. Berg, ed.). Oxford: Pergamon Press.
O'Connor, N. and Yonge, K. A. (1955). *J. genet. Psychol.* **87,** 89.
O'Connor, N. and Tizard, J. (1956). 'The Social Problem of Mental Deficiency'. London: Pergamon Press.
Penrose, L. S. (1938) (Colchester Survey). 'A Clinical and Genetic Study of 1,280 Cases of Mental Defect'. *Sp. Rep. Ser. Med. Res. Coun.* No. 229. London: H.M.S.O.
Pinel, P. (1806). 'Treatise on Insanity', translated by D. D. Davies. London: Cadell and Davies.
Pringle, M. L. J., Butler, N. and Davie, R. (1966). '11,000 Seven-year-olds'. London: Longman.
Richards, B. W. (1960). *Brit. med. J.* **2,** 714.
Richards, B. W. (1963). *Develop. Med. Child. Neurol.* **5,** 65.
Richards, B. W. (1964). *Ibid.* **6,** 175.
Richards, B. W., Donnell, G. N., Wilson, W. A., Stowen, D. and Perry, T. (1965). *Amer. J. Dis. Child.* **109,** 185.
Richards, B. W. and Rundle, A. T. (1959). *J. ment. Defic. Res.* **3,** 33.
Rowan, D. (1958). 'Sentenced Without Cause'. Publisher unknown.
Rutter, M., Graham, P. and Yule, W. (1970a). 'A Neuropsychiatric Study in Childhood'. London: Spastics International Medical Publications.
Rutter, M., Tizard, J. and Whitmore, K. (1970b). 'Education, Health and Behaviour'. London: Longman.
Seguin, E. (1846). 'Traîtement Morale, Hygiène et Education des Idiots'. Paris: Baillière.

Sheridan, M. (1956). *Brit. med. J.* **1**, 91.
Tizard, J. and Grad, J. C. (1961). 'The Mentally Handicapped and Their Families'. London: Oxford University Press.
Wing, J. K. (ed.) (1966). 'Early Childhood Autism'. Oxford: Pergamon Press.
Woodward, M. (1955). *Brit. J. Delinq.* **5**, 281.
Woodward, M. (1962). *J. ment. Subnormality* **8**, 1.

DISCUSSION

Holt (Chairman): Thank you, Dr. Kirman. I think we all have waited for you to clarify this classification status. I gathered when we began that you wanted us to concentrate upon the milder handicapped child, but later as I followed you, you were wanting us to consider all those children where the aetiology is not yet apparent, and you were suggesting that a large majority of these may have a multifactorial cause rather than a single one. Presumably on this basis the histological effects of the multifactorial causes may not be quite so readily apparent. This paper is now open for discussion.

Crome: I wanted to protest against your last statement that pathological changes might not be quite so apparent. I will try to prove to the contrary tomorrow!

O'Connor: Although, Mr. Chairman, you say there is no precise relationship between mild subnormality and the group we are considering, I suppose it is more likely, obviously, that pathology might be demonstrated in the classified group. I wonder if Dr. Kirman would like to comment on the frequent association that people make between mild subnormality and the term 'familial' which was used in America widely to describe the group about which we are talking and which suggested a genetic origin? Also would he like to take into account the suggestion of associated inherited level of intelligence in this general concept?

Kirman: I think we are getting away from the slightly sterile discussion of these dichotomies. They seem to be less evident now, but people are still influenced by them. If their approach was multidisciplinary they would have to take account of the findings of a difference in the neurological state of mildly handicapped children coming from different classes of parent, and parents with different levels of intelligence. This kind of observation has repeatedly been made and it emphasises the genetic and cultural aspects of the determination of intelligence, and likewise of the impact of brain damage and neurological factors in the broadest sense. So that if the family is disadvantaged and if the parents are not very intelligent, it's perhaps according to pattern that we would expect a proportion of the children also to be not very able. But when one gets the opposite pattern of advantaged and intelligent parents with mildly retarded children one expects pathology. Clearly these are not discrete processes, there is an interplay, and I think the British perinatal follow-up study and the American counterpart bring this out very well. They show the nice interplay of these factors, which do not separate discrete groups, but show there is a matrix of factors.

Jellinger: Dr. Kirman, I don't fully agree with your scepticism and negativism. Perhaps the pathologist can keep a certain control over some of the factors, which I can demonstrate tomorrow, on the history of perinatal distress. In a certain number of cases you know there is perinatal damage. Taken as controls, it is found that in 38% of mongols there are histories of more or less severe perinatal distress, and almost the same percentage in developmental disorders. The pathologist can perhaps clarify certain, although a limited number, of these cases.

Laurence: It's surprising how infrequently one finds anoxic lesions in babies who have suffered very well documented anoxic episodes. I suspect that the neonate is well able to withstand more anoxia than the older child.

Jellinger: Perhaps we can modulate the clinician's view, particularly on perinatal distress. We do not fully agree that this might have the importance it was formerly given.

Laurence: I think perhaps perinatal distress is not only concerned with anoxia. Anoxia *per se* is surprisingly hard to substantiate in sections.

Crome: To complement this observation, one might again quote Dr. Saugstad's work in Oslo (Saugstad and Woolf, L. I. (1971) in 'Phenylketonuria' (H. Bickel and F. P. Hudson, eds., Stuttgart: Thieme) who found in the history of cases of phenylketonuria that there was a significantly raised incidence of perinatal difficulty.

Richter: One of the bases of classification is response to treatment, and where social and cultural factors are clearly important one can expect some kind of response, but I would particularly like to ask about the group described as autistic.

Holt: Are you asking about children described as *autistic* as an adjective, or about children with autism?

Richter: With autism.

Kirman: Perhaps Dr. O'Connor can answer this better, but from my own experience and the reported studies, the results have been uniformly bad when published objectively, although a minority have done well. Any objective study over a long term shows very poor results. However, there is a basis for saying that this group is qualitatively distinct, on the behavioural side, and there is some evidence that their physical side may be different too; for instance, their stature may be less affected.

O'Connor: What Dr. Kirman says is essentially correct. The follow-up studies of Rutter (Rutter, M. (1966) Behavioural and cognitive characteristics 'Early Childhood Autism' (J. Wing, ed.). Oxford: Pergamon Press) suggest that only about 15% ever enter a normal school. As to stature, there is one study only, on bone growth, that gives unfortunately rather similar results to those of Rundle on subnormal children. There are many other ways, e.g. psychologically, in which they are similar. It took us a very long time to prise out one or two tiny differences from comparative studies. For example, their long digit-span, or remembering a lot of numbers, is about normal. Also their EEG's in our study showed certain peculiarities different from those of mongols. The only treatment that is claimed to rate success, apart from the analytic treatment, is that of Lovaas (Lovaas, O. I. (1966) A programme for the establishment of speech in psychotic children 'Early Childhood Autism' (J. Wing, ed.). Oxford: Pergamon Press) in California, who reckons to change their capacity to talk over a short time, but there is some doubt as to whether he is using the classification in the same way as in England. They can certainly benefit from the sort of education given to other handicapped children, e.g. in social behaviour, ability to read in a limited way, etc.

Holt: This is a condition which is extremely hard both to define and to diagnose, and one would want to have the criteria very carefully analysed. I have seen two children with autism being specially trained who in fact were undiagnosed phenylketonurics, but who showed autistic features. There is a lot of misdiagnosis among so-called autistic children.

Laurence: In this family study of unclassified mental retardation, one with a mentally retarded child is really a handicapped family. We have studied the siblings of cases of spina bifida, with matched control families, and we find that the siblings perform below the expectation of function. Some of the E.S.N. incidence in your families is, perhaps, related to this deprivation factor, or, perhaps, the emotional effect of having this defective child in the family.

Kirman: The question we were asking ourselves was what is the risk that another equally retarded child would be born to this mother, and Table 4 of my paper sums up the answer to this. This refers to children with I.Q.'s under 50, and we were not primarily concerned with the mildly retarded.

Laurence: I appreciate that, but I was trying to point out that the rest of the family may suffer considerably.

Kirman: While accepting this to be generally true, I would like to qualify that. There is a spectrum here and the impact on the children is determined largely by the way in which the parents adapt to this situation. At one end is the rejecting parent, and at the other is the over-protecting parent who neglects the normal children; these then suffer psychologically. Most, in fact, fall in the middle of these two categories who manage surprisingly well, although there may be a class difference in the pattern of response.

Since meningomyelocoele has a class distribution, could not this in part be responsible for these findings?

Laurence: No, the control families are matched for those class factors, and family size.

Kirman: If there is some factor operating at the biological level in those families to cause the meningomyelocoele, is it not conceivable that it might disadvantage the nervous system of the other siblings?

Laurence: No. I don't think so. If one looks at the individual problems in the families, it is not difficult to see why these children do not do well.

Stern: At Sutton, it is clear that there is also the cumulative effect of deteriorating physical health together with the physical strain of repeated visits to hospital.

Laurence: Another point is the implication from your Table 3 on family study and genetic counselling. How much genetic counselling is there in fact arising spontaneously from the parents themselves? How aware are they that this family problem is a genetic problem? In spina bifida from our cohort study, the situation is rather lamentable. Very few sought genetic advice, and when given it was universally very misleading and usually grossly over-optimistic. What is the situation with severe mental handicap?

Kirman: Just the same. Most have not spontaneously sought advice. Where they have, what is given is often incorrect, and in the minority it has been over-pessimistic. With the majority of parents they are concerned with the burden of the handicapped child, and this in itself prevents them from having further children. When the question is broached they are usually very interested, but did not like to mention it.

Laurence: This is exactly our finding. Their worries are always there, but are not voiced. The time when they come for genetic advice is when the child dies, and they think about other children.

Holt: I can add some quantitative information from our study in Sheffield with a population of half-a-million. Only 7% of families with a handicapped child had had adequate advice. Although done 16 or so years ago, I doubt whether the situation is any different now.

The other point is that such families coming to the Wolfson Centre have usually seen a number of doctors before they arrive, and over 50% have not had an adequate discussion of the genetic problem.

Laurence: Comparable figures for our spina bifida group is that a quarter have asked their G.P., and all but one got the wrong advice, a quarter did not dare to ask, and the rest put if off.

Balázs: May I ask a rather naïve question? From what Dr. Kirman has said a high proportion of these cases have a multifactorial origin, so statistically, social conditions will play a role in a high proportion. Is it better that the State should take care of these children, or what alternative is there?

O'Connor: Can I complicate that question? It is common experience to go to a school for the subnormal to find two groups of the same I.Q., one where the parents are foreign with language problems, the other group of more genuine E.S.N. children. The only way I can distinguish those groups is in their reaction times, which always differ, the former always being normal. This shows the sort of problem you might be hinting at.

Laurence: In your paper you hinted at rejection. The amount of rejection is very variable from one part of the country to another, and is very dependent upon the morals of the community with which we are dealing. In South Wales rejection is uncommon for a number of reasons. One is that there is a close family grouping, another is that the community is very close-knit, and thirdly there is nowhere to reject to. I suspect that all three factors are different in the London area.

Kirman: Number three is not different, I think, because it is possible to admit only about 10% of patients coming to hospital. We manage by providing day- care and out-patient advice and by bringing pressure to bear on the local authorities and others to provide some kind of community support. I think, therefore, that this problem does equally exist in London. The groups we deal with differ very much, but we find in general that Asian parents tend not to reject, this isn't part of their approach to this problem, and neither on the whole do our Irish families. There is also a class difference, in that the middle class look at this more objectively and may decide that this is not a burden they would wish to carry. But they are influenced by professional guidance. Advice is changing and people are being encouraged to continue to look after their children, and this advice seems to carry much weight.

Laurence: This trend towards the family looking after the handicapped in my opinion is very good, provided there is sufficient community support, and that is usually not forthcoming.

General Discussion

K. S. HOLT

I think we can now turn to a more general discussion of the afternoon's topic, which is the aetiology and epidemiology of unclassified mental retardation. I wonder if it is by accident or not that this is the midpoint of the symposium. Yesterday we heard about the experimental work and tomorrow we will hear more about the investigations of the case material. This afternoon we have been exposing some of the really basic problems, because fundamentally we are all concerned with trying to prevent mental handicap in humans and to improve the health of all individuals; and to achieve optimal survival for all people. So this in a way is the nub or focus of the whole symposium.

We have had a clarification of what we mean by the term unclassified mental retardation. It seems to me that it is not so much the mental retardation which is unclassified, but rather the aetiology which is unknown. We have not yet really touched upon the description of the different patterns of behaviour of the children with different manifestations of mental retardation. Yesterday, Dr. Richter was suggesting that we ought to pay attention to this, and should be describing some of the clinical features and behavioural aspects in more detail, hoping to find correlations with the pathological findings.

But are we expecting too much to be able to determine the aetiology in all these cases? Dr. Kirman suggested that it might be difficult to determine the aetiology in many cases because of complex multifactorial influences. This should not be beyond our capacities, but what may be even more difficult is to determine the importance of the timing of various insults. There may at one time be episodes which predispose towards damage by other influences later on. Examination of the child's brain shows only the end picture. This timing of insults in relation to subsequent damage and of mental retardation is something we have not touched upon anywherc near enough yet.

It is quite clear that we need to learn much more and it is also quite clear that there is a limit to what we can learn from studies which are biased in one way or another. We need to have studies on carefully selected groups of individuals, more longitudinal studies, and careful documentation. There is a lot of clinical information available which could and should be tapped, if only it was documented adequately and reliably. The possibility of this was hinted at yesterday by Dr. Harris who asked whether we could not use the 'At Risk' registers for learning more about mentally retarded children, and the factors that may be operating. You probably know, however, that the 'At Risk' registers have been a failure and that they are about to be abandoned officially. Although the 'At Risk' concept is excellent and has been helpful and stimulated a lot of interest in the examination of young children, the keeping of the registers has been carried out without sufficient definition of the various parameters so that in practice the registers have become unsatisfactory. The concept is so valuable, however, that we cannot just cast it aside along with the registers, but we have to replace it by more accurate methods of recording.

It is desperately important that if we are going to monitor the health of children, we must have satisfactory recording methods, and must accept the responsiblity for saying how this can best be done.

Now, I hope that for the rest of our time this afternoon there will be suggestions about how in the future we can carry out long-term longitudinal studies to explore further the aetiology and epidemiology of unclassified mental retardation.

Earlier we heard about some experimental studies involving massive pharmacological insults to experimental animals, but this is not necessarily related to the physiological variations and influences which may affect our children. There is a real need for us to define the clinical problems and to hope that the experimental scientists will be able to help us and say how we should go forward in the future.

We have talked about the multifactorial approach which suggests that many small insults might produce the final picture, and this leads beyond the realms of pathology and biochemistry, and makes us begin to wonder about the results of deprivation, cultural influences, and so forth. Now, these are factors which apply in all cases of mental retardation, and even if there is a very definite single insult, its clinical effects and expression are likely to be determined by many factors. So this exploration of multifactorial influences applies to all forms of mental handicap and not just to those in whom there is no single cause.

Parents of mentally retarded children want to know why did this happen to their child, but quite often we have to say that we just do not know. One approach which I find useful is to say: 'if only you think about the immense complexity of the human brain, and realise its development from minute origins to reach the complex function we see in ordinary individuals, you will perhaps begin to wonder not why it has gone wrong, but why it does not go wrong more often'. And having heard all the discussions today, I am still wondering why things do not go wrong more often than they do. I think we should look at the wonderful mechanisms of homeostasis which enable some children to survive insults which would be damaging to others, as well as looking at children who are retarded.

Drillien: I think that the timing of the insult is particularly important in the low birth weight babies. Was the thing that went wrong in early or late pregnancy? One thing we are doing in our present series is to look at the deciduous teeth. These structures are present at about 35 days of gestation and are presumably subject to adverse influences affecting general growth. My dental colleagues are hopeful that they will be able to date adverse incidents, although they will not be able to say what they were. So we are going to compare the ground sections of deciduous teeth of low birth weight children who are normal with the teeth of those that have defects. At the moment they can only look at enamel, but there are differences in enamel hypoplasia that are related to status.

Laurence: You say that we must know more about epidemiology of this problem, but as far as I know there are very few community studies on the total problem of mental retardation. There should be far more in different communities, to show us various ways in handling the child and the neonate which might point the way to possible differences in aetiology.

Harris: There is in fact a survey going on at the moment of all severely subnormal children in Camberwell. If this meeting had taken place before it started, we might have asked a few more correct questions. I am only dealing with the EEG side, but it seems to me that why more of this work is not being done is because two important things are needed. One is time and the other is money. They are really very essential, and perhaps we ought to press for more of this sort of work.

Kirman: I am sure that is true. The Kushlick and Tizard (Kushlick, A. (1969) *Lancet* ii, 1196; (1970) *Roy. Soc. Hlth J.* **90**, 255, Tizard, J. (1964) 'Community Services for the Mentally Handicapped', O.U.P. London) surveys are epidemiological and are concerned with numbers and degrees of handicap and with social problems, but they are not particularly concerned with aetiology, and Innes (Innes, G., Kidd, C. and Ross, H. S. (1968) *Brit. J. Psychiat.* **114**, 35) study was only able to make a limited approach to this. I am not sure how far the Camberwell Survey is going in this direction, but time and money are the limitations.

Laurence: I was thinking of detailed complete studies in various ethnic groups, and this may help to highlight some of the genetic factors. For example, I do not know of a study on an Indian community in this country.

Kirman: I must confess that I am sympathetic to the point of Dr. Bamford (Bamford, F. N. (1971) *Brit. Med. J.* **i**, 276) in Bradford that the problems of an Asiatic community are not essentially dissimilar from native-born children at a similar disadvantage.

Zlotnik: It has occurred to me that when we are worrying about mental retardation without any evident underlying pathological process, whether this is not just part of the normal scale of human variation. Perhaps you should also study mental excellence. Maybe there is exactly the same number born with unclassified mental excellence, and no matter what you do you will not find the cause of it.

Kirman: This point of view has been put forward, but there are many other aspects of this phenomenon. I think that to look at this distribution in pathological terms, if the brain is functioning very well, it is unlikely that any obvious pathology will be seen. But it is the extra bump on the bottom end of the curve we are studying and then qualitative changes begin to appear with gross pathology, such as tuberous sclerosis, homocysteinuria, etc.

Zlotnik: But if there is no pathological background may be you will find in the upper scale of the cases of mental excellence the percentage is exactly the same.

Kirman: Everybody says it is not the same.

Zlotnik: But there may be physiological subnormal brains where the intellect is not developed and the I.Q. not so high. Perhaps this is the minus variation of the normal.

Kirman: But this is only one aspect of the phenomenon, and anyhow there must be an explanation, accepting the principle of causality, as to why an individual had such a position. It may be genetic, physiological, background, etc. But there is not a pure reason why he should be where he is.

Holt: I think we should point out that tests of ability are all comparative, and there is no absolute measure of this. If we had absolute tests, I might agree with this point of view. Moreover, the criteria for growth and other parameters have changed over the last 50 years and the mean is now much higher than before.

Woollam: As an embryologist, I would like to ask, Dr. Kirman, whether the patterns of mental retardation are determined at birth or not.

Kirman: Below an I.Q. of 50% a high proportion of them already have something wrong with the brain at birth, but this is only a guess.

Woollam: Is there any place, in fact, for embryology in the study of these things?

Kirman: I am sure there is a big place, both in the neonatal period and early infancy as well as earlier.

Harris: Is it not true that children with severe subnormality even though not classified have a greater incidence of other problems, such as squints, or minor movement disorders, etc. This suggests that it is not just the other end of the scale.

Kirman: Yes, the great majority, as Dr. Jellinger showed, do have structural abnormality of the brain, indicating that they have a high proportion of somatic defects.

Zlotnik: I was interested in those with no pathological changes.

Kirman: In 1932 we did not know about phenylketonuria, and now this has come out of the simple unclassified group.

Zlotnik: Do you consider those cases which were born normal, but who deteriorated over 2-3 years?

Kirman: Unless one can demonstrate a disease process, one must call them unclassified.

Clayton: Of course it is very hard to know whether an infant at birth is normal or not.

Kirman: Yes, but so long as no cause for deterioration is found a case remains in the unclassified group.

Zlotnik: How do we know that certain viral infections have not been overlooked completely? It is difficult to look for serum antibodies, since one does not know where to look.

Holt: We know that in about 45% of babies affected as a result of maternal rubella that there is no definite history of illness during pregnancy. It is subclinical. But the clinical problem which is baffling us at the moment is that of the 'odd man out'. In families with high intelligence, e.g. I.Q. levels of 120 and above, with several children in the family equally well endowed, there may be one who is the 'odd man out'. He may have an I.Q. of 95-100. This, of course, is average, but this child is so discrepant by comparison with his parents and siblings that he suffers tremendously, and he is relatively retarded and also emotionally disturbed. Now, it could be that this is chance variation. The parents often say his birth was a little difficult, he had measles at six months and so on, which might have contributed. We have to find out whether he is suffering from something which could have been prevented. But how do we explore this?

Zlotnik: You get the same problem where one child is brilliant in a family.

Kirman: I would like to know what is the normal variation due to, is it a biochemical change or what is it?

Rundle: One of the most exciting developments recently is work on biochemical variation and individualism in relation to enzyme polymorphism. Something like 30% of all enzymes are polymorphic and this gives us about 10^9 possibilities of individual variation. When thinking in these terms, one will begin to consider that it might be possible to measure what is causing individual variation, and certainly this should be looked at in mental retardation. We mean to know why these cases are at the lower end of the normal range and what the mechanism is.

Holt: We seem to be really just at the beginning of our enquiries and we must clearly continue the discussion through the months and years ahead.

5

Psychological, Electrophysiological and Biochemical Aspects of Unclassified Mental Retardation

Clinical Biochemistry and Unclassified Mental Retardation

BARBARA E. CLAYTON

The care of all mentally retarded patients should include general biochemical investigations and in some a definitive diagnosis will be reached, such as a specific amino acid disorder, hypoparathyroidism or leucine-sensitive hypoglycaemia, etc. However, it is only our ignorance which causes us to label a patient 'unclassified' and the unclassified patients of today are likely to become the specific syndromes and biochemical disorders of tomorrow.

Our routine survey of these children includes chromatography of urinary amino acids and it is not unusual to find that a mild generalised aminoaciduria is present or alternatively one amino acid may be raised, especially alanine or glycine; on repeating the investigation the finding is frequently not confirmed and it is apparent that in these children there may be fleeting abnormalities of which the significance is unknown. A similar situation occurs with plasma amino acids. Of particular interest is the occasional presence of increased levels of branch chain amino acids in plasma and this finding too may be transitory. For example, amongst the 449 children with unclassified mental retardation described by Roberts (1966), there were 11 with raised levels of leucine, valine and isoleucine, but these were not investigated further. From studies on a further 17 children with unclassified mental retardation it is apparent that considerable daily variation occurs in these levels, even though the blood is collected under standardised conditions. In Roberts' (1966) series there were a further three children with raised levels of the branch chain amino acids, who were studied in some detail. Two retarded sibs, a girl aged five years and a boy aged three years, consistently had slightly raised serum concentrations of leucine and isoleucine and the boy had a raised concentration of valine too (Heeley *et al.*, 1966). This was shown to be linked with an abnormal handling of a tryptophan load. This type of study in depth is so time-consuming that only an occasional patient can be examined in this way.

During the investigation of these children a generalised increased excretion of glucose, galactose, fructose, sucrose and lactose may be found in the urine (e.g. Roberts found 10 in 150 retarded patients). This generalised pattern is very characteristic of unclassified mental retardation and occurs with normal diet as well as when a specific loading test with disaccharides is performed. In intestinal biopsies performed on nine such children, reduced disaccharidase activity was found in five of them (see Table 1). The significance of the relationship between mental retardation and excessive excretion of several sugars in the urine is not at all clear, nor is it known whether the sugars are present from early life or only arise later as a secondary effect. There is however experimental evidence to suggest that unhydrolysed lactose and sucrose may not be harmless when circulating in the body. As part of a more extensive study on the actions of circulating lactose, the effects of this carbohydrate on the concentrations of pyruvate, glucose-6-phosphate and metabolites of the citric acid cycle were measured in the brains of rats that had received regular injections of intraperitoneal lactose from the 5th to the 20th days of life (McLean and Clayton, 1970). The mean concentration of isocitrate was significantly raised whereas those of the other metabolites showed no significant change compared with controls. Preliminary studies *in vitro* with a commercial preparation of isocitrate dehydrogenase showed 16 and 23% inhibition by 1 mM- and 6 mM-lactose respectively. Glucose, galactose and maltose did not have this effect but sucrose gave 10% inhibition. It is known that sucrose has a damaging effect on lysosomes (Wattiaux *et al.*, 1964) and more recently Bender and Thadani (1970) have been studying the effect of feeding large amounts of sucrose to rats. Presumably at the high concentrations being fed unchanged sucrose would be entering the circulation. They found that sucrose depressed the rate of oxidation of glucose and of lipogenesis from glucose in both liver and adipose tissue. They suggested that sucrose might stimulate the formation of glucose-6-phosphatase and glucose-6-phosphate dehydrogenase.

Routine investigation of retarded children should include the determination of three fasting blood sugars. At birth the blood sugar is usually within the adult range but it then falls rapidly and may not regain adult levels for several days or more depending upon the feeding regime. Individual babies often have levels of 15-30 mg/100 ml or even below 10, and these values may be unassociated with clinical findings though at levels <20 these are more likely. Shelley and Neligan (1966)

TABLE 1

Jejunal Biopsies in Mentally Retarded Children

	Disaccharidase activity (units/g wet wt.)*				
Age (year)	*Lactase*	*Sucrase*	*Palatinase*	*Maltase*	*Histology*
1.4	–	0.6	–	–	Villous pattern normal; abnormal distended mucus cells
1.5	9.4	8.8	3.0	19.9	–
1.6	0.2	0.8	–	–	–
2:25	0.8	0.9	–	–	–
2.25	1.1	2.5	–	–	–
2.6	7.7	3.5	–	–	Minimal changes consistent with malabsorption
2.6	0.6	1.9	0.4	6.7	Severe partial to sub-total villous atrophy
3.0	8.8	9.2	2.9	22.1	–
3.75	8.1	5.5	2.4	24.5	Normal
Normal range	> 2.5	> 3.0	> 1.0	> 10.0	

– Indicates insufficient material for study.
* Assayed by the method of Arthur (1966).

have suggested that asymptomatic hypoglycaemia is unlikely to cause cerebral change in babies, but nevertheless careful observation of infants from this point of view is essential. When assessing a retarded child, there may be little information about the possibility of hypoglycaemia in early life. In an attempt to see whether unclassified (and ultimately undiagnosed) patients exhibit mild biochemical abnormalities as a group, a number of studies have been made (Grant, Shepherd and Clayton, unpublished observations). Fasting blood glucose was determined in 62 such children. The results fell within the same range and showed the same distribution as the values for 86 'normal' children (i.e. surgical patients without mental retardation). In all but one of them, fasting serum insulin was estimated. Again the results fell within the range for the 86 surgical patients and showed the normal significant correlation with age (Grant, 1967). Serum insulin was measured also in 21 unclassified retarded children during leucine tolerance tests (Grant, 1968). There was no evidence that as a group these children showed any abnormal response with respect to blood sugar or insulin levels.

Abnormalities of tryptophan metabolism are common in children with brain disorders. A detailed study of this was made by Heeley, Piesowicz and McCubbing (1968) in 59 children with mental retardation unrelated to any recognisable inborn error of metabolism. Fifteen of them metabolised tryptophan abnormally but were otherwise indistinguishable from the other children. Pyridoxine supplements altered the metabolism where it had previously been abnormal but it had no effect clinically. The metabolism of tryptophan, via the degradation of the indole ring, is dependent on enzymes which require the co-factor pyridoxal phosphate for activity. Perhaps unexpectedly, in this survey the excretion of metabolites differed from the pattern expected for a deficiency of pyridoxine for the kynureninase reaction. It seemed that the abnormal metabolism might be the result of an imbalance of the mechanisms that regulate tryptophan pyrrolase activity in response to a tryptophan load (Feigelson *et al.*, 1962). Heeley *et al.* (1968) suggested that a biochemical defect at this level might explain why the administration of large amounts of pyridoxine failed to alleviate the convulsive state which some of these children had. It was certainly a striking finding that so many of the children studied had an abnormality.

With the reduction in breast-feeding and the increasingly better care of infants with small birth weights, the possibility of diet leading to brain damage has to be considered. For example, in infant rats Chase and O'Brien (1970) have shown that a number of parameters of brain metabolism including the formation of brain sulphatide are markedly inhibited by excessive amounts of phenylalanine, methionine, tyrosine, arginine and to a lesser extent by leucine and valine. The more general use of screening tests on infants is leading to the recognition of such conditions as neonatal tyrosinaemia, transient tyrosinaemia and transient methioninaemia for example, but their significance in clinical terms is largely unknown. From a careful study of newborn babies receiving various protein intakes, Avery *et al.* (1967) concluded that high serum tyrosine levels are generally harmless and that no consistent clinical syndrome is associated with the finding. Similarly no more developmental or neurological defects were found in infants of low birth weight with tyrosinaemia compared with those with normal tyrosine levels, during a follow-up of 56 months (Menkes and Avery, 1963; Menkes *et al.*, 1966; Partington *et al.*, 1968). There are reports however describing individual patients with various signs and symptoms in association with a high tyrosine level (e.g. Wong *et al.*, 1967). In my view the relationship between diet in early life, biochemical findings and mental development requires further study. Such information cannot come from retrospective studies on retarded children since information about plasma amino acids in early life is, as yet, not generally available.

Perhaps we pay insufficient attention to the mother during our investigation of mental retardation. Experimental work on the effect of maternal diet on the central nervous system of offspring has of necessity to be done in animals, though some natural biochemical 'experiments', such as maternal phenylketonuria, also throw light on this problem. Already a number of nutritional variables during pregnancy are known to alter the rate of cell division in the brain of the developing foetus. One of these is galactose which can be fed to the pregnant rat in large amounts (Haworth *et al.*, 1969). Protein restriction results in similar changes (Zamenhof *et al.*, 1968) and malnutrition affects myelin deposition in developing brain (Dobbing and Widdowson, 1965). Newberne *et al.* (1970) fed groups of rats on diets with varying methionine and choline content with and without B_{12}. If choline and methionine intakes were low and B_{12} was given no abnormality was seen; if B_{12} was deficient and yet choline and methionine intakes were normal, congenital anomalies, alterations in nucleic acids and protein of brain and liver were seen. It is well recognised that the children of women with untreated phenylketonuria are likely to have a variety of severe abnormalities including mental retardation (Yu and O'Halloran, 1970). The high circulating phenylalanine in the mother, or one or more of its metabolites damages the developing foetal brain. By feeding phenylalanine to pregnant rhesus monkeys hyperphenylalaninaemia and tyrosinaemia were produced though, of course, the condition was not phenylketonuria. When this was done throughout pregnancy the offspring had a reduced birth weight though no other abnormalities were seen but, in general, learning ability was most reduced in infant monkeys who were exposed to maternal hyperphenylalaninaemia throughout the entire pregnancy and who had the lowest birth weight (Kerr *et al.*, 1968).

Our detection of heterozygotes for a variety of disorders is rudimentary and we have little knowledge about metabolism in women heterozygous for a particular disorder when they are pregnant. Since amino acids for example are normally found in greater concentration in the foetal blood than in the maternal circulation (Widdas, 1961), not only may the high levels in the mother lead to damage, but the normal placental transfer may make the situation worse.

Mentally subnormal children are often small. In the series reported by Dutton (1958, 1959) he described a group who were significantly retarded with respect to height, weight, skeletal development, onset of puberty and development of genitalia. He also demonstrated increased faecal fat and reduced absorption of nitrogen. A particular study of growth was made by Roberts and Clayton (1969) in their survey (Roberts, 1966). They found a great excess of children who were on or below the third percentile for height and weight and the overall frequency distributions were consistently bimodal. Detailed studies were made in 15 of those below the third percentile. From a study of their infant welfare records it was seen that in some growth was retarded from birth and in others it did not fall off until after several months of age. The more severe the mental retardation the greater was the retardation of growth, the number of children below the third percentile with severe subnormality being no less than 11 times the expected figure. They also found that 8 out of 13 whose skeletal ages were measured had scores below the 10th percentile. Amongst the very short children were the three described by Creak *et al.* (1964) as 'Three mentally retarded children of similar appearance'. These children who were 25-33 months of age had a series of tests to assess endocrine function (unfortunately before radioimmunoassays were available) and they all showed a deficient response to adrenocorticotrophic hormone (ACH) probably secondary to a lesion of the anterior pituitary gland. One of them, R.W., was retested at the age of nine years and then had a normal response to ACH, and another eight-year-old seen by Dr. Creak elsewhere also had a normal response. Systematic endocrine studies were performed on three of the other short children and one of them had an impaired ACTH response.

Though it is clear that acute plumbism leads to recurrent seizures, cerebral palsy and mental retardation, it is not clear whether less severe exposure with only slightly elevated blood-lead levels can cause damage. In 1964, Moncrieff *et al.* published a paper on blood lead levels in 122 children aged 6 months to 14 years who had mental retardation or severe behaviour disorders, and found that 45% of them had lead levels greater than in 'control' children. The authors stated that 'due consideration should be given to the fact that a child may have mild lead poisoning on top of mental retardation due to other causes. Preconceived ideas about the level of blood lead at which toxicity occurs should be abandoned'. Since then a number of workers have repeated such a study, and the reported overall incidence of raised blood lead levels has varied greatly. The probable reasons for such variations include the amount of lead in the environment of any particular patient, the degree of mental handicap and behaviour disturbance, and the level of blood lead considered to be abnormal. In a further attempt to elucidate this problem Bicknell *et al.* (1968) examined 330 children in a hospital for the severely subnormal and used an oral load of calcium disodium ethylenediamine-tetraacetic acid (CaEDTA) to give additional information. The children were divided into three groups (a) with pica (b) severely physically handicapped without pica (c) mobile children without pica. It was found that there was excessive ingestion of lead by 70% of the pica group.

The work by Moncrieff *et al.* (1965) sparked off a lot of argument and the controversy as to the importance of excessive ingestion of lead has still not been finally settled nor is the extent of the danger of a persistently raised blood lead level in a retarded child known as yet. A most important contribution to this problem has been made recently by Millar *et al.* (1970). Lead inhibits enzymes which require sulphydryl groups, and these workers investigated the relationship between blood lead and δ-aminolaevulinic acid dehydratase (A.L.A.-dehydratase) in normal and retarded children, and also the effect of lead on A.L.A.-dehydratase in the brain of suckling rats. None of the children had blood leads above 50 μg/100 ml but significant decreases in enzyme activity occurred at lead levels considered to be in the upper range of normal, i.e. 20-40 μg/100 ml. In addition, lead produced a reduction in the enzyme in both the blood and brain of the suckling rats. Millar *et al.* (1970) suggested that even these modest rises in blood lead might be associated with biochemical abnormalities in the child's brain. Evidence to date therefore suggests that the raised blood lead levels are the result of pica by patients in a lead-contaminated environment and that modest ingestion can cause biochemical changes, though the relationship of this to actual clinical findings is still inconclusive. This problem is an important one. In the U.S.A. for example lead ingestion is a significant public health problem where it is most prevalent in those aged 1-3 years. As many as one-quarter of this age group may have evidence of excessive ingestion in areas where there is old housing and up to 5% may show clinical features of frank intoxication (Chisholm, 1970). In Baltimore 50-70% of old housing in certain slum areas contained dangerous quantities of lead in places accessible to young children (Schucker *et al.*, 1965).

The study of these patients is frequently unrewarding and frustrating, yet general biochemical studies are essential in order to identify patients with known disorders. In addition mild, possibly transitory, biochemical disorders may be detected. Staff and facilities are available to study only a few of these in depth. Another frustration is that the biochemical episode leading to brain damage may have occurred some time in the past.

ACKNOWLEDGEMENTS

I gratefully acknowledge the help of my colleagues, particularly those in the Department of Chemical Pathology, who made many of these studies possible. The Nuffield Foundation provided much of the finance for this work.

REFERENCES

Arthur, A. (1966). *Arch. Dis. Childh.* **41**, 519.
Avery, M. E., Clow, C. L., Menkes, J. H., Ramos, A., Scriver, C. R., Stern, L. and Wasserman, B. P. (1967). *Pediatrics* **39**, 378.
Bender, A. E. and Thadani, P. V. (1970). *Nutr. Metabol.* **12**, 22.
Bicknell, J., Clayton, B. E. and Delves, H. T. (1968). *J. ment. Defic. Res.* **12**, 282.
Chase, H. P. and O'Brien, D. (1970). *Pediat. Res.* **4**, 96.
Creak, E. M., Roberts, G. E. and Clayton, B. E. (1964). *Arch. Dis. Childh.* **39**, 384.
Dobbing, J. and Widdowson, E. M. (1965). *Brain* **88**, 357.
Feigelson, P., Feigelson, M. and Greengard, O. (1962). *Recent Progr. Horm. Res.* **18**, 491.
Grant, D. B. (1967). *Arch. Dis. Childh.* **42**, 375.
Grant, D. B. (1968). *Arch. Dis. Childh.* **43**, 69.
Haworth, J. C., Ford, J. D. and Younoszai, M. K. (1969). *Pediat. Res.* **3**, 441.
Heeley, A. F., McCubbing, D. G. and Shepherd, J. (1966). *Arch. Dis. Childh.* **41**, 652.
Heeley, A. F., Piesowicz, A. T. and McCubbing, D. G. (1968). *Clin. Sci.* **35**, 381.
Kerr, G. R., Chamove, A. S., Harlow, H. F. and Waisman, H. A. (1968). *Pediatrics* **42**, 27.
McLean, A. and Clayton, B. E. (1970). *Biochem. J.* **118**, 41P.
Menkes, J. H. and Avery, M. E. (1963). *Bull. Johns Hopk. Hosp.* **113**, 301.
Menkes, J. H., Chernick, V. and Ringel, B. J. (1966). *J. Pediat.* **69**, 583.
Millar, J. A., Battistini, V., Cumming, R. L. C., Carswell, F. and Goldberg, A. (1970). *Lancet* **2**, 695.

Moncrieff, A. A., Koumides, O. P., Clayton, B. E., Patrick, A. D., Renwick, A. G. C. and Roberts, G. E. (1964). *Arch. Dis. Childh.* **39**, 1.
Newberne, P. M., Ahlstrom, A. and Rogers, A. E. (1970). *J. Nutr.* **100**, 1089.
Partington, M. W., Delahaye, D. J., Masotti, R. E., Read, J. H. and Roberts, B. (1968). *Arch. Dis. Childh.* **43**, 195.
Roberts, G. E. (1966). *Develop. Med. Child. Neurol.* **8**, 26.
Roberts, G. E. and Clayton, B. E. (1969). *Develop. Med. Child. Neurol.* **11**, 584.
Schucker, G. W., Vail, E. H., Kelley, E. B. and Kaplan, E. (1965). *Pub. Health Rep. (Wash.)* **80**, 969.
Shelley, H. J. and Neligan, G. A. (1966). *Brit. med. Bull.* **22**, 34.
Wattiaux, R., Wattiaux-de Coninck, S., Rutgerrts, M. J. and Tulkens, P. (1964). *Nature, Lond.* **203**, 757.
Widdas, W. F. (1961). *Brit. med. Bull.* **17**, 107.
Wong, P. W. K., Lambert, A. M. and Komrower, G. M. (1967). *Develop. Med. Child. Neurol.* **9**, 551.
Yu, J. S. and O'Halloran, M. T. (1970). *Lancet* **1**, 210.
Zamenhof, S., Marthens, van E. and Margolis, F. L. (1968). *Science* **160**, 322.

DISCUSSION

Rundle: May I say how refreshing it is to hear a biochemist who is not spending all her time looking for more rare inborn errors of metabolism. My first question is on the generalised disaccharidase deficiency.

Clayton: We do an enormous number of urine chromatograms for sugar, and you certainly do not get this picture in 'normal' children, for example, those who come to hospital for tonsillectomy. You do of course get disacchariduria in children with malabsorption but the picture is quite different. In malabsorption there is a characteristic preponderance of one or two sugars. The picture in mental retardation however is readily recognisable, and in seeing the report on urine sugars one can be fairly certain that it belongs to a retarded child, more likely than not, with fits.

Rundle: My second question is on lead. In those cases with elevated lead, have you been able to detect any lead-lines in the bones?

Clayton: Yes, in some of them you can. With the co-operation of Dr. Jean Bicknell, we were able to perform oral EDTA tests on three groups of children (i) those who were retarded and had severe pica (ii) those who were retarded with no pica, and (iii) those who were so severely physically handicapped as to barely be able to get hand to mouth (J. Bicknell *et al.* (1968) *J. ment. Def. Res.* **12**, 282). The blood levels of lead were closely related to whether pica was present or not. When EDTA was given it could be clearly shown that lead was chelated and excreted in the urine in large amounts in the pica group. There is clearly a heavy lead load in such patients, but we do not know whether this matters very much.

Rundle: On the basis of your published work on this I went back on 200-300 X-rays, but in no case could I detect bone changes. I was wondering how often you saw this and how elevated the lead has to be before you see such changes.

Clayton: Some of our children had lead lines, but it was a small number. I cannot say how elevated the blood lead must be since lead lines depend upon excessive ingestion over a long time.

Giroud: You have quoted the noxious influence of phenylalanine in the blood, but according to the literature, there may be other amino acids doing the same thing. Thus, lysine may induce disturbances during pregnancy, and the foetal weight may be disturbed associated with suppression of anabolic metabolism in the mother. But we did not study the brain.

Many biochemical disturbances may be relevant. There are, however, the same disturbances found in newborn or children in which the mental retardation is suspected to be correlated with a genetic condition, or those which are suspected to be connected with trauma at birth.

Clayton: You are thinking of phenylketonuria? These findings of yours are of course on animals, but we do not know about women in these disorders, particularly the effect on the offspring of heterozygotes of these disorders.

Davison: Professor Clayton, the finding of disaccharides in urine and the changes in amino acid pattern does suggest to me that this is likely to be an impairment of absorption. I wondered whether, just as intellectual development is retarded, some difference in absorption may not also occur. Have you also looked at babies, as well as tonsillectomy cases, for the excretion of disaccharides in the urine? Is there any other evidence of generalised developmental retardation from a biochemical point of view, e.g. the haemoglobin pattern, or isoenzyme changes?

Clayton: We have a lot of data on disaccharides in normal infants. I would agree with you, and I was trying to say this earlier, one does not know whether this process occurs because of general changes in the body, or whether it relates in any specific way to the mental retardation. It is an abnormality which may be secondary.

Davison: You have no other biochemical data on retardation?

Clayton: I have not looked specifically at haemoglobin, but in general most of the investigations are depressingly negative.

Kleihues: I was wondering if there was any information on the half-life of the lead in the serum after single exposure, that might indicate a failure to excrete it normally.

Clayton: No, I do not think it is that.

Kleihues: But does one know the half-life of lead after a single exposure?

Clayton: No, I do not know the answer. I am not suggesting, however, that lead is the primary cause of brain damage in the bulk of the children.

Wigglesworth: Is there any evidence that blood lead levels are higher than in the past? Does the motor car play a role here?

Clayton: I have no doubt that for inorganic lead it is old paint which is the major source. In our own children, I have seen no evidence that the levels are rising, and it may even be falling. The paint industry has been very responsible in this country, and it is largely a matter of old paints now.

Cavanagh: Is there any evidence that lead in any form interferes with the maturation of the brain? Are there any animal experiments over the critical periods on this?

Clayton: Yes, it does.

Dobbing: Lead acetate certainly has an effect on the young in animal experiments.

Zlotnik: In Scotland there is a disease in lambs, where there is a lot of lead in the soils, and bone, kidney and liver troubles are the main features. There is very little change in the nervous system (Butler, E. J., Nisbet, D. I. and Robertson, J. M. (1957) *J. comp. Path.* **67**, 378). It would be interesting to look at the blood levels of children in this area.

Clayton: Professor Goldberg is concerned about this, I believe.

Jellinger: Have you any idea of the incidence of rare metabolic disorders which might be correlated with mental retardation? What percent can be expected?

Clayton: It will vary according to the region. At Great Ormond Street we run a screening service for all newborns in the North Eastern and North Western Metropolitan regions of London. In 14 months we tested more than 110,000 infants and the incidence of classical phenylketonuria was about 1 in 14,680 births. We saw only one with atypical phenylketonuria, and one with homocysteinuria. A few had persistent raised methionine levels, but we do not know the significance of this finding.

Jellinger: And in 400 mentally retarded children a year, how many do you expect to find?

Clayton: Our patients come from many areas, of course. In the survey with Roberts we found about 7% with some sort of chemical disorder, but not all were properly defined or understood.

Balázs: I would like to take up the question of transient changes in growth hormone output. One must take this rather seriously, since the consequence of a transient change will depend on the time when it occurs. A transient change can have a rather powerful effect on developing nervous system particularly when the neuronal circuitry is produced. You may end up with the wrong 'wiring-pattern' if your disturbance comes at a certain period. One ought to pay quite a lot of attention to those transient changes, and one ought to define the period when this might have an important organising effect on the CNS. Dr. Dobbing's finding of cell proliferation continuing in the human brain for one-and-a-half years, give the limit of the period when one ought to look for this type of change. Giving cortisone to animals in early life will affect the activity of the growth hormone-releasing factor in the hypothalamus for good. Determining the activity of the hormone-releasing factor will give an indirect indication of how neurones will behave in the long run.

EEG Aspects of Unclassified Mental Retardation

RUTH HARRIS

Introduction

This paper examines some of the EEG (electro-encephalographic) findings in a group of children with severe, unclassified mental retardation. An extensive literature has now accumulated about the EEG in many known disorders that has led to some useful diagnostic criteria in the EEG assessment (Eastham and Jancar, 1968; Gibbs and Gibbs, 1965). The present series of EEGs have been assessed, bearing in mind these published EEG and clinical correlations in an attempt to see if the routine EEG recording can offer further help in the diagnosis and management of these children.

Material and Methods

A total of 148 EEGs were reviewed from 101 children. They were all severely mentally retarded and were selected from a larger group of children who from a previous survey were considered to have an unclassified encephalopathy. The EEGs were taken either as part of a general assessment or because of the onset or persistence of epilepsy.

As far as possible no child was included who might have had some additional cerebral trouble in early infancy. In a group of such gravely handicapped children it is not easy to find patients without other physical defects or retardation in motor skills. Thirty-eight children had some additional problem including squints, cataracts, blindness, minor deformities of the limbs, hypotonia, movement disorders, small head circumference and behavioural problems. Epilepsy was a common complication and occurred in 66, nearly two-thirds of the children. This of course is a well-known association with mental retardation (Donoghue *et al.*, 1970). The age range of the patients was from seven

TABLE 1

	Number of patients	Number of EEGs
1. Without epilepsy	35	45
2. Epilepsy	50	80
3. Previous infantile spasms	16	23
Total	101	148

months to 14 years. Many of the younger children were referred because of associated epilepsy and serial recordings were mostly obtained from these children (Table 1). In 16 of the children with seizures the syndrome of infantile spasms had occurred. It was not always clear from the history whether or not the child had been retarded before the onset of the spasms, but none had any of the numerous possible associated conditions (Millichap *et al.*, 1962). The cause of this state is not known but is distinguished by the peculiar form of the initial clinical onset. They must form a sizeable percentage of the severely retarded population and although they do represent a special group one feels justified in considering them alongside children having other forms of epilepsy associated with mental retardation. Nine of the 16 who had had infantile spasms were still having various other types of epilepsy at from 3 to 10 years of age.

The difficulties of obtaining EEGs from the severely retarded children should not be underestimated. It is often a severe problem to communicate with them, they are often restless and usually resent the placing of recording electrodes. They thus present a formidable task to the technician (Tizard, 1968). These difficulties probably explain the relatively small literature on the EEG in the older, severely retarded child. In many instances it proved impossible to carry out the test without giving sedation and 66 of the records in this survey were taken using either Seconal, Nembutal, chloral or Vallergan. In these, recording in the waking state was not often feasible even after a period of sleep.

Silver/silver-chloride disc electrodes were used, attached to the scalp with collodion. The electrode placement used was that described by Pampiglione (1956). Photic stimulation was carried out routinely but a period of hyperventilation was rarely possible.

The records were then graded into three main categories. (1) Those without any special EEG features. (2) Those showing a minimal abnormality and (3) those which were definitely abnormal.

(1) A normal group was not designated as so many of the records were limited in one way or another. Some of the recordings were taken in either only the waking or sleeping state so that full assessment of the

appropriate rhythms could not be made and the facilitating effect of sleep in producing abnormalities was not always tested. The first category was therefore one in which no definite abnormality was found within the restrictions of the test. No attempt was made to carry out any sophisticated analysis of the EEG rhythms other than by counting wave frequencies with the aid of a simple cursor and by making general statements about the amplitude of the activities present in light of experience.

(2) Mild abnormalities included slight but consistent asymmetries in the distribution of the various activities, unusually low voltage activity, a mild excess of either generalised or focal theta activity (in relation to the child's age), an excess of fast activity in a child who was not taking any medication and occasional sharp waves which were not seen repeatedly over a single region of the head.

(3) The definitely abnormal group showed one or more of the following features: a consistent marked asymmetry between the activities of the two hemispheres, a marked excess of theta or delta activity either focal or generalised in distribution, sharp waves, spikes or complex wave forms (mixtures of slow waves with sharp waves or spikes), these spike or sharp wave discharges were either repeatedly focal over one region, multifocal or generalised. The severity of the abnormality was not graded but a few records were particularly noted because of their bizarre appearance.

These EEG abnormalities were then charted with regard to age and the incidence of seizures or previous infantile spasms. No statistical analysis was made, however, because of the selected nature of the case material. There was naturally a greater proportion of children with associated epilepsy than would be expected in a group of severely retarded children, Donoghue *et al.* (1970), for example, found 36% with epilepsy in their unselected series compared with 65% of the present group.

Results

EEG Features Related to the Incidence of Epilepsy

(a) NO HISTORY OF EPILEPSY

Figures 1, 2 and 3 show the distribution of EEG abnormalities in relation to age and the incidence of epilepsy. Most of the children who did not have seizures had no special EEG features or only mild abnormalities. Three of the eight children in the abnormal group had

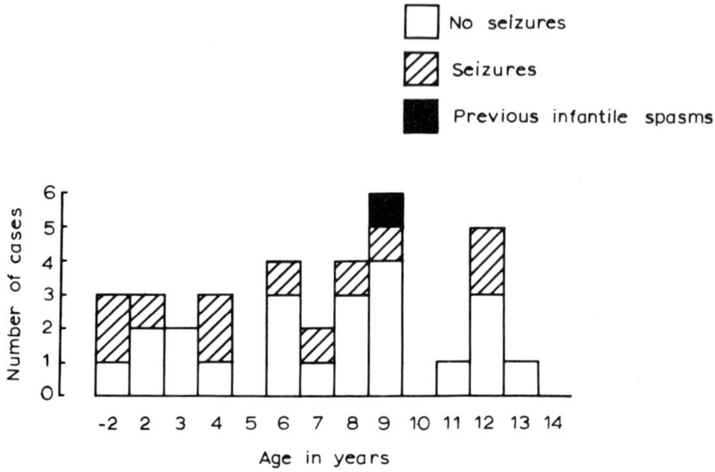

Fig. 1. No special features in the EEG.

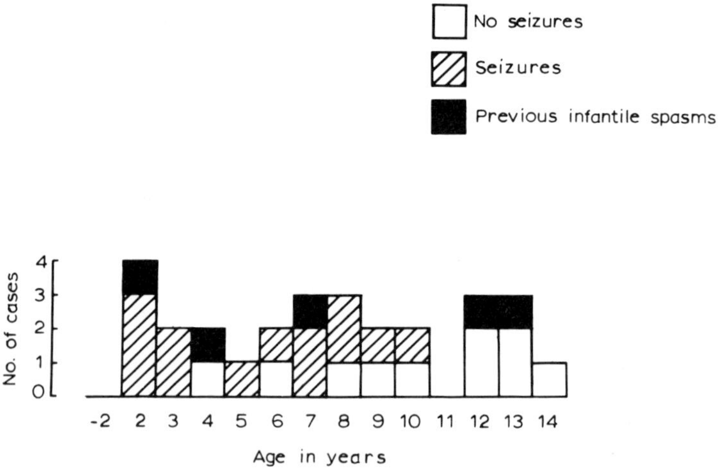

Fig. 2. Mild EEG abnormality.

rather unusual records. They all had some additional anatomical or neurological abnormality apart from their severe retardation. None showed any biochemical or chromosomal abnormality. The EEG abnormalities were generalised but dissimilar. The tracings from one of the children with limb deformities showed the repetitive slow waves in the sleep record similar to some of the abnormalities found in subacute

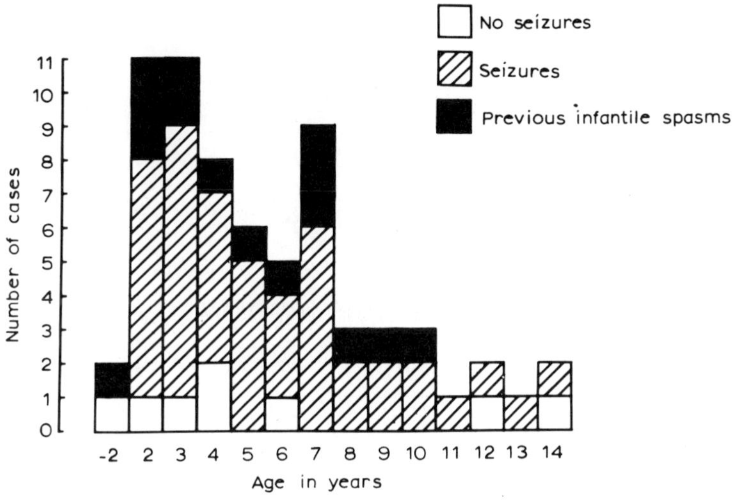

Fig. 3. Abnormal EEGs.

sclerosing leuco-encephalitis (Cobb and Hill, 1950), but there were no clinical features to suggest that this condition was present. Repetitive generalised sharp wave-forms were seen in a later record and were difficult to relate to any known pathological process. The other child with mild deformities showed persistent theta activity at 5-6 c/s in her EEG, unaffected by eye opening or closure or sleep (Fig. 4). The third child had generalised episodes of very large amplitude delta waves in the sleeping record lasting several seconds. Normal type of EEG patterns were seen in the intervening period. No waking trace was obtained.

(b) EPILEPSY

No special features, or only mild abnormalities were found in some of the children with epilepsy (Figs 1 and 2). These children were among those in whom only a few seizures had occurred. In a few instances the EEG had been taken before the onset of seizures or after a good clinical response to anti-convulsants. Those with epilepsy who had abnormal records showed the same variety of phenomena to be expected in children with epilepsy regardless whether mental retardation was present or not.

Two patients had episodes of minor epileptic status with persistent slow wave-and-spike activity which largely disappeared whenever thc

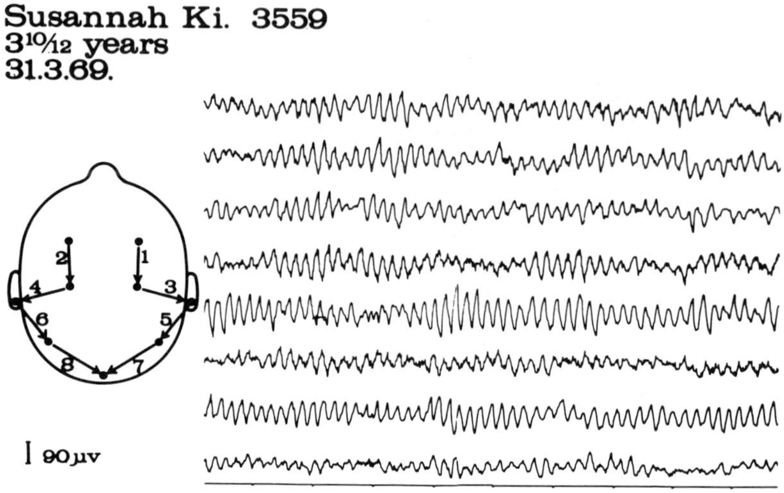

Fig. 4. Generalised rhythmic 5-6 c/s activity which persisted during sleep and was unaffected by eye opening and closure. The amplitude is smaller over the left than over the right side posteriorly.

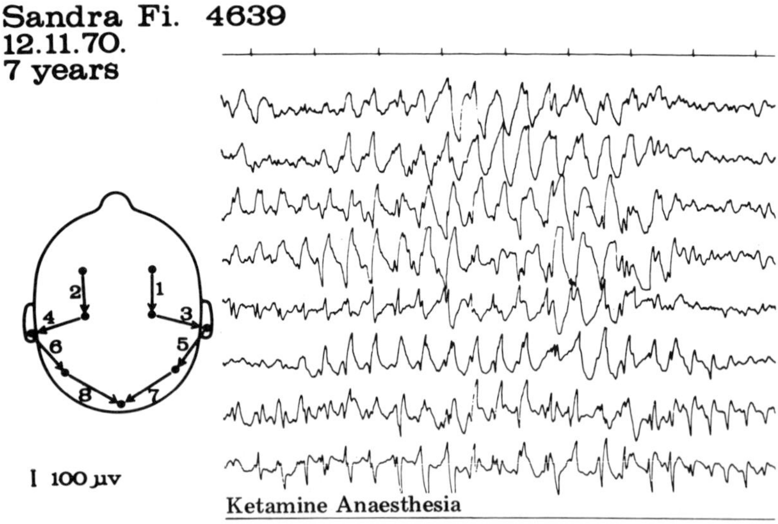

Fig. 5. Continuous, generalised, fairly rhythmic slow waves and spikes in the record of a child who had only infrequent seizures. The EEG abnormality remained unchanged over an interval of four years.

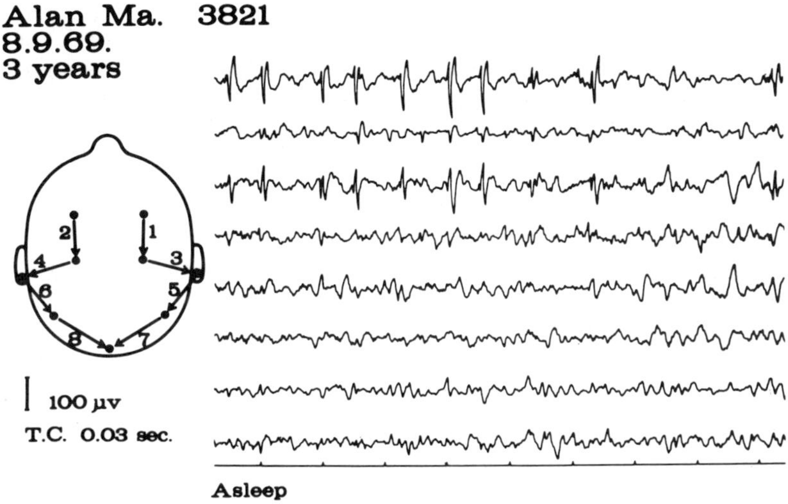

Fig. 6. Almost continuous slow waves and spikes over the right central region and occasional independent sharp waves over the left side. This child had had one dubious seizure at 10 months and had no localised neurological abnormality.

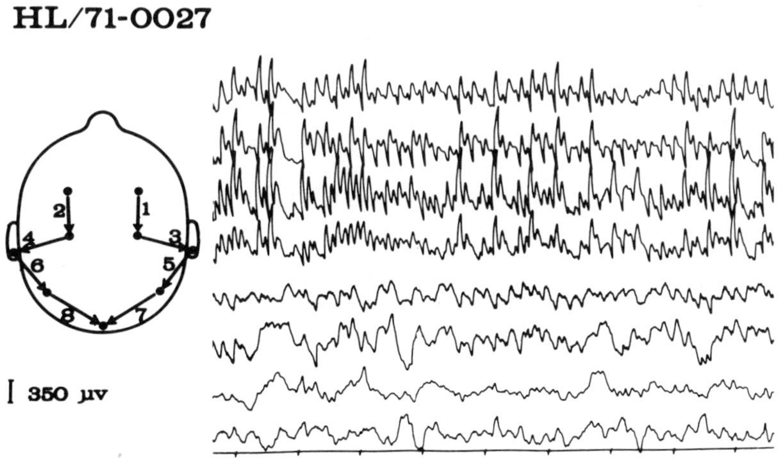

Fig. 7. Runs of very large amplitude 6-10 c/s activity over the anterior regions of the head, sharp in outline and mixed with spikes. These prolonged episodes occurred when the child was drowsy and preceded a fretful type of arousal. This fluctuating state continued for a long while before the child finally fell asleep (Julia St., 8 years, 1.2.71).

epilepsy improved (Brett, 1966). Almost continuous slow wave-and-spike complexes were also seen in three other children who did not suffer from episodes of minor epileptic status. These records were not unlike the findings in some cases of neurolipidosis (Cobb and Pampiglione, 1952). One girl with infrequent seizures showed this type of EEG abnormality which did not get worse (Fig. 5) at three and seven years of age. A distant relative was said to have had Tay-Sachs disease, but investigations (not a brain biopsy) failed to show any cause for her serious mental defect.

Persistently focal spikes or slow wave-and-spike complexes were seen in 13 of the children with epilepsy. None had any focal neurological abnormality or localising clinical phenomena during seizures. Five of these had infrequent attacks in spite of marked EEG abnormalities and in one of them, there was some doubt about the only seizure which occurred at 10 months of age. This boy's EEG at three years showed almost continuous spikes and slow waves over the right central region together with occasional independent discharges on the left (Fig. 6).

Frequent multifocal discharges were seen in the records of two girls aged six and seven, and both records were suggestive of multiple potentially epileptogenic lesions but there were no other clinical clues as to the underlying pathology.

Many of the children with epilepsy had generalised bursts of slow waves and spikes in their EEG. In three, paroxysmal EEG features were associated with clinical changes that were not previously thought to be seizure phenomena. Thus in one child nocturnal screaming attacks from the age of four were followed by generalised seizures at five years. The EEG abnormalities, seen with irritability and upsetting arousal episodes in the drowsy state, suggested that the screaming attacks might be related to some form of epilepsy (Fig. 7). There was both clinical and EEG improvement following medication with Valium. Another child had numerous odd mannerisms but it was not until her EEG was recorded that it was realised that some of these episodes of eye fluttering and chewing movements were in fact brief seizures and were associated with generalised discharges (Fig. 8). These features improved after anti-convulsant therapy. The third child also had numerous odd mannerisms and had suffered earlier from infantile spasms. At two-and-a-quarter years he showed a patchy distribution of slow waves and spikes with brief runs of large amplitude fast activity posteriorly, most marked over the left posterior temporal region. Such episodes resembled the changes which occur in babies suffering from infantile spasms and often accompany the clinical attacks (Samson-Dollfus, 1958). In this child, the fast wave activity often coincided with a sudden jerk of his head to the left. This type of attack had been noted

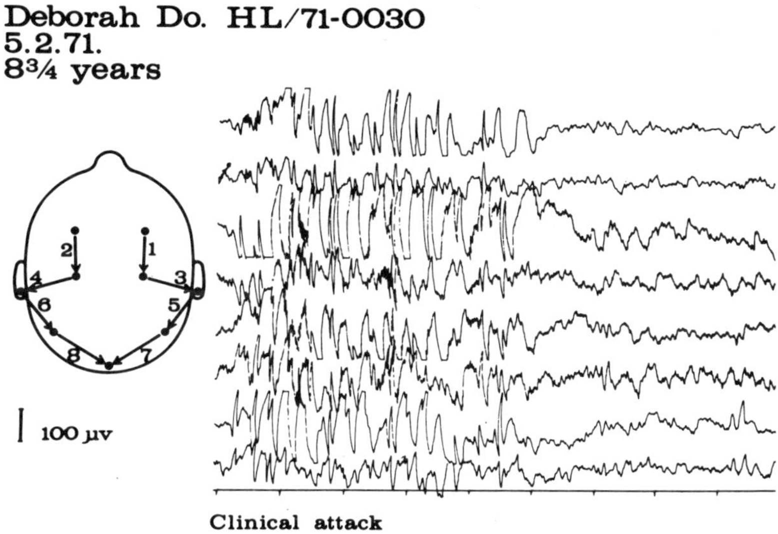

Fig. 8. A generalised burst of irregular slow waves and spikes accompanied by slight eyelid flutter and chewing movements. It was not realised that this child had epilepsy.

by Féré in 1883 as a variant of 'tic de salaam' (infantile spasms), but it was not easy clinically in this child to distinguish the head jerking from other peculiar movements.

Odd mannerisms were seen in an eight-year-old girl associated with episodes of twitching and the possibility of epilepsy was considered. In addition to these mannerisms she had an abnormal respiratory pattern with episodes of hyperventilation followed by breath-holding. There were considerable fluctuations in the amount of theta and delta activity in her EEG which were probably related in some way to this respiratory disturbance and there were no EEG patterns appropriate for the child's age. Jerking and twitching tended to occur in a random fashion but were not accompanied by any cerebral spike discharges.

(c) PREVIOUS INFANTILE SPASMS

It has been shown that the natural evolution of the EEG abnormalities in this syndrome is towards recovery (Janz and Mathes, 1955). It is not surprising therefore that six of these children, all free from seizures and between 2 and 13 years of age had relatively normal EEGs with perhaps only a slight asymmetry between the activities of the two hemispheres or a minimal excess of theta activity. All the other children had severe EEG abnormalities and only one of them, a three-year-old girl was said to be free from epilepsy. Another, described above had brief episodes of head jerking but all the others had severe and easily recognisable seizures of various types. The EEG abnormalities consisted of a generalised excess of slow activity mixed with spikes showing an asymmetrical distribution in some children. The oldest patient having a marked EEG abnormality was a 10-year-old girl who suffered from grand mal seizures. Her record, taken during Nembutal-induced sleep was indistinguishable from many of the sleeping records obtained from babies during the florid clinical stage of infantile spasms (Harris, 1966).

Some Particular EEG Variations

(a) THE ALPHA RHYTHM

Fourteen children between 6 and 14 years of age showed an alpha rhythm in their EEG which although stable in appearance and of an appropriate frequency for their age, was of a rather small amplitude (Fig. 9). In this type of EEG there also tended to be less rhythmic activity over the anterior part of the head than would be expected. None of these children had epilepsy and all their records were graded into either the first or second category.

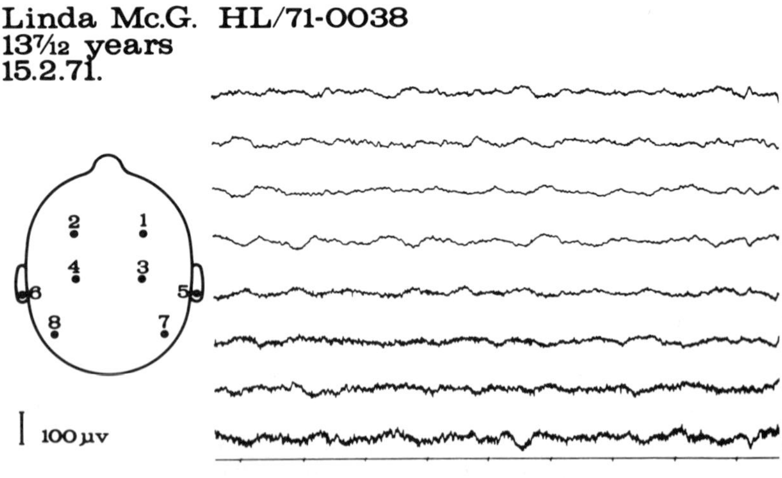

Fig. 9. An example of the rather small amplitude type of EEG record seen in many of the children without epilepsy. The alpha rhythm is well formed although of small amplitude.

(b) LAMBDA WAVES

One child with epilepsy had peculiarly large amplitude lambda waves.

(c) ABNORMAL RESPONSES TO PHOTIC STIMULATION

Spike discharges, facilitated by photic stimulation were only seen in the EEGs of two children. One was a two-year-old boy who had only had a single seizure at about one-and-a-half years of age. There was no clinical evidence of photosensitivity and his EEG was generally abnormal with generalised bursts of slow waves and spikes in addition to focal spikes over the posterior temporal regions. The second child was a 13-year-old with epilepsy and several other clinical problems. He had had pyloric stenosis and a congenital largyngeal stridor. His face was odd and he had a systolic murmur in addition to a minor foot malformation. Investigations, including chromosome studies, had failed to reveal any cause for his various defects. His EEG showed generalised bursts of spikes during photic stimulation associated with momentary 'blankness'. There was an excess of theta activity in his resting record.

(d) SLEEP RECORDS

Waves corresponding morphologically to the phenomena of 14 and 6 positive spikes (Gibbs and Gibbs, 1951) were seen in the sleep records of three boys aged 4, 9 and 12 years. The eldest and the youngest were free from epilepsy and the nine-year-old had had seizures from the age of 15 months to 3 years. The frequency of the spikes was not exactly 14 or 6 per second in any of these children. Sleep records from some of the children failed to show some of the expected fluctuations in EEG activity that would have been expected in relation to drowsiness and sleep. These changes were difficult to assess, particularly in EEGs with relatively short periods of sleep, where the sleep was drug-induced or where the records were abnormal in other respects. Eleven children had rather inappropriate sleep patterns, the most notable feature being the absence of sleep spindles. The ages of these children ranged from 1 to 12 years and seven of them had epilepsy.

Two Cases with Post-mortem Examinations

Post-mortem studies were available in only two children. One severely retarded boy developed generalised seizures, each lasting 2-3 min from six months of age. At two years there was a marked excess of delta activity particularly over the left temporo-occipital region where, in addition spike discharges were seen. Attacks of generalised jerking were accompanied by bursts of slow waves and spikes over both hemispheres. He died seven months later of broncho-pneumonia. The brain showed changes due to non-specific terminal anoxia (Dr. L. Crome). The second boy was normal at birth and in the neonatal period, but blindness and retardation became evident at two months. Generalised fits began at two years and continued until his death at 12 years from broncho-pneumonia. A Seconal-induced EEG sleep record at 10 years showed continuous bursts of generalised slow waves and spikes and none of the expected sleep patterns. Investigations had not shown any cause for his retardation and epilepsy. At post-mortem the brain showed cortical atrophy in the occipital lobes with gliosis and demyelination of the occipital white matter. The anterior parts of the hemispheres were intact apart from some unevenness of neuronal staining and central chromatolysis. The brain stem showed microglial clusters, extensive atrophy and gliosis of the cerebellar folia and a diagnosis of congenital gliotic encephalopathy was made (Dr. L. Crome).

Serial EEG Recordings

Twenty-five children had serial EEGs over periods of up to six years. Six of them were free from seizures and remained so. They matured normally with respect to the appearance of the alpha rhythm in those where recordings were taken in the waking state.

Fourteen of the children with epilepsy had repeated EEGs and in four there was an improvement over a period up to three years. Some of the others showed fluctuations in the frequency of spike discharges or more dramatic changes related to the occurrence of minor epileptic status but only one child showed a definite deterioration with an increase in slow activity in three records taken between two and five years of age, associated with deterioration in her clinical state but without evidence of a progressive cerebral disorder.

Repeated EEGs were obtained in five children who had had infantile spasms over intervals of up to six years. They were all still suffering from various types of seizures and their records showed persistent, severe generalised abnormalities

Discussion

The EEG may be regarded as a technique which demonstrates one aspect of brain function but the genesis of the various cerebral electrical events shown and their relationship to cerebral development and function are still poorly understood. The correlations with clinical, biochemical and pathological defects are unclear and it would be naïve to search for any easily identifiable EEG feature which could be related to intelligence. In addition, in any EEG survey it must be remembered that in children, as well as in adults, a proportion of apparently normal subjects will show EEG abnormalities. Petersen *et al.* (1968) found that 99 out of nearly 1000 normal children showed abnormal paroxysmal activity.

The high incidence of EEG abnormality in the retarded children who also had epilepsy would be expected (Gibbs and Gibbs, 1965). These authors commented, that the EEG abnormality correlated with the epilepsy and not the retardation. The unusual EEGs seen in a few of the children without epilepsy however remain unexplained. Records showing bizarre or curious features can be produced from the shelves of every EEG department and it is difficult to argue about the significance of isolated peculiarities in the EEGs of mentally retarded children. From the EEGs taken from this series as a whole, examples can be selected where a particular EEG resembles the abnormalities described in some known cerebral illness but there have been few claims about the absolute specificity of particular EEG features with regard to underlying neuropathological processes.

The importance of the EEG evolution in a number of progressive cerebral disorders, including the inborn errors of metabolism, has been stressed by Pampiglione and Papatheophilou (1961), della Rovere *et al.* (1964), Pampiglione and Lehovský (1968) and Mastropaolo *et al.* (1971), and it is perhaps the relatively static nature of the EEG abnormality or trend towards spontaneous improvement which distinguishes the records found in these retarded children with unclassified encephalopathy.

Interpretation of the focal abnormalities found in the records of 13 children is especially difficult owing to the usual variability of the location of focal spike discharges in childhood. Trojaborg (1968) in a longitudinal study of 242 children with spike foci in their records found that there was a change in the localisation of the discharges in 85% of the children, so it is clear that such discharges are of limited value as an indication of focal cortical damage in children.

One practical use of the EEG in this series was in the diagnosis of epilepsy in a few cases. It is not uncommon in paediatric EEG work to find the combination of some slight clinical change, with paroxysmal features in cases where the clinical features had not previously been recognised as seizures. In retarded children with peculiar mannerisms or behaviour disturbances the EEG assessment, especially of four children in this series, could be helpful in their management.

The group of children with infantile spasms showed the expected EEG evolution (Janz and Mathes, 1955), but why the evolution follows a particular trend in some children and not in others is an interesting question. Jeavons and Bower (1964) have shown that clinical and EEG recovery is unrelated to the therapy during the early stages of the illness. In general there was no particular feature in the persistent EEG abnormalities in children that continued to have epilepsy when compared with those with frequent seizures, but no infantile spasms.

Abnormal responses to photic stimulation with, or without associated clinical changes are found in normal children (Petersén, 1968), in epilepsy and in various abnormal metabolic states such as barbiturate withdrawal (Wulff, 1959), Tay Sachs disease (Pampiglione and Lehovský, 1968) and Type I hyperprolinaemia (Effron, 1965). The incidence of photosensitivity is less than the 13.4% reported in normal children (Petersén, 1968) and is probably unrelated to their retardation.

Apart from these definite abnormalities the incidence of low voltage EEG activity and variations in the alpha frequency are particular EEG features which have been described in retarded children. Low voltage activity was found in 14 children as also has been noted by Gibbs and Gibbs (1965) and Berger (1932). The basic problems in the assessment of low voltage in mentally retarded patients had already been presented by Berger (1932) together with a realistic account of the practical difficulties in obtaining EEGs. The last four patients Berger studied included two six-year-old boys and all showed low voltage traces.

Unusual sleep patterns have been reported in retarded patients including Mongolism and hypothyroidism (Ellingson, 1970). Many of these studies describe less sleep spindle activity than would be expected, particularly in the hypothyroid patients, even after treatment. Gibbs and Gibbs (1965) on the other hand have also described a significantly high proportion of retarded children with 'extreme spindles', a characteristic and persistent high voltage rhythmic activity at a similar frequency to normally occurring sleep spindles. This was not found in this series, but this may be partly due to recording technique and possibly to the method of sedation. The proper assessment of sleep patterns requires repeated all night recordings to determine the proportion of the various sleep stages compared with normal subjects. Such studies are tedious, time-consuming and expensive, and not perhaps an attractive research prospect in these difficult patients.

No attempt has been made to correlate the EEG variables found with the level of intelligence by sophisticated and complicated methods of analysis (Ellingson, 1966; Vogel and Broverman, 1966). Ellingson concluded (1970) that, 'if there are relationships between intelligence test scores and EEG variables, they are slight and evanescent'.

Neuropathological findings were only available in two cases. In one with severe retardation, epilepsy and a gross EEG abnormality, in keeping with a marked abnormality of cerebral function of unknown cause, was not associated with equivalent structural change. The second child had focal cerebral abnormalities with some appropriate clinical findings (blindness and occipital lobe atrophy), but the EEG abnormality was diffuse and did not show a particular location over the occipital regions. It is probable that examination of cerebral visual evoked responses would have given more information about the occipital lobe defect (Ellingson, 1970).

Summary and Conclusions

EEGs have been studied from a group of 101 children with severe mental retardation of unknown cause. Most of the 66 patients with associated epilepsy had abnormal EEGs, but there were a few patients without epilepsy who had peculiar and severe EEG abnormalities. From the abnormal EEGs as a whole, a small number showed features similar to those described in known cerebral conditions. The EEG was of practical help in the clinical assessment of the occurrence of seizures. In 25 children with serial records, the EEG features tended in general to remain unchanged over a period of time or to improve, unlike many known progressive cerebral disorders.

Variations in basic EEG rhythms and sleep patterns were not uncommon but examination of these aspects of the EEGs was limited by the practical difficulties encountered in obtaining the records.

With increasing correlative studies on the clinical, biochemical, neuropathological and EEG aspects it is hoped that a greater understanding will be obtained of the various EEG phenomena described, but at present, apart from some help in the management of coincidental epilepsy, the EEG findings in unclassified retardation pose more questions than can be answered.

ACKNOWLEDGEMENTS

My thanks are due to the physicians of Queen Mary's Hospital, Carshalton and to Dr. John Corbett of the Hilda Lewis Unit, Bethlem Royal Hospital, and Dr. Peter Woolf, Darenth Park Hospital, for allowing me to study patients under their care. I am indebted to Dr.

Emily Angeli who carried out a clinical survey of the children with unclassified mental retardation at Queen Mary's Hospital.

The task of obtaining the EEGs was carried out by Mrs. Burrows-Peakin, Mrs. Emly, Mrs. Gibbs and Staff Nurse Simpson.

REFERENCES

Berger, H. (1932). In 'Hans Berger on the Electroencephalogram of Man' (P. Gloor, ed.) *Electroenceph. Clin. Neurophysiol.,* 1969, Suppl. 28, p. 168.

Brett, E. M. (1966). *J. Neurol. Sci.* **3**, 52.

Cobb, W. and Hill, D. (1950). *Brain* **73**, 392.

Cobb, W., Martin, F. and Pampiglione, G. (1952). *Brain* **75**, 343.

Della Rovere, M., Hoare, R. D. and Pampiglione, G. (1964). *Develop. Med. and Child Neurol.* **6**, 149.

Donoghue, E. C., Abbas, K. A. and Gal, E. (1970). *Brit. J. Psychiat.* **117**, 531.

Eastham, R. D. and Jancar, J. (1968). 'Clinical Pathology in Mental Retardation'. Bristol: John Wright.

Effron, M. L. (1965). *New Eng. J. Med.* **272**, 1243.

Ellingson, R. J. (1966). *Psychological Bulletin* **65**, 91.

Ellingson, R. J. (1970). In 'Mental Retardation' (J. Wortis, ed.), Vol. 1, p. 164. U.S.A.: Grune and Stratton.

Féré, Ch. (1883). *Bulletin du Progrès Médical* **11**, 970.

Gibbs, E. L. and Gibbs, F. A. (1951). *Neurology* **1**, 136.

Gibbs, F. A. and Gibbs, E. L. (1965). In 'Medical Aspects of Mental Retardation' (C. H. Carter, ed.). U.S.A.: Charles C. Thomas.

Harris, R. (1966). EEG changes in children with infantile spasms treated with ACTH, p. 65. London University: M.D. Thesis.

Janz, D. and Mathes, A. (1955). *Bibl. Paediat. Fasc.* 60, Suppl. ad Ann. Paediat.

Jeavons, P. M. and Bower, B. D. (1964). 'Infantile Spasms'. Clinics in Developmental medicine No. 15, p. 56. London: Heinemann.

Mastropaolo, C., Pampiglione, G. and Stephens, R. (1971). *Develop. Med. and Child Neurol.* **13**, 20.

Millichap, J. G., Beckford, R. G., Klass, D. W. and Backus, R. E. (1962). *Epilepsia* **3**, 188.

Pampiglione, G. (1956). *Proc. Electrophysiol. Technol. Ass.* **7**, 20.

Pampiglione, G. and Papatheophilou, R. (1961). *Electroenceph. Clin. Neurophysiol.* **13**, 143.

Pampiglione, G. and Lehovský, M. (1968). In 'Clinical Electroencephalography in Children' (P. Kellaway and I. Petersén, eds), p. 287. Stockholm: Almqvist and Wiskell.

Petersén, I., Eeg-Olofsson, O. and Selldén, U. (1968). In 'Clinical Electroencephalography in Children' (P. Kellaway and I. Petersén, eds), p. 167. Stockholm: Almqvist and Wiskell.

Samson-Dollfus, D. (1958). *Rev. Neurol.* **99**, 126.

Tizard, B. (1968). *Amer. J. Ment. Defic.* **73**, 34.

Trojaborg, W. (1968). In 'Clinical Electroencephalography in Children' (P. Kellaway and I. Petersén, eds), p. 213. Stockholm: Almqvist and Wiskell.

Vogel, W. and Broverman, D. M. (1966). *Psychological Bulletin* **65**, 99.

Wulff, M. H. (1959). 'The Barbiturate Withdrawal Syndrome'. Copenhagen: P. Munksgaard.

DISCUSSION

Crome: I wanted to ask how often do you find perfectly normal EEG's in very severely subnormal children? And how do you explain this?
Harris: I cannot give you an answer in numbers, but after the Camberwell Survey I might be able to. The children I usually see are sent for EEG for a particular reason, but it isn't an uncommon finding, provided there is no history of epilepsy.
Jellinger: Perhaps I might draw further attention to the true correlation between the fit patterns and the morphological findings. In 220 children a correlation between these was attempted, but we could not find any correlation between fit patterns, aetiology and the morphological findings, except that unilateral lesions almost or never occurred in vascular encephalopathies which may be due to the multifocal lesions of this process, whereas myoclonus was often associated with metabolic disorders, e.g. lipidosis, spongy dystrophies and so on. One point of particular interest is infantile spasms. We have collected 15 necropsy cases and found all the possible cerebral lesions known which may be associated with infantile spasms. We, therefore, thought that this might be a non-specific response of the infantile brain to a variety of insults. Anatomical changes cannot be any more conclusive therefore in this matter, than the EEG.
Laurence: Dr. Pampiglione and I looked at the EEG's of 50 hydrocephalics, none of whom had fits, although there were spike-and-wave patterns and some focal features in those with acquired lesions rather than those with spina bifida. It was only a tendency, however.
Giroud: It would be interesting to follow the later evolution of these changes. I remember the study of Platt and Stewart (Platt, B. S. and Stewart, R. J. C. (1968) *Dev. Med. and Child Neurol.* **10**, 3) working on protein-deficient diet in dogs, in which they did the EEG at various times and showed that when return to a normal diet was sufficiently early the abnormal EEG features disappeared.
Harris: I think that to follow the evolution of the EEG may not be of great help, for instance in infantile spasms they ultimately have a reasonable EEG state, but remain grossly retarded. There is something more here than just the electrical activity.
Jellinger: Most cases of infantile spasms have very severe morphological lesions and they must be severely retarded.
Harris: Not all, there are some without abnormal pathological findings.
O'Connor: Has Dr. Harris any observations on the percentage alpha in cases of this kind?

Harris: I haven't, in fact, looked at this aspect. One has to do special. analysis of the EEG which perhaps one ought to do. But the technical difficulties are probably insurmountable.

O'Connor: We did a little work with autistic children, with mongols and siblings control groups and the results were extremely difficult to get, but oddly the percentage of alphas bore rather little relationship to the state at the time.

Dobbing: May I ask a more general question? To what extent are the changes which you see always originating in the brain? What I was thinking of was to what extent do your EEG changes reflect systemic changes rather than changes in brain function?

Harris: I certainly think they do, and this is very important indeed. The EEG pattern will be even more abnormal when there is an electrolyte disturbance, for example in hypocalcaemia the EEG's are very abnormal which is quickly reversed by treatment. One has to take this into account constantly when assessing the EEG's which is only an expression of brain function at that moment of time.

Dobbing: You take steps to standardise the metabolic state, as far as possible?

Harris: Not ordinarily. But if they are ill one tries to. Certainly for the Camberwell survey one will know their biochemical state.

Kirman: I do not know whether one ought to call infantile spasms a syndrome or not. I have always thought that it forms part of the expression and evolution of a whole variety of pathological processes in the brain leading to severe mental retardation, and that it was not specific.

Harris: I think one must label it, because it is so dramatic an incident. It might indeed be part of the evolution of a process, and I agree that it occurs in many states, but it does stand out as a separate clinical illness, at least at its beginning.

Jellinger: I would say it is a special type of reaction of infantile brains.

Harris: Yes. I agree.

Brain Injury and Mental Subnormality

N. O'CONNOR

Introduction: Statement of the Problem

The Psychology of Subnormality in relation to brain injury has a long and apparently respectable history. The early work of Goldstein (1939, 1942) and others gave rise to studies concerning rigidity by Strauss (1941) and to much experimental work involving concepts of arousal by Berkson (1960a, b, c), Berkson *et al.* (1961) and O'Connor and Berkson (1963). The main themes of this work can be summarised as pointing on the one hand to greater rigidity, i.e. tolerance for repetition or redundancy and a greater tendency to deficits of attention in the subnormal. Essentially, therefore, neurologists turned psychologist in this phase of research drew on their speculative concepts of neurological damage to render accounts of psychological or more strictly cognitive deficits. This interesting and perhaps even rewarding work drew heavily on clinical observations and in the end amassed considerable evidence concerning deficits of perception and problem solving in the subnormal.

For example, the later work of Strauss and Lehtinen (1947) suggested that defects due to brain injury resulted in confusions of figure and ground. That is, the brain-injured were supposed to be unable to detect partially hidden figures. It was claimed that familial subnormals could do this more easily. It was also alleged that the imitation of visual patterns was easier for familials. Strauss and his colleagues claimed that more systematic solutions were offered by familials who were better able to organise complete patterns. However, in this work a special meaning is given to the phrase 'brain-injury'. It has the meaning of local damage in a person of subnormal as distinct from severely subnormal ability, i.e. brain damage in someone of about

I.Q. 70 or above. In addition, the criteria of injury are poorly defined so that a close reading of the reports leaves the reader undecided about the basis on which decisions are reached. Sometimes one thinks that neurological criteria are being used, for example soft signs, presence of squint, etc. and sometimes it seems as if the diagnosis of brain injury is made on the basis of the psychological deficit which it is supposed to explain. Extensive criticisms have been offered of this work by Wortis (1956) and O'Connor (1958) chiefly on the grounds of this circularity of criteria.

Obviously the problem of brain injury applied in a holistic and uncritical fashion to all kinds of subnormality without specification can end by explaining everything and nothing. Apart from the question of criteria, this neurological approach of the inter-war and post-war periods treated the central nervous system too generally, making no concessions to localisation theories, although interestingly most of the claimed deficits were visuo-spatial. Thus this approach relied on psychology when neurology failed, using psychology to define brain injury instead of explaining the former by the latter. But additionally it confined the meaning of brain injury to visuo-motor defects leaving out many other possible deficits, for example, speech deficits, which are perhaps more marked in the subnormal.

The second line of study arising from the early speculations of Goldstein is both more general and less objectionable. This is the work on concepts of arousal. Berkson's (1960) and our own work are examples of this kind of study but very significant speculations concerning learning deficits have been developed by such authors as Ellis (1963). Our own theory implicating input deficits may also be beholden to concepts of arousal.

The basic theory can be expounded by describing an experiment carried out by Berkson *et al.* (1961). Imbeciles were asked to lie down on a couch in complete darkness. When alpha rhythm was normal a flash of light was presented. The alpha interruption time was measured and recorded. The same process was gone through with a normal control group. Results demonstrated that imbeciles were less 'alerted' by the stimulus than normals. Perhaps an even simpler way of demonstrating this inert character of the CNS in the subnormal is to test their slower reaction time which is about half normal speed in the case of simple uncomplicated reaction times.

Inferences from this aspect of subnormal 'arousal' can be made and have been made concerning attention (Zeaman and House, 1963), short-term memory (Ellis, 1963), and perception (Spitz, 1963) and more complex concepts (Das, 1970). Deficits in each have been attributed to a low state of arousal. However, as we know (Claridge and O'Connor, 1957) some subnormals are not under-aroused, but over-aroused and the state of arousal in one system does not necessarily reflect that in another. Thus even this more plausible neurophysiological account of psychological subnormality leaves something to be desired. Nonetheless, it does reflect the slowness, lack of dexterity and general lack of CNS alertness of some severely subnormal patients. In being both more realistic and in offering somewhat more plausible explanations of psychological events, it deserves recognition.

From a number of points of view, however, it is as unsatisfactory as the brain injury hypothesis. Firstly, it may not be reasonable to suppose that all subnormals have deficient activating systems without further study. Second, it is unlikely that the deficiencies which may exist will be uniform across sub-diagnoses and thirdly, arousal systems in themselves seem unlikely to provide adequate explanations of, for example, the relative lack of abstracting capacity shown by the subnormal. On the other hand, some of the advantages of the approach, as seen from the point of view of cognition, should be appreciated, the chief of these being the uniform character of the cognitive deficit shown by many subnormals. The nature of the psychological deficit in other words is what we have called developmental, i.e. characteristic of all functions and not, as in the case of aphasia, confined to one function like spoken or written language.

There are no completely satisfactory solutions to the attempt to associate brain and behaviour in the subnormal, however. Most psychologists know, for example, that in some instances patterns of disability can be found. So subnormals with poor verbal and high performance ability exist. It has been said that this pattern can be detected in mongolism although the evidence is insecure and was not reflected in Mein's (1961) and in Mein and O'Connor's (1960) findings for example. It is certainly true of autistic subnormals, however, and was mentioned as a common occurrence in mildly subnormal adolescents by Duncan (1942). The reverse pattern is found in some epileptic subnormals according to Blundell (1966) and Sylvester (1966).

Unfortunately the amount of research in this area is limited and few adequate studies are available. As a result the key issue as I see it is the description firstly of patterns of psychological deficit whether cognitive or otherwise, and the association of these patterns either with sub-diagnoses or known pathology or both. A second major problem is the explanation of development deficit as distinct from specific or localised deficits.

Review of Studies

Perhaps one of the most systematic investigations of brain injury in the subnormal is that of Strauss and Lehtinen (1947) and Strauss and Kephart (1955). They preserve a tradition of studies with its origins in Europe and in the work of Goldstein (1942) and in Gestalt studies. Another group of studies which reflects an origin in Gestalt work is that of Spitz (1963). This work is primarily concerned with the concept of arousal and its perceptual consequences. A third group of studies, that developed by Reitan (1966) is based on Halstead's (1947) earlier experiments which also have their origins in the copying of block designs. It will be instructive to outline each of these groups of studies before trying to estimate the success of the work in this field.

The work of Strauss *et al.* is concerned primarily with perception and arose from Goldstein and Scheerer's (1941) development of tests involving the copying of block designs. The concept of block design imitation is one of two or three sources of analysis of brain injury in man, a second being the Hunt-Minnesota involving a vocabulary and word design test and a third being the Pietrowski-Rorschach signs technique. The third test group which we mentioned above, that of Halstead (1947), the Halstead Impairment Index was intended as a measure of frontal lobe injury. However, as the two groups mentioned previously, Strauss *et al.* and Hunt-Minnesota, are also in a sense measures of localised injury, the Halstead in its original form is no exception.

Unfortunately for our specialised topic, much of the work mentioned was designed to cover cases in which subnormal intelligence was not taken into account. As a result I was able to make the following kind of criticism of this work in a chapter which I wrote on brain injury in Clarke and Clarke (1958), p. 205, 'The majority of these studies have not included groups of mental defectives and it should be remembered that several of the signs said to be characteristic of brain-damaged patients are also commonly found in the records of the feeble-minded in whom organic pathology is not suspected.' Another observation made in the same chapter quotes directly from Strauss and Lehtinen (1947).

'One question concerns the differential diagnosis between malformation of the brain, a developmental defect of brain substance, and the acquired defect of brain injury. Children with malformation of the brain usually show gross motor disturbances. They show definite brain defects on pneumo-encephalogram, and they do not show the slight behaviour abnormalities of the brain-injured child either in regard to mental development (they belong quasi-exclusively to the group of imbeciles and idiots) or with respect to the slight deviations of emotional behaviour as described....' It is clear therefore that their work, even if it covers studies of what we now call subnormality, does not extend to the group of the severely subnormal. This point is of some importance in assessing the significance of the approach to brain injury made by the two other groups mentioned, Spitz and his colleagues, and surveys such as that of Reitan (1966) based on Halstead's tests.

The work of Strauss and his colleagues purports to show two main effects. The first connected with the copying of geometric patterns, such as those made on a marble board with marbles placed in indentations on the board. Strauss claims that the copying of such patterns will be lacking in coherent intention and will be made spasmodically with many restarts and without reference to the overall design. The second effect is an alleged failure to distinguish figure and ground in situations in which an outline drawing of a common object is presented against a complete background with which it might merge.

In the experiments of Strauss *et al.* brain-injured children saw tachistoscopically exposed figure-ground combinations as ground only whereas normals and subnormals saw the figure. So long as one considers only the one-fifth second exposure of such figure-ground phenomena, it might be said that we are dealing with a decision or input phenomenon. In fact other tests mentioned by others and referred to by Strauss elsewhere, include for example, flicker-fusion tests. If we are concerned with a phenomenon of speed of comprehension, the phenomenon is likely to be a different one from that which might affect direct visual discrimination. Strauss reasoned that figure-ground confusion and marble board pattern imitation deficits were similar phenomena, but capacity for visual discrimination and speed of detection of visually presented phenomena may well be quite distinct processes. One-fifth of a second is a short exposure time as O'Connor and Hermelin (1965) showed in a short-term memory experiment and is much shorter than the average R.T. characteristic of subnormal or severely subnormal patients. Venables (1960) has developed the concept of the two-flash threshold from the original flicker-fusion test into an accurate measure of perceptual latency. His work shows that for schizophrenics, fusion time is abnormally slow. The same is true of subnormals. This general phenomenon of slowed response whether dependent on a visual or a motor component or both, seems to characterise many of the subnormal or the mentally ill. It may therefore represent a psychological result of all disability whatsoever, whether acute or chronic, pathological or developmental, and whether resulting from genetic or other causes.

This observation arose from the concern with Strauss's interpretation of his results with experiments on pattern perception. The problem of imitation of patterns, however, remains, and constitutes a separate problem in itself. This capacity to imitate patterns may reflect two abilities, a capacity to discriminate (and name) shapes which many experiments with children show to be a developmental ability, and the capacity to discriminate and reproduce shapes, which may be affected by injury, presumably in the right temporo-parietal cortex in dextrals. There is no adequate information on shape perception in the severely subnormal which would justify any classification according to sub-diagnosis. Some studies by O'Connor and Hermelin (1963) have suggested that short-term memory and capacity to draw shapes presented to the subject visually, may be more affected than the perceptual process itself, although few studies except those of Bryant (1970) have contributed further to this problem. Bryant's work indicates once more the importance of a developmental component. However he was not oriented towards studies of brain damage and does not discuss specific brain injury. Few replications of the Strauss and Lehtinen work have been attempted, and the effects in those studies which have been made usually reflect the effects of lack of measured intelligence rather than those of known brain injury. Examples are the studies of children who have suffered arrest of mental development as a result of veningitis, such as that of O'Connor and Haritos (1953).

If we now consider further work on perception by Spitz (1963), it will be seen that the concept of perceptual deficit takes a different form. This investigation explores the tendency for subnormals to show a slower oscillation of perspective in such visual phenomena as the Necker Cube perspective change. He attributes this observed phenomenon to the presumedly greater inhibition present in the CNS and resulting from brain injury. However, Spitz does not confine his observations to brain-damaged defectives, but assumes a degree of inhibition in all retarded subjects. He thus infers from a variety of visual gestalt phenomena observed in the subnormal a condition of the CNS characteristic of this group. The nature of this condition is described as follows (Ellis, 1963, p. 29).

'Let us assume from the satiation studies as previously described that–when compared with equal C.A. normals–retardates as a group can be physiologically categorised by the following four postulates:

Postulate I. In retardates it takes longer to induce temporary, as well as permanent, electrical, chemical and physical changes in stimulated cortical cells . . .

Postulate II. Once stimuli induce temporary chemical and electrical modifications of cortical cells, it takes longer for these cells to return to their previous state . . .

Postulate III. In retardates, over-stimuli induce permanent chemical, electrical and/or physical changes in cortical cells. It will be more difficult and take a longer period of time to switch consequent like–or relatively similar–stimuli away from these particular cell traces or current patterns so as to form new, or different, traces or patterns . . .

Postulate IV. In retardates, there is less spread of electrochemical activity from stimulated cells into the surrounding cortical field . . .'

Spitz acknowledges that the postulates are based on a certain sluggishness or torpidity of cortical cells in subnormals and regards this as part of a general picture of lowered metabolic efficiency.

Obviously this position is theoretically somewhat sounder than one which differentiates brain damage and the kind of malformations noted as occurring frequently in severe subnormality by Crome (1954) for example. Although the two types of damage may differ in many ways, most other research workers tend to overlook the abnormal condition of the central nervous system frequently found in subnormals. It is, or was, a common practice among psychologists to contrast familial and brain-injured subnormals. This classification usually meant a comparison of SN and SSN, in itself a division which ignored a considerable difference in intellectual level. The term endogenous usually meant someone with a genetic basis for subnormality, or no known cause, whereas the term exogenous was used to mean an injury associated with a circumscribed event. Furthermore the problem of Down's syndrome, in some sense familial and yet certainly showing considerable cortical malformation, is completely ignored.

Spitz's results, he himself observes, are confined to a limited set of visual phenomena and do not generalise easily beyond the narrowly defined concept of rigidity.

The work of Reitan (1966) is based on Halstead's (1947) work, and a brief description of the Halstead tests battery is necessary. This battery of tests includes a concept appreciation test, a test of flicker fusion, a tactile formboard test, a test of appreciation of rhythms, a coding test, i.e. recognising the written form of a spoken sound, a tapping speed test, and a test of time estimation. Additionally, Reitan uses a test of aphasia and one other test. The only comment that springs to mind concerning this heterogeneous group of probes is that its selection is based on a principle of catholic eclecticism.

The results of the application of this standardised neurological procedure are hard to assess because control groups often included paraplegic and neurotic patients. The justification for this procedure is given as an attempt to allow for the effects of hospitalisation. Brain-damaged subjects in one study were diverse and details are not given here but nonetheless the differences between the groups on the tests cited above were considerable with some notable exceptions. For example, critical flicker frequency was not a good discriminator, and tactual test memory was not as good as some other indexes. Good discriminators included the concept appreciation or category test, touch localisation and time taken to complete a tactile formboard.

Reitan's work addresses itself to one interesting problem, i.e. the difference between specific abilities and the ability to abstract. Goldstein and Scheerer (1941) made this distinction and thought that abstraction was in principle a completely separate ability from concrete behaviour. Reitan reasoned that if this were so, the abilities used by brain-damaged patients and controls would differ, and that this would be detectable in a different pattern of inter-test correlations in the two groups. An analysis of results showed that this result could not be found. In fact, the correlation matrices were closely similar. Reitan (1966) considers (p. 176) '. . . the results provided a strong argument that the effects of cerebral lesions are not, as claimed by Goldstein a "totally different activity of the organism" but instead seem to represent quantitative deviations from normal levels of the same kind of abilities as measured in subjects with normal brain functions.'

Much of the work reported by Reitan is not based on studies with subnormals but he sees the work as applicable in so far as he claims to be able to distinguish localised and general lesions including localised lesions of right and left hemispheres and frontal or non-frontal lesions and including a sub-division of general lesions. His method was to collect patients with intrinsic tumours, extrinsic tumours, cerebral vascular lesions and traumatic focal lesions in each of the frontal and non-frontal areas of each hemisphere. Sixty-four patients, 16 in each area were collected in this way. Each of four different types of lesion was thus represented in each of the four areas. Three additional groups of 16 subjects were collected, one with cerebral arteriosclerosis, one with closed head injuries, and one with multiple sclerosis but each showing diffuse cerebral damage.

Blind categorisation of subjects by both neurologists and psychologists as to area of lesions and into types of general or diffuse damage was reasonably good—better in fact for the latter than the former. The results are instructive for any over-simplified approach to a concept of brain damage in psychology. It should be pointed out, however, that in a follow-up study solely concerned with focal lesions, Reitan was less successful and felt bound to emphasise the importance of more refined statistical techniques. The upshot appears to be the usual tantalising variability of test results in this area.

Most important for the present discussion is the possible application of this work to studies with subnormals. Reitan sees a possible connection with studies of impaired cardiovascular function. He observes that ageing subjects show the same tendencies on the Halstead impairment index as are shown by subjects with brain damage. He also notes an interesting finding which might be disputed, that retarded groups show considerable impairment on verbal tests whereas subjects with a normal history prior to a cerebral injury tend to show performance impairment. He also points out that lateral differences are equally likely to occur against a background of retardation as against a background of otherwise normal ability.

It is clear from consideration of the three sets of studies described that the major trend of results would appear to justify an inference of generalised injury with an overlay of specific, frequently lateralised lesions. None of the researches can account for the frequently assumed abstraction deficit in the subnormal group.

Miscellaneous Studies

Heath (1942, 1949), Malpass (1959), Ellis and Sloan (1957) and Berkson (1960) have all carried out studies which reveal the involvement of motor function. They also drew attention to relatively slowed function in the subnormal. Bensberg and Cantor (1957) showed that the brain-injured subnormal was slower than the familial and Berkson (1960) by ingenious experiments, indicated that the slowed RT in the subnormal was chiefly a matter of response rather than input. The relevance of these studies to brain injury is the possible association between motor inefficiency and CNS lesions. Extensive and recent studies by Clausen (1966) with subnormals showed that those with severe neurological impairment differed from the familials on motor dexterity measures. Other measures failed to discriminate the groups. Clausen concludes that most of his evidence supports an hypothesis of general deterioration of association mechanisms rather than of distinct elements of behaviour. Clausen's as well as Semmel's (1965) and Folkard's (1971) studies suggest an attentional or vigilance deterioration. A possible cause for this basic association defect is suggested by the ingenious experiments of Belmont *et al.* (1966), and Birch and Belmont (1965) who measured the capacity of hemiplegics to integrate sensory input within or across modalities. Their results indicate once more a deterioration of association mechanisms or inter-sensory or sensory-motor integration.

Conclusions

In any statement concerning the psychology of brain damage in the subnormal and especially in the context of an audience of neurologists, anatomists and biochemists, it should be said firstly that psychologists have seldom been fully aware of the complexity of the field when formulating their theories and reports. The attempt to differentiate organic and familial types of mental deficiency is naive. It ignores the most obvious cases such as Down's syndrome with translocation of chromosomes. Secondly, the psychologist frequently compares the subnormal with the severely subnormal, ignoring the possible effects of intelligence and the association of brain damage with intelligence. As a result, much of the work of Strauss and his colleagues appears to me to be irrelevant to the problem of brain damage and mental deficiency. Over all most research reveals generalised damage which is just what would have been expected.

Whether patterns of test behaviour can be found superimposed on general diffuse lesions remains to be established. It is fairly clear that verbal, non-verbal differences occur and may reasonably be assumed to indicate hemisphere differences. On the other hand, these are the only clear differences established by test. Most so-called visual deficiencies seem to be more often associated with deficits of attention or vigilance or motor skills, as in reproduction of pictures from memory. Few actual errors of visual interpretation occur which could not be explained in terms of speed of intake or loss of memory trace.

Thus although attention and arousal may vary from system to system and be unequally affected by brain damage, most subnormals seem to show overall deficits of attention which may be explicable in terms of over or under arousal. Clausen, Spitz and Heath might well agree with this view. Such a theory would accord well with the slowed reaction times demonstrated by Bensberg and Cantor, and by Berkson, and would be similar to the slowed intake described by Venables for psychiatric patients. Our own work also showed that input for rapidly presented material was poor in severely subnormal children. There might therefore seem to be good evidence for a general effect of brain damage in severe subnormality, resulting in deficits of attention and as Semmel and Folkard have shown of vigilance. The case for such a condition is well made, and needs no further emphasis. An association with sub-diagnosis might be a real possibility, although no adequate evidence is available.

Unfortunately this general finding does not account for Goldstein's poverty of abstracting ability and no results of any research appear to be able to provide an explanation for this deficiency. If one analyses the concept of abstraction, it could be described as capacity to think of something in its absence, i.e. recall, capacity to encode incoming signals by using concepts, i.e. availability of a conceptual structure, or capacity to infer principles of solution. The first seems to be undamaged in subnormals, but the two latter are undoubtedly poorly developed, although the presence of the latter has been demonstrated in our own experiments. Reitan's work, however, does not demonstrate defects of abstraction, and it may be unscientific to presume them. A possible outline may be seen in Birch's experiments showing lack of sensory integration. If so, the explanation might be sought once again in defects of arousal.

Finally, therefore, the most consistent effect of the brain damage found in subnormality would appear to be an arousal deficit and an attentional deficit. The possibility of patterns of specific deficits as indicated by Sylvester and by Blundell, remains to be demonstrated on a wider scale among subnormals, although aphasia on the one hand, and perceptual deficiencies on the other, are easily demonstrable in brain-damaged normals.

REFERENCES

Belmont, I., Birch, H. G. and Karp, E. (1966). *J. Nerv. Ment. Dis.* **141**, 4, 410-418.

Bensberg, G. J. and Cantor, G. N. (1957). *Amer. J. ment. Defic.* **62**, 534-537.

Berkson, G. (1960a). *J. ment. Def. Res.* **4**, 51.

Berkson, G. (1960b). *J. ment. Def. Res.* **4**, 59.

Berkson, G. (1960c). *J. ment. Def. Res.* **4**, 69.

Berkson, G., Hermelin, B. and O'Connor, N. (1961). *J. ment. Def. Res.* **5**, 30.

Birch, H. G. and Belmont, L. (1965). *Devel. Med. and Child Neurol.* **7**, 135-144.

Blundell, E. (1966). *J. ment. Def. Res.* **10**, 141.

Bryant, P. E. (1970). 'Mirror Image Comparisons by Young Children'. B.P.S. London Conference (abstract).

Claridge, G. S. and O'Connor, N. (1957). *J. ment. Def. Res.* **1**, 16.

Clarke, A. M. and Clarke, A. D. B. (eds) (1958). 'Mental Deficiency: The Changing Outlook'. London: Methuen.

Clausen, J. (1966). 'Ability Structures and Subgroups in Mental Retardation'. Washington: Spartan Books.

Crome, L. (1954). *J. ment. Sci.* **100**, 894-912.

Das, J. P. (1970). *Amer. J. ment. Defic.* **75**, 253.

Duncan, J. (1942). 'The Education of the Ordinary Child'. London: Nelson.

Ellis, N. R. (1963). In 'Handbook of Mental Deficiency'. (N. R. Ellis, ed.). New York: McGraw-Hill.

Ellis, N. R. and Sloan, W. (1957). *Perceptual and Motor Skills* **7**, 65-67.

Folkard, S. (1971). 'Vigilance Performance and Attentional Selectivity in Educable Subnormal and Normal Children'. B.P.S. Exeter Conference (abstract).

Goldstein, K. (1939). 'The Organism'. New York: American Book Co.

Goldstein, K. (1942). *Charac. & Person.* **11**, 209.
Goldstein, K. and Scheerer, M. (1941). *Psychol. Monogs.* **53**, No. 2.
Halstead, W. C. (1947). 'Brain and Intelligence'. Chicago: Univers. Chicago Press.
Heath, S. R. (1942). *Amer. J. Psychol.* **55**, 240-247.
Heath, S. R. (1949). *Motor Skills Res. Exchange* **1**, 34-36.
Malpass, L. F. (1959). 'Responses of Retarded and Normal Children to Selected Clinical Measures. 1. Perceptual and Response Abilities of Retarded Children'. South University Press, Carbondale, Illinois.
Mein, R. (1961). *J. ment. Def. Res.* **5**, 52.
Mein, R. and O'Connor, N. (1960). *J. ment. Def. Res.* **4**, 130.
O'Connor, N. (1958). In 'Mental Deficiency: The Changing Outlook' (A. M. Clarke and A. D. B. Clarke, eds). London: Methuen.
O'Connor, N. and Haritos, M. (1953). Unpublished study.
O'Connor, N. and Hermelin, B. (1963). 'Speech and Thought in Severe Subnormality'. Oxford: Pergamon Press.
O'Connor, N. and Berkson, G. (1963). *Amer. J. ment. Def.* **68**, 1, 85.
O'Connor, N. and Hermelin, B. (1965). *Quart. J. expt. Psychol. XVII* **4**, 323.
Reitan, R. M. (1966). In 'International Review of Research in Mental Retardation' (N. R. Ellis, ed.), Vol. 1. New York: Academic Press.
Semmel, M. I. (1965). *Amer. J. ment. Defic.* **70**, 38-47.
Spitz, H. H. (1963). In 'Handbook of Mental Deficiency' (N. R. Ellis, ed.). New York: McGraw-Hill.
Strauss, A. A. (1941). *Amer. J. ment. Defic.* **45**, 548.
Strauss, A. A. and Lehtinen, L. E. (1947). 'Psychopathology and Education of the Brain-injured Child'. New York: Grune and Stratton.
Strauss, A. A. and Kephart, N. C. (1955). 'Psychopathology and Education of the Brain-injured Child', Vol. II, Progress in Theory and Clinic. New York: Grune and Stratton.
Sylvester, P. E. (1966). *J. Neurol. Neurosurg. Psychiat.* **29**, 176.
Venables, P. H. (1960). *B.J. Psychol.* **51**, 37.
Wortis, J. (1956). *Amer. J. ment. Def.* **61**, 204.
Zeaman, P. and House, B. J. (1963). In 'Handbook of Mental Deficiency' (N. R. Ellis, ed.). New York: McGraw-Hill.

DISCUSSION

Rundle: One aspect of growth that I was unable to touch on yesterday, which must also apply to psychologists in this field is that a lot of the previous results were probably due to bias in the sample, caused by tendency not to measure those difficult to measure. Is this true in psychology? Are you going to measure attention in a very hyperactive brain-damaged child?

O'Connor: It would obviously be rather difficult to do this, but we have done it. In autistic children, who may or may not be brain damaged, but who are very hyperactive we have used transmission techniques coupled with simple EEG. From this we have results suggesting that autistic children have a very short period of visual fixation, whereas on the other hand they show a failure to adapt to auditory signals. Another approach is to measure vigilance, that is to say the capacity with which a subnormal child can detect signals in different parts of the visual field over a long period of time. We are not in fact rejecting the possibility of examining the disturbed child in this way, and attention is getting, one might say, a lot of attention! It is complicated by the fact that attention is not only arousal, but is selective curiosity.

Harris: On the matter of flicker fusion tests, in a normal series something like 13.4% of children have, in fact, abnormal electrical responses to photic stimulation. I wonder if this does not play a part in some of these tests, that if you were not monitoring electrical changes it might make assessment of the test rather more difficult.

O'Connor: I think that would be so. Nowadays, people use the two-flash technique where there is not much danger of inducing a fit. Usually, with one flash, we just measure alpha interruption.

Balázs: In defence of our hormone-treated animals, what I tried to say in my talk was that there were two major ways in which the organisation of the CNS can be affected by hormones. One is by deletion of certain cells, and most of those are non-cortical, such as the microneurones in the hippocampus, the olfactory bulb and the cerebellum that are formed post-natally. The other effect related to differentiation of the neurones is not so specific. For example, treating animals with thyroid hormone, produces an acceleration of spine formation on the cells in the cerebral cortex. This means that differentiation can be affected in the cerebral cortex in a lower animal, and presumably in man. The other factor which is probably important is that cell migration, which may be related to connections between cells, can be definitely affected by hormones.

O'Connor: There are one or two points that I missed making. The strength of the generalised arousal approach is that it reflects the general lack of CNS alertness in this group, and thus appears to account better for the developmental retardation. It is a uniform response and not like, say, receptive aphasia in childhood where there is one specific disability. On the other hand, one of its bad points is that it cannot explain the more complex processes like coding, language formation, in the subnormal. Although it might account for a lot of the phenomena we observe in the subnormal, it does not account for these patterns we are talking about, and for phenomena like abstractions and coding. So that I agree with Dr. Balázs that we ought to look for it, but unless we go a lot further with the sort of thing he was talking about, the kind of cells affected at particular stages of development, we will not get anywhere near the connection between behaviour and the cell, and we will have to go on using the well known 'black box' which psychologists on the whole have resorted to. Sad to say I feel that the field is not much use to psychologists, so I work elsewhere. I very much hope we could come closer together, but it depends a bit on how worthwhile it is going to be.

Wigglesworth: If the EEG is of no use in determining intelligence, can I ask whether it is helpful in determining grouping with psychological tests, apart from epilepsy?

O'Connor: If you consider whether or not there is a longer alpha interruption-time, or when we took autistic children and tested them in conditions where we equated them on mental age and other things and on percentage alpha with control groups, and then measured their response to continued or interrupted visual signals. If you have this sort of approach with EEG you can get results which differentiate, for example, the autistic child, diagnosed psychiatrically, and an equivalent subnormal or normal child. There are other approaches using the EEG, such as the unexplained finding I made with Prof. Venables many years ago, where we got a very strong inverse relationship between skin conductance and intelligence, which remains unexplained, but has been confirmed.

Dobbing: I would like to underline what Dr. Balázs has said. We have recent findings that make it clear that certain layers of cerebral cortex are deficient in neurone numbers following very mild undernutrition.

What I would like to ask is that it seems that you can be descriptive about mental retardation in your discipline. One can also be diagnostic. Is it possible to say that you can be preventive?

O'Connor: I have usually felt that this was something that psychologists could not be, and if they wanted to become effective in any way, they had better get out of that field. But of course that is not entirely true. Thus, I suppose, if their techniques were refined enough, they could detect early on possible deficiencies and suggest a special training that might prevent the maldevelopment of, say language. We are currently studying 'babbling' in mongols and in normal children, and we find that 'babbling' at nine months is normal, although we know that language is going to become defective at some point. One might on this basis begin certain regimens of training that might be effective. But I can't think of any way at the moment of going much further than this. You have raised an important issue, namely that of cell population and cell size. Whether it will be possible to look at those where these differences have occurred, and their possible psychological results, I cannot say.

Dobbing: Personally, I think cell size in the brain is a pretty poor thing to talk about. What do you mean by cell size when you have axons a yard long?

O'Connor: I just wondered whether, on whatever theory of association and learning one might have, that association might be more possible in one instance, whereas attention night be affected by the other condition. In relation to Dr. Zlotnik's paper, attention is usually affected by the state of the hippocampus.

Prestige: Is it possible to distinguish whether in a subnormal child this was due to real retardation in the sense of elongation of the developmental process, or whether it was due to dysfunction? One could say that a lesion is present, of a certain sort, and ask whether this has caused retardation or dysfunction?

O'Connor: I toy with this question all the time and currently I am trying to see whether one can find a phenomenon or two which is the general result of a specific disability, such as when three digits are presented to a certain group, either visually or auditorially. The result will depend to some extent upon the input defect, and there may be other phenomena of that sort. On the whole, in subnormality, it is difficult to find specific phenomena. In autism, one phenomenon is the large digit-span which may be up to six or seven digits, whereas in the severely subnormal this might be only three or two. These are specific deficits, or specific abilities, because the I.Q. is often as low in autism as in the severely subnormal child. The sad thing about the subnormal is that development does occur, but why does it not occur more selectively? This is my number one question. Why does everything appear to be retarded equally?

Kirman: Would it underline what you said if you also mentioned Mary Woodward's work as well as Len Crome's, in as much as Dr. Crome finds that the great majority of the severely retarded do show structural abnormality. Therefore, they presumably have pretty gross cerebral dysfunction. Yet, as Mary Woodward showed the order of development, on the Piaget approach, is normal, although the timing of the stages is greatly delayed.

O'Connor: In a sense that is true, but on the other hand, it is also worrying. In the obvious case of the mongol, where there is a normal incidence of epilepsy, if a similar phenomenon is found as with Dr. Sylvester, would not one expect a pattern of this kind as compared with a non-mongol that is affected at the same level, or might not one begin to look for differences between these two groups. What about the brachycephalic development of the cortex? Isn't this relevant say to short-term memory for instance? What is it that accounts for the supposed lack of verbal facility in the mongol, which probably may be a false presumption? What effects does the cerebellar defect have? What might one expect in mongolism from the defect in frontal lobe development? Should not one expect differences between mongol and non-mongol children to appear more clearly because of these differences in development of the CNS?

Prestige: But this, in fact, is the interesting point to an outsider like myself. If the child is growing up with some external function to be achieved, and it is presented with the wrong or inadequate materials to achieve this, although it does so but more slowly, then one could argue that treatment and assistance is going to be very valuable. Whereas in a genuine dysfunction, one has to treat each particular case for the type of dysfunction present.

O'Connor: I have laid a lot of stress on this kind of thing because it does occur and one might expect in low performance cases one is getting dysfunction connected with their visuo-spatial, or visuo-motor function. This presumably is going to be lack of development of the right temporo-parietal side. Is one to look for special deficiencies in these and try to compensate for them? I think one can do it to some extent. Professor Tizard's and others' work has shown the possibilities of special treatment for certain groups of handicapped children. Their expected I.Q. of 80 may rise to well over 100. I happen to be somewhat sceptical about those results, but it might be a case in point. One needs rather more precise information.

Laurence: When there is handicap, there is usually some form of compensation to get round it. One would expect some similar compensation in mental retardation, and careful education might to some extent achieve this. I wonder how far the mental retardation we used to see in institutions may in fact be deprivation. How far do newer methods get round some of the gross retardation?

O'Connor: There is obviously only a beginning in this respect. The groups brought up in training schools should lead to some changes. There are certainly compensatory skills that we do not always become aware of. We studied the capacity to recognise shape visually and tactually, and although the visual capacity of the severely subnormal was very retarded, their capacity to recognise shape by touch was equivalent to the normal, except in the case of mongolism. There is another dramatic one, namely the genuine 'idiots savants' although their I.Q.'s are around 70.

Harris: About low performance. Dr. Gamstorp (Gamstorp, I. (1964) *Acta paediatrica* **53**, 408) studied nerve conduction velocity in lower and upper limbs of retarded children and found that the velocities were at the lower limits of the normal range in the upper limbs. She suggested that this might be linked with their clumsiness and so forth.

Kirman: One should mention briefly here that Dr. O'Connor is being unduly modest on behalf of the psychologists, who have made the major social contribution in this field. Apart from bringing into this field of behaviour, a scientific discipline, he with Tizard did a major job in showing the impact of these factors of deprivation, and that simple measures of rehabilitation could dramatically alter the lot of many retarded children.

Laurence: As I was hinting at, one hopes that mental subnormality with more education and training is going to be a shrinking problem.

General Discussion

OPENED BY J. STERN

Yesterday's speakers repeatedly stressed the multifactorial approach, for in so many instances it has been found that not one, but many aetiological factors come to play a part. In this connection, the emphasis is shifting further and further towards pregnancy about which more information is now becoming available, and it is furthermore quantitative information. Thus, for instance, the oestrogen and progesterone levels of the 'at-risk' pregnancy are being monitored. When the infant is born data on glucose, calcium and blood gases will be available, so that if, for example, a child's retina is damaged by excess oxygen, the problem can be related to pO_2. The case histories we see now refer not to 'jaundice', but to bilirubin levels and so forth. Now, looking at these children at Queen Mary's Hospital, who die or survive to be mentally retarded, the multifactorial nature of the disease process is again apparent. Thus, for instance, if a child has hypernatraemia solely due to deficient water intake, it may recover completely, while another with, perhaps, lower sodium levels, but also with an infection and hypothermia, may become mentally retarded. The same holds for bilirubin levels, where an association with prematurity septicaemia and acidosis may lead to kernicterus at bilirubin levels well below 20 mg/100 ml.

Another topic in the paper by Prof. Clayton is that of amino acid disturbances in the neonatal period and in the older child with mental retardation. A large number of environmental factors can affect these. Infections and even a circadian rhythm for example in the case of methionine (Feigin, R. D. (1969) *Amer. J. Dis. Child.* **117**, 24). Moreover, high levels of methionine may also be associated with abnormality, such as liver disease or simply a high protein intake. Another problem is amino acid imbalance and toxicity, mentioned by Prof. Giroud, which has been reviewed by Harper (Harper, A. E., Benerenga, N. D. and Wohlhueter, R. M. (1970) *Physiol. Rev.* **50**, 428). Professor Clayton and her group first drew attention in this country to the grave risk of the artificial diets given to children. For instance, if there is an imbalance in protein and calorie intake, there may be a detrimental effect on the liver, and abnormal findings have been recorded by morbid anatomists in the liver of mentally retarded cases that could conceivably arise from this cause. This field is not yet fully explored.

What should perhaps also be stressed is the iatrogenic effect of the prolonged use of antibiotics, anticonvulsants, and tranquillisers which can affect the clinical chemistry. The adverse effects on learning of large doses of barbiturates may well complicate the findings of the psychologists.

With regard to hormones, I would like to mention the classic study of Weil-Malherbe (Weil-Malherbe, H. (1955) *J. Ment. Sci.* **101**, 733) on the blood catecholamines in a variety of psychiatric disorders. He found that in mental subnormality there was a significantly low level which perhaps linked up with the lack of arousal which one finds in such cases. There was, moreover, a specific effect in phenylketonuria, where the levels were much lower still. There will always be a search for substances that can be related more directly to brain metabolism. Here one might mention the 5-hydroxyindoles in CSF or 3-methoxy-4-hydroxyphenyl glycol, a catecholamine derivative which is disproportionately representative of brain metabolism.

Enzyme polymorphism, as mentioned by Dr. Rundle, is of great interest, particularly its possible links with mental retardation. This certainly illustrates how inextricably heredity and environment are linked. Certain abnormalities in the enzyme patterns which are in themselves harmless, may become serious when the patient is confronted with an adverse environmental situation.

The hazards of lead intoxication have long been known but in the work of Prof. Clayton and her group lead poisoning was for the first time systematically related to the psychiatric state of the patient. A major unsolved problem is how to get rid of lead in the environment, and short of pulling down all the old hospitals, this is very nearly impossible. Even then other sources of lead are likely to be found by the children. The same almost certainly applies, of course, to other environmental hazards. Perhaps we should look to the psychologists to apply various conditioning behaviour-shaping techniques to stop the children taking in these substances, as well as improving the environment.

Professor Clayton's observations on sugars in the urine were of interest to me personally, because our findings have been very similar. Dr. Sylvester studied with us a case of sucrosuria, originally described by Moncrieff, and we found that the sucrosuria had disappeared. Later when the child died the neuropathology was quite different from that described in another case by Moncrieff (Stern, J. and Sylvester, P. E. (1962) Proc. London Conf. on Scientific Study of Mental Deficiency, p. 153. Dagenham: May & Baker; Moncrieff, A. A. and Wilkinson, R. H. (1954) *Acta paediatrica* **43**, Suppl. 100, 495). It seemed that this was not a syndrome in the sense of phenylketonuria. The possible toxic effect of sucrose is yet another aspect of this matter. Also, as a terminal change in very sick children, we have sometimes found disaccharides in the urine, particularly in gastrointestinal disorders.

At the Fountain Hospital we had the same dilemma as Dr. O'Connor for there, too, it was found that no matter what the aetiology or pathology, the patients, as demonstrated by Mary Woodward, went through the Piaget stages in exactly the same way. But I feel that both psychology and electrophysiology have the advantage over the morbid anatomist, because they can do serial studies. To be unable to do this is a distinct drawback in understanding virus infections of the type described by Dr. Zlotnik. One valuable new technique for electrophysiological studies is the evoked auditory response technique which offers a new approach to the study of non-communicating children. It involves, however, a great deal of expertise from the electrophysiologist, and the help of anaesthetist, recordist, technicians, nurses etc. This may limit the application of the method.

Crome: Dr. Stern has outlined a feast of possibilities, but I would like to ask Dr. Jellinger and the biochemists this question. The Viennese paediatrician called Rett (Rett, A. (1966) 'Uber ein Zerebral-atrophisches Syndrome bei Hyperammonaemie'. Vienna: Hollink) investigated a large number of cases of unclassified mental retardation, and found a significant increase in blood ammonia in many of the girls. He thought it to be a special syndrome, but without the usual progressive course of hyperammonaemia. How can this be explained?

Jellinger: I am not familiar with biochemical studies of Dr. Rett and his associates, but I have examined seven brains. In two we could exclude hyperammonaemia, for one had a gliotic encephalopathy and the other had severe chronic myositis. I suspect that part of his cases are symptomatic hyperammonaemia associated with other diseases. In four or five or these cases, one of which came from Innsbruck, there was a decreased activity of arginase and ornithine-carbamyl transferase. In these cases, ranging from 11 months to 12 years, one a boy, there was a certain degree of cerebral atrophy, but more important there were spongy lesions with hyperplasia and Alzheimer II changes in the astroglia. There was also some delayed myelination in one case and severely retarded pigmentation of the substantia nigra, as is also found in phenylketonuria. The majority do not, however, fulfil the criteria of hyperammonaemia and the CNS lesions are non-specific.

Cavanagh: If a woman with chronic liver disease becomes pregnant, does the foetus become affected?

Wigglesworth: I was interested in this. In advanced cirrhosis it is of course uncommon for them to become pregnant. From the literature, however, it appears that those with liver disease tend to have slightly low birth weight infants, but this seems to be the only finding.

Jellinger: We have looked at the brains of two foetuses whose mothers were in an advanced stage of liver disease, but there was nothing to be seen with the light microscope.

Wigglesworth: In inborn errors of metabolism, one of the problems is the ingestion of normal articles of diet which cause the damage. One thinks of this as a rather chronic process. However, in two recent cases from one family this was an acute effect. The first child had severe liver necrosis with subarachnoid and gastro-intestinal haemorrhages. The second child was found to have fructosaemia with liver damage. Both these were artificially fed and neither would have developed these symptoms if they had been breast fed. Such acute cases may be missed when causing trouble in the perinatal period.

Jellinger: I saw a very similar case with galactosaemia.

Stern: Many fructosaemics are said to be self-selective in their diet, according to the Swiss workers (Froesch, E. R. (1969) *J. clin. Path.* **22**, Suppl. Disorders of Carbohydrate Metabolism, p. 7).

Dobbing: We have been loading normal guinea pig foetuses with galactose, but found the same reduction of birth weight and of brain weight in the glucose-fed controls. The brains of the galactose-fed animals were, however, found to be lower than was appropriate for their body weight.

Cremer: Is the galactose and fructose competing with glucose or are these sugars harmful to the brain?

Dobbing: Our current feelings are that it is something specific to the galactose.

Hanefeld: Do they develop cataracts?

Dobbing: One animal did, but it was in the glucose group!

Balázs: It was mentioned that methionine was sometimes increased, and this seems probably to be the worst of the amino-acids in this context. It certainly stood out in schizophrenia as being the amino-acid that made things much worse. There seems to be a circadian rhythm for methionine levels, so that one ought to standardise the time of sampling.

Clayton: In a big screening programme, one cannot really standardise the time of sampling. But the raised methionines referred to were so high, you cannot really miss them. Later you can standardise the time as you investigate them in more detail.

Davison: We have repeated some of our work using methionine instead of phenylalanine and its effects on brain protein synthesis, and it seems that these large amounts of methionine prevent the entry of other essential amino-acids into brain. A unifying hypothesis might be that an imbalance of any one of those amino-acids is going to affect brain protein and amino-acid metabolism.

Dobbing: We know that the transport mechanisms into the brain are shared by two or three amino-acids. Is it these that show a common carrier mechanism that are affected or are they all affected?

Davison: It is the sharing of the common carrier mechanism that leads to the inhibition.

Stern: According to Udenfriend (Udenfriend, S. (1963) *Amer. J. Clin. Nutrit.* **12**, 287), there are also carrier mechanisms that are not common to other tissues.

Clayton: Transient rises in plasma amino-acids are common in premature babies. I would be interested to know Dr. Drillien's view on the feeding of these children.

Drillien: I am sure that breast milk is best. The artificial diets to keep the amino-acid intake satisfactory are not particularly successful.

Stern: Harper (loc. cit.) particularly stresses methionine toxicity and also that it is affected both by threonine, and by carbohydrate-protein balances.

Dobbing: Reducing calorie intake to levels of frank malnutrition does effectively produce a low protein situation.

Is it not better to think of amino-acids in groups when considering how to maintain a good balance for these cases?

Clayton: Before one embarks on artificial diet for these purposes, one has to have good evidence that the findings are harmful. I do not think we have this at present. The artificial diet might produce far worse results than letting the thing run its habitual course. Personally I would hesitate selectively to reduce groups of amino-acids in the diet.

Dobbing: I was thinking rather of the balance of the amino-acids within the groups.

Clayton: But this would lead to a very artificial type of feed.

Hanefeld: Many of the inborn errors of metabolism produce mental retardation in the new born, but how can one explain the apparent onset of the known metabolic disorders at very much later ages?

Balázs: Genetic factors probably come in here, don't they? Some of the mutants in mice with myelin deficiency are well until 16-17 days of age, and then they begin to show defects.

Davison: The point is, surely, that the patient is mentally quite normal and then suddenly things go wrong. The reason is that in metachromatic leucodystrophy, say, sulphatide is accumulating at that time. But why is it that in this case, where sulphatide is preferentially located in myelin, that the effects are on mental ability?

Jellinger: Is this in part at least a question of the reduction of enzyme activity? In heterozygotes there may be some retardation, but this does not cause symptoms.

Davison: In metachromatic leucodystrophy it seems to be a failure of catabolic enzymes, and altered balance. It comes later because at this time regulatory balance between synthesis and breakdown is important in the brain. But why should dysmyelination have any effect upon intellect?

Laurence: But surely there is a gradation of effects. The first change is often a behaviour disorder. Later intellectual deficit occurs. That is, the most sensitive functions get noticed first.

Magee: It is not quite clear to me when do we know that these children have got mental retardation? When looking for a causal factor, it would be helpful to know at what time to concentrate one's attention.

Kirman: This is a fundamental question. Any one of a number of diseases lie somewhat outside this discussion because of the timing. It is important to contrast this with, say, acrocephalosyndactyly which seems to be a genetically determined disturbance of development when at a very early stage some as yet unknown enzyme is at the peak of its activity. There is no straight answer to this question in fact. Some appear at birth while others may be as late as five years of age or later with milder mental retardation.

Harris: In some of the inborn errors one can say from the EEG point of view that the child has got it earlier than from other standpoints. This becomes apparent particularly in sibling studies.

Zlotnik: There is the 'reeler' syndrome in mice connected with cerebellar and hippocampal developmental failure. In spite of this, even though it is controlled by a single gene, it may be at least six weeks before they show the specific disturbances of function.

Crome: There are many human parallels of this. Hydrencephaly for instance, where the cerebral hemispheres may be completely absent, the baby may appear to be quite normal for 12 weeks or so.

Rundle: May I make a plea for the normal person? The late onset of chemical and other changes is not restricted to the abnormal. Puberty, for instance, begins very much earlier than the crude external characters would suggest, and may even be laid down at birth.

6
Morphological Aspects of Unclassified Mental Retardation

Defects in CSF Pathways and Unclassified Mental Retardation

K. M. LAURENCE

Before the development of the ventriculo-atrial shunts, made possible by the introduction in the middle of the 1950's of the newer plastics and inert silicone rubbers, most children who developed hydrocephalus died with progressive head enlargement, but sometimes not before this reached the grotesque proportions. However, in some without any surgical treatment, the condition would arrest spontaneously, but not usually before head enlargement and intellectual deficit had occurred (Laurence and Coates, 1962). Even today, with the modern surgical techniques available, treatment is far from satisfactory, and many patients suffer from mental retardation not only as a result of the hydrocephalus which brought the child to surgeon, but also from complications of treatment, such as valve infections or acute episodes of progressive hydrocephalus resulting from blockage of the valve system.

In this paper it is intended to examine the causes and effects of hydrocephalus and see how far it is possible to relate the degree of hydrocephalus to the amount of intellectual deficit.

Causes of Hydrocephalus

Hydrocephalus may be defined as the excessive amount of cerebrospinal fluid within the cranial cavity. The variety secondary to brain atrophy or abiotrophy, 'hydrocephalus evacuo', where excessive amounts of cerebrospinal fluid replace the volume within the cranial cavity which should have been occupied by the brain, will not be discussed in this paper. This apart, hydrocephalus may be due to three different causes (Table 1).

TABLE 1

Causes of Hydrocephalus

Overproduction of C.S.F.	—	Choroid plexus papilloma
Underabsorption of C.S.F.	—	Venous thrombosis
Obstruction of the pathways	—	Within the ventricular system
	—	In the subarachnoid space
	—	by skull abnormalities

Overproduction of Cerebrospinal Fluid

Overproduction is present in a large proportion of the rare choroid plexus papillomata. These tumours, of which about 500 are on record, form about 3% of childhood intracranial tumours, but are less common in adults (Laurence, 1972). They are usually large (Fig. 1) and have a microscopic structure indistinguishable from the normal choroid plexus; although these papillomata, when situated in the lateral ventricle, do not cause obstruction, they give rise to a symmetrical and often quite severe hydrocephalus affecting the whole of the ventricular system and the basal cisterns as well. Cerebrosopinal fluid production in excess of 1000 ml per day (i.e. 30 times the normal amount) may be precipitated by such procedures as ventricular punctures which disturb the internal milieu. Such amounts can be drained at continuous ventricular drainage. This production is undoubtedly caused by the greatly increased bulk of functionally normal choroid plexus tissue. These cases are, however, not quite straightforward, for many have a co-existing obstructive hydrocephalus due to basal cistern block, probably as a result of minor haemorrhage from the excessively vascular tumour.

Underabsorption

This is a theoretical possibility when the venous return from the brain is impaired in such conditions as cortical vein and sagitttal sinus thrombosis. Although underabsorption is probably present in the acute phase of these conditions, it does not seem to persist for any length of time. Another cause for any ventricular dilatation present can usually be found, such as the co-existent obstruction to the cerebrospinal fluid pathway or atrophy of the brain following interference with its blood supply.

Obstruction to the Cerebrospinal Fluid Pathway

Nearly all cases of hydrocephalus seen clinically fall into this group

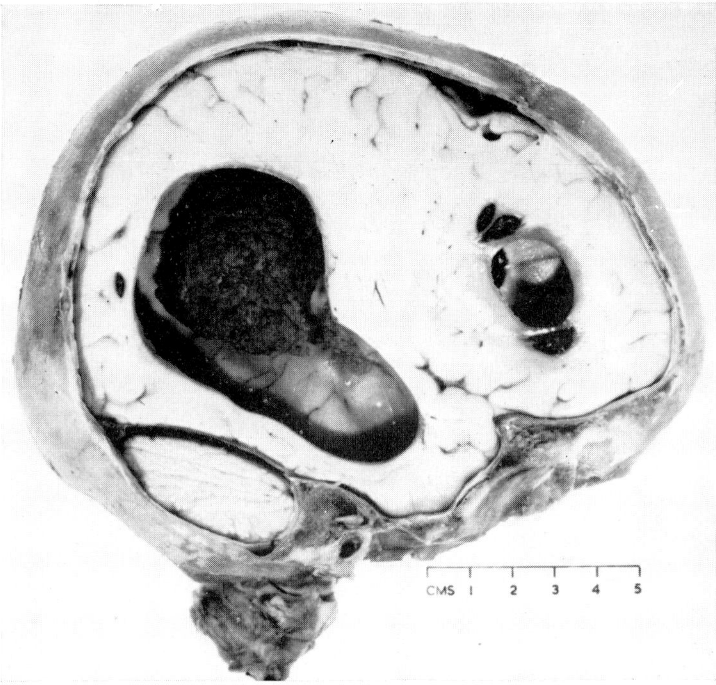

Fig. 1. Parasagittal section of a skull of a 9 months old boy. A large rounded papilloma of the choroid plexus is situated in the posterior horn of a dilated lateral ventricle.

[*To face p. 270*

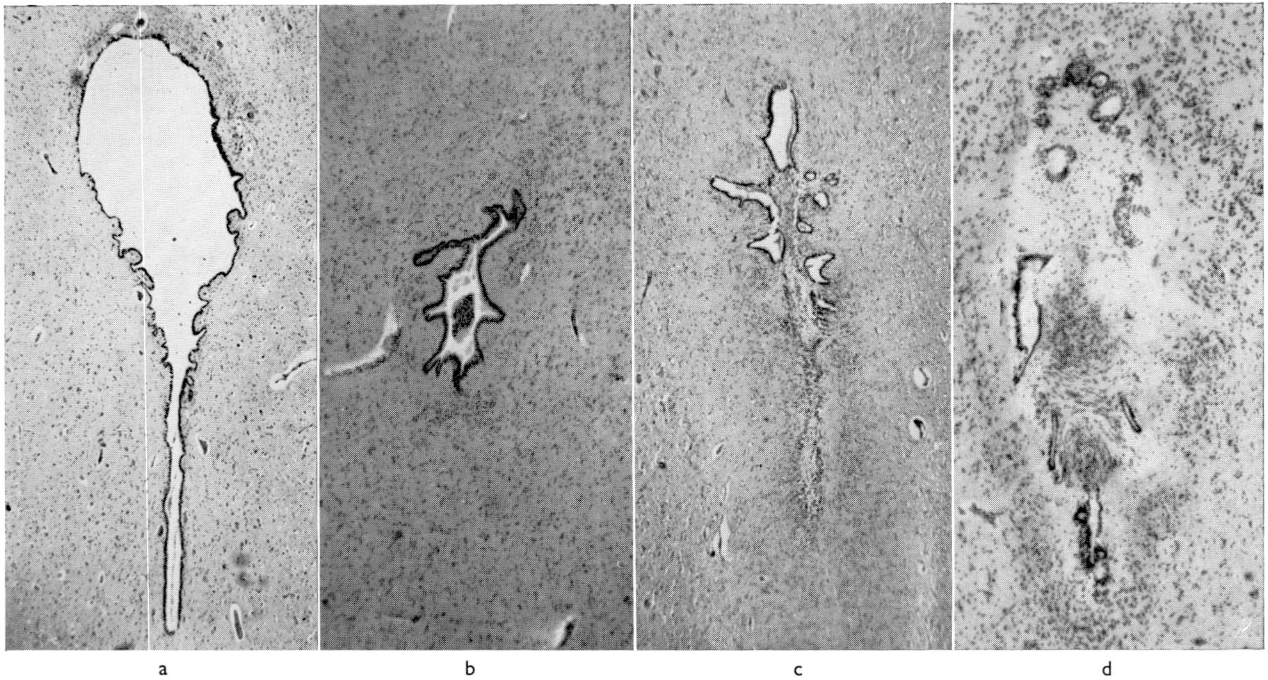

Fig. 2. Photomicrographs of the aqueduct at the level of the inferior colliculus (H & E × 60)

(a) Normal aqueduct in a newborn. This is a single ependymal lined channel 1 mm. in diameter.

(b) Aqueduct stenosis in a 1 year old girl. The narrow channel is irregular in outline, lined with intact ependyma and is surrounded by normal brain tissue.

(c) Congenital aqueduct forking in an 8 week old girl. The several small ependyma-lined channels are separated by brain tissue free from gliosis.

(d) Post-inflammatory aqueduct gliosis in an 8 year old boy. The channel has been broken up into a number of small ones partially lined by ependyma and by dense glia.

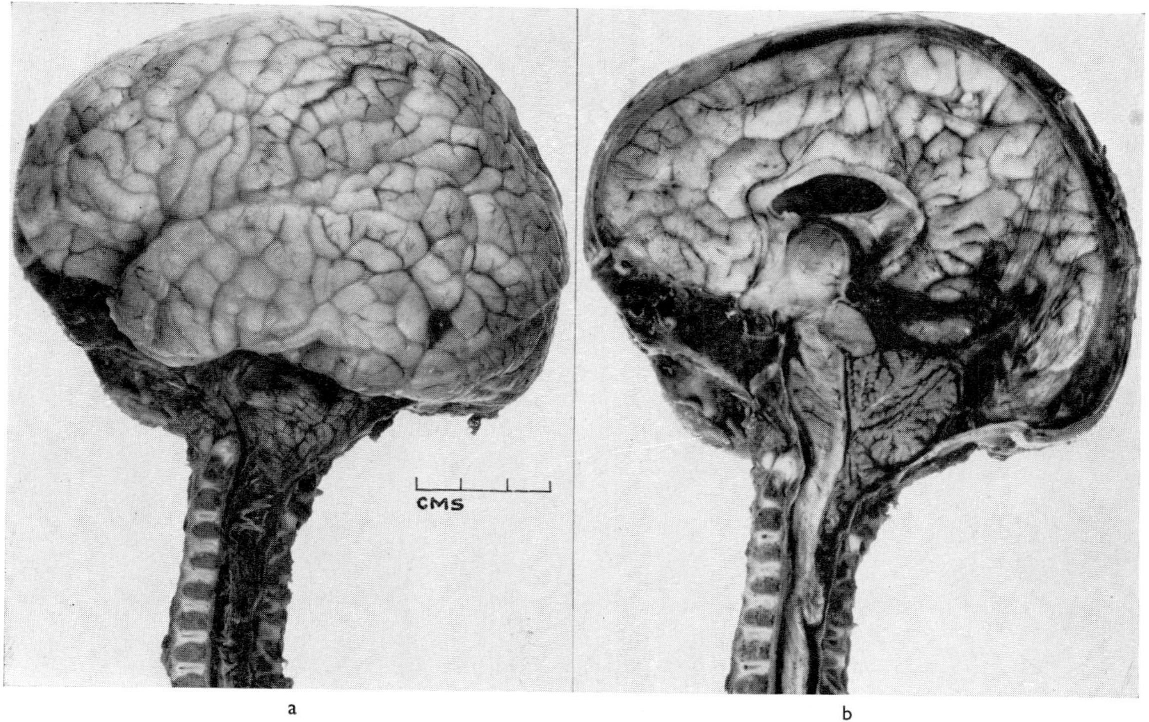

Fig. 3. A dissected skull and vertebral column of a one week old girl.

(a) The surface of the cerebral hemisphere has flattened convolutions, and the hind brain which is closely moulded by the contours of the skull is covered by thickened congested meninges. Note the cranial direction of the upper spinal nerve roots.

(b) Midline section. The cerebral hemisphere with a dilated lateral ventricle (seen through the defect in the septum pellucidum) and the Arnold-Chiari malformation, with its cerebellar extension down the spinal canal. The elongated and kinked medulla and elongated fourth ventricle are well illustrated.

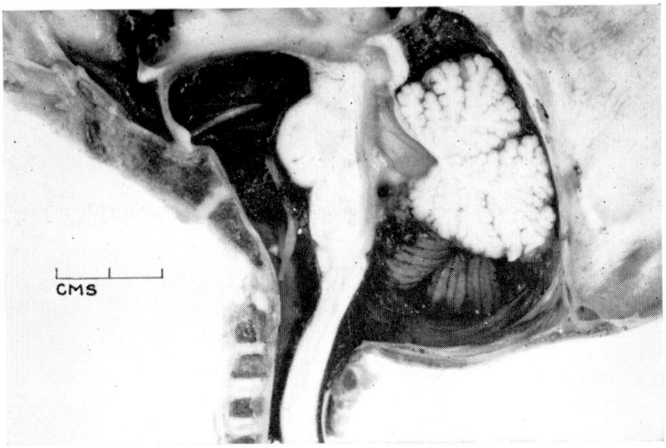

Fig. 4. Hemisected skull in a case of basal cistern block in a 6-months-old girl. The dilated lower half of the third ventricle, aqueduct and fourth ventricle are illustrated. Indian ink had been injected into the distended basal cisterns which has outlined the cisterna magna posteriorly and the cisterna interpeduncularis and chiasmaticus anteriorly. The pituitary stalk has been stretched and the anterior lobe of the pituitary gland has almost been detached from the posterior lobe.

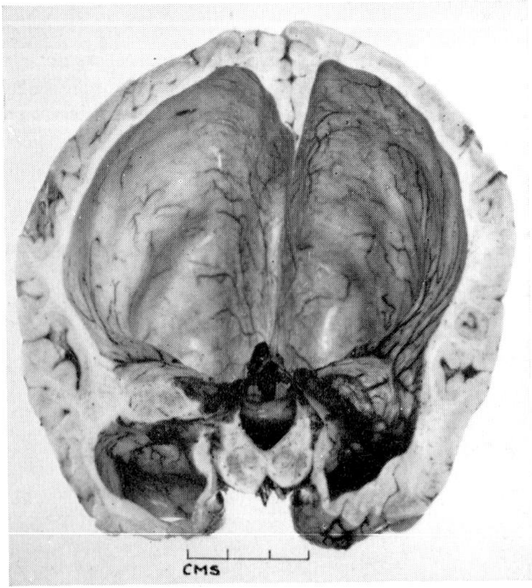

Fig. 5. A coronal section through the brain of a severely hydrocephalic 1 year old boy. There is considerable unfolding of the cerebral convolutions. The lateral ventricles are severely and symmetrically dilated, and the cerebral mantle has been greatly reduced in thickness but largely at the expense of the cerebral white matter, while the grey matter has retained its normal thickness except in the temporal lobes.

(Laurence, 1959). When obstruction is present the ventricular system proximal to the obstruction dilates as the choroid plexuses in the ventricles usually continue to form cerebrospinal fluid. Thus, if the lateral and third ventricles are dilated while the remainder of the pathways are of normal dimensions, the obstruction will be found in the aqueduct of Sylvius. When the whole of the ventricular system is enlarged and the basal cisterns are normal, then an exit foramina block will be present. However, as there are two sets of choroid plexuses, one within the lateral ventricles, the other within the fourth ventricle, dilatation of the fourth ventricle may be associated with an aqueduct block if there is also a block of the exit foraminae or of the basal cisterns present.

Obstructive lesions to be considered may be due (a) to maldevelopments or (b) to inflammatory lesions.

MALDEVELOPMENTS

The aqueduct of Sylvius, normally a single narrow channel about 1 cm in length with a cross-sectional diameter of less than 1 mm that links the third and the fourth ventricle and is completely lined by ependyma and is surrounded by normal brain tissue free from gliosis, may be the site of two abnormalities: namely, stenosis and forking. *Stenosis* is an uncommon condition usually found in isolation. In this the channel may be completely obliterated, or the cross-sectional diameter may be very grossly reduced and have a crenated outline, but still possessing a complete ependymal lining (Fig. 2a). There should be no gliosis in the surrounding brain tissue. *Forking,* on the other hand is fairly common and is usually found in association with myelocoeles. Here the aqueduct is split into a number of separate irregular channels, some of which end blindly, but all are lined with intact ependyma. There is often one larger dorsal and a number of smaller ventral channels, but the effective channel has been grossly reduced. Normal brain tissue free from gliosis usually intervenes between these channels (Fig. 2b).

The most important malformation associated with hydrocephalus is *spina bifida cystica,* which is seen in about 2.5 out of every 1000 babies born in the United Kingdom (Laurence *et al.*, 1968). The myelocoele, the commonest form of spina bifida cystica, is where the neural tube has failed to close and spina cord tissue is exposed on the surface as the *zona vasculosa.* This is usually associated with a hind brain malformation, known as the *Arnold-Chiari malformation.* The latter consists of a poorly formed and often small cerebellum with an elongated vermis which usually extends down the spinal canal, an elongated pons, and an abnormal elongated medulla that may also extend below the level of the foramen magnum. An elongated fourth ventricle, with its choroid plexus tissue, lies between these structures. The whole malformation within its small posterior fossa is closely moulded by the bony structures and is covered by congested and often thickened meninges (Fig. 3). The basal cisterns may be obliterated. Apart from the Arnold-Chiari malformation other anomalies may be found in the brain, such as micropolygyria, porencephalic cysts, ectopic subependymal grey matter, fusion of the two thalamic bodies, upward herniation of the cerebellum, and, of course, aqueduct abnormalities.

There are three main causes for the hydrocephalus associated with spina bifida cystica. Aqueduct forking is seen in about 25% of the cases and leads to hydrocephalus, often severe and progressive, which may be obvious at birth. The Arnold-Chiari malformation, by virtue of the overcrowding of the structures within the posterior fossa, also leads to hydrocephalus that is seen in about 80% of all cases of myelocoele. In such instances the hydrocephalus tends to be less severe and may indeed arrest spontaneously. Hyperaemia and eventual fibrosis and thickening of the meninges that surrounds the Arnold-Chiari malformation may further interfere with the already embarrassed cerebrospinal fluid circulation and lead to progression of the hydrocephalus. However, most serious of all, is the effect of ascending infection from the raw spina bifida sac. Thus, an inflammatory obstruction to the aqueduct or to the exit foramina, less commonly the foramina of Munro or basal cisterns, may be superimposed on the congenital malformations that may already be present. This usually will lead to a rapidly progressive hydrocephalus, which because of active inflammation is not often readily amenable to surgical correction.

INFLAMMATORY CHANGES

In this large and important group the commonest cause is bleeding into the cerebrospinal fluid pathways following delivery. Such deliveries need not be obviously traumatic nor need there have been any signs of intracranial mischief at birth. When a subdural haematoma is found, it is likely that the same injury will have also produced bleeding into the cerebrospinal fluid pathways and probably parenchymal brain damage as well. Other causes of bleeding, such as haemorrhage from a berry aneurysm, from operations, or from head injuries in childhood, may also give rise to hydrocephalus.

Infection is the other important cause. This may be acute or chronic, and be bacterial, viral, or parasitic. Usually the milder infections produce the worst effects, for such cases may be missed, may receive only late treatment, or on occasion receive none at all. On the other hand, a fulminating *B. coli* meningitis in the neonatal period may be completely silent. With all these meningeal infections, associated parenchymal brain damage must be borne in mind, for these conditions are often more akin to a meningoencephalitis. However, in a considerable proportion of cases where in retrospect some inflammatory process must have occurred no actual aetiological factor is found.

A variety of anatomical lesions may follow such inflammations. The severest, usually following neonatal meningitis, may result in an organising pyocephalus in which the ventricular system may be converted into a series of intercommunicating cysts. In less severe inflammation the aqueduct may become blocked by pus or by a blood clot, while inflammatory damage involving the ependymal lining may lead to denudation of the ependymal cells. Once lost these cells will not regenerate, and the sub-ependymal glia will proliferate and eventually may completely block the aqueduct (Fig. 2c). In the majority of cases, however, the inflammatory reaction takes place in the meninges producing either a block of the exit foramina of the fourth ventricle, or more commonly in the basal cisterns (Fig. 4). Any combination of these lesions may be present in a particular case; thus inflammatory aqueduct stenosis may well be associated with block of the exit foramina and of the basal cistern as well.

Other causes of hydrocephalus, such as the rare septum of the aqueduct, the Dandy-Walker syndrome, the extremely rare hamartomatus gliosis of the aqueduct, and tumours of the brain and skull abnormalities will not be considered here.

Anatomical Effects of Hydrocephalus

In the infant the distensible skull and the soft brain enlarge to accommodate cerebrospinal fluid, but the weight of brain tissue remains relatively normal for the age until the hydrocephalus becomes severe. As the cerebral mantle becomes stretched and reduced in thickness, the cerebral convolutions become progressively unfolded. This is usually most pronounced in the occipital and temporal lobes, while the parietal lobes seem to be relatively spared. Nor does the loss of tissue, when it occurs, fall equally on grey and white matter, for the grey matter, both cortical and in the basal nuclear complex, remains relatively normal in extent while the white matter becomes rapidly reduced and stretched until it is represented by a grossly attenuated strip, a mere millimetre or so in depth (Fig. 5). It is only when the hydrocephalus becomes gross that the grey matter also becomes reduced in extent. However, long before this happens the number of neurones are reduced and those that remain may be anoxic (Granholm and Siesjo, 1970) probably from interference with the blood supply for the cerebral vascular bed is considerably reduced as the hydrocephalus progresses (Hassler, 1964).

Structures such as the corpus callosum and the septum pellucidum become stretched and reduced, while the latter may largely disappear, eventually leading to a single lateral ventricular cavity. The choroid plexuses remain normal for some time, but as the condition becomes chronic they tend to atrophy and ultimately become reduced to small fibrous nodules. This change may, in fact, be part of the mechanism in spontaneous arrest. The ventricular ependyma becomes stretched and partially denuded and the subependymal glia proliferate leading to the familiar granular ependymitis (Russell, 1949). Occasionally the ventricular walls rupture to produce white matter cavitation (Granholm and Radberg, 1965) and cystic dilatation along needle tracks at ventricular punctures may dilate markedly giving appearances akin to porencephaly (Lorber and Grainger, 1963).

With successful surgical treatment of hydrocephalus there may be considerable recovery in the thickness of the cerebral mantle, especially if the condition had not advanced too far before operation (Grotte and Lundberg, 1961). However, most of the damage to white matter and neurones is likely to be irreparable, and probably accounts for much of the neurological abnormalities and intellectual deficits shown by patients with advanced hydrocephalus.

Incidence

Reliable figures of the incidence of hydrocephalus are not available. This is probably because of the variable pathology and aetiology of the condition and because in so many instances the hydrocephalus is not the only major problem. In addition, different criteria seem to have been used. McKeown and Record (1960) in their investigation of CNS malformations in Birmingham list spina bifida unassociated with hydrocephalus at birth in 1.76 per 1000 births, while the South Wales investigation (Laurence *et al.*, 1968) list hydrocephalus without spina bifida cystica (i.e. uncomplicated hydrocephalus) in only 0.45 per 1000 births. It is likely that the Birmingham survey included some cases associated with spina bifida cystica, some chromosome abnormalities, and also cases with acquired hydrocephalus. It is possible that macerated stillbirths which sometimes give the impression of hydrocephaly may well have been included. It seems that 'uncomplicated' congenital hydrocephalus is a relatively rare condition.

Most cases of hydrocephalus in the United Kingdom, with its high incidence of spina bifida cystica, are associated with this abnormality; fewer are acquired mostly due to birth trauma or meningitis.

Most cases of the congenital hydrocephalus have severe dilatation of the ventricular system at birth, many are stillborn and few survive (Table 2). Hydrocephalus associated with spina bifida cystica, especially if at all severe, seems to have the gravest prognostic significance for survival in that condition (Laurence, 1964). However, with atrioventricular shunt operations employing modern valve systems, such as the Holter or the Pudenz valves, and with the vigorous use of antibiotics for ascending meningitis and valve infections, 60% or more of the cases of spina bifida cystica with hydrocephalus should be enabled to survive.

TABLE 2

Incidence of Hydrocephalus

Causes of hydrocephalus	*Incidence per 1,000 births*	*Percentage survival*
Congenital (excluding Spina Bifida Cystica)	0.5	20%
Associated with Spina Bifida Cystica	2.0*	60%
Acquired	0.7**	90%

* 80% of the incidence of myelocoele.
** According to McKeown and Record (1960).

There seems to be no reliable figures available for the incidence of acquired hydrocephalus. In any case the incidence is likely to vary considerably with the quality of obstetric care and the incidence of meningitis. Probably the most useful figures are those of McKeown and Record (1960) which suggest an incidence of about 0.7 per 1000 births. These cases have a much better prognosis for survival, some 90% reaching school age. With an estimated total incidence of all forms of hydrocephalus at 3.2 per 1000 births, one would expect over 3000 new cases to present each year. Of these, about 2000, mostly associated spina bifida cystica, would be expected to reach school age.

Degree of Hydrocephalus and Performance

To examine the performance of hydrocephalics, 70 cases of hydrocephalus without spina bifida cystica were examined neurologically and psychologically. The degree of hydrocephalus was divided into slight, moderate, severe and gross (i.e. a cerebral mantle of more than 4 cm, 2-4 cm, 1-2 cm, and less than 1 cm respectively) at the time of the acute phase of the condition. It was found that there was a highly significant relationship between intelligence quotient and the degree of hydrocephalus ($p < 0.001$), with those who have more severe thinning of the cerebral mantle tending to have lower intelligence scores (Table 3). Exceptions included six patients who had only slight or moderate hydrocephalus scoring less than 49, who probably suffered severe parenchymal brain damage independent of the hydrocephalus.

TABLE 3

Intelligence and Hydrocephalus without Spina Bifida

Degree of hydrocephalus	*Mean*	*Intelligence quotient* < *20*	*49*	*84*	*99*	> *100*	*Totals*
Slight	92.2 (113.0)	1	–	–	1	3	5
Moderate	82.7 (96.3)	4	1	4	8	10	27
Severe	64.0 (70.7)	2	3	11	4	1	21
Gross	45.1 (64.6)	6	3	6	2	–	17
Total	–	13	7	21	15	14	70

Mean given in brackets is computed without one case with an I.Q. of less than 20.

Their clinical histories, namely of severe birth anoxia in two, meningitis not diagnosed before some days in two more, and the finding of unilateral neurological signs in a further case, would be consistent with such a view. Six of the eight patients with severe or gross hydrocephalus who had intelligence quotients of less than 20, also had some unilateral signs, suggesting that they too suffered from parenchymal brain damage.

A further 41 cases where the hydrocephalus was associated with a myelocoele from two investigations (Laurence, 1964; Laurence and Tew, 1971) were examined in a similar manner (Table 4). The same relationship between intelligence quotient and the degree of hydrocephalus was found, but in this group the mean intelligence quotient was considerably greater for each degree of hydrocephalus than in those cases with acquired hydrocephalus. The most striking difference between the two series was that where hydrocephalus was due to a malformation, there was less evidence of parenchymal brain damage, borne out by the finding of only one patient who had an intelligence quotient of less than 20, a case who suffered from intracranial infection which responded only slowly to treatment. If all cases with intelligence quotients less than 20 (i.e. those who almost certainly suffered from severe parenchymal brain damage independent of their hydrocephalus) are excluded the mean intelligence quotients in relation to the degree of hydrocephalus in the two series are almost identical. This supports the contention that there is probably little difference in the quality of the intellect, between acquired and congenital hydrocephalus, provided the patient has not suffered from focal parenchymal brain damage.

TABLE 4

Intelligence and Hydrocephalus with Myelocoele

Degree of hydrocephalus	*Mean*	*Intelligence quotient* < 20	49	84	99	> 100	*Totals*
Slight	106.1	–	–	3	6	5	14
Moderate	91.0	–	–	8	3	3	14
Severe	68.3 (78.2)	1	1	1	3	1	7
Gross	62.2	–	1	4	1	–	6
Total		1	2	16	13	9	41

Mean given in brackets is computed without one case with an I.Q. of less than 20.

Contrary perhaps to the theme of this symposium, hydrocephalic patients, with non-specific mental retardation, in the absence of spina bifida cystica or focal brain damage, show quite characteristic neurological and intellectual defects. They tend to have spasticity which is more marked in the legs and the arms, tremor of the hands and feet, clumsiness of the fine finger movements, ataxia and imbalance. All these neurological features are not only much more frequently present when the hydrocephalus is more marked, but tend to be also more severe. In the more markedly affected individual the neurological deficit amounts almost to a combination of a cerebellar ataxia with a spastic diplegia (Ingram and Naunton, 1962). Intellectually, too, the more severe hydrocephalics tend to have a significantly greater incidence of scatter in the results of the various sub-tests of the intelligence examination, to have a shallow intellect somewhat more frequently, to function more often below expectation, and to be more emotionally labile. These features, too, tend to be more pronounced the more severe the hydrocephalus (Laurence, 1969). Indeed, one of the most characteristic intellectual features is the 'cocktail party syndrome', as it is called by Hadenius and her co-workers (1962). This is more often found in girls than boys and in those who have limited intelligence (I.Q. range 50-75). They tend to be sociable, pseudo-bright, love to chatter and to have a vocabulary level well above their general psychometric level. Their language development is usually within normal limits, if not in advance of expectation, in contrast to the delayed motor development. There is a specific memory at an early age, but they have little appreciation of the content of their talk, they have illogical thought processes and little ability to reason. Hagberg and Sjögren (1966) regard these features, both motor and intellectual, of such hydrocephalic patients to be so typical that they have designated them as the 'chronic brain syndrome of infantile hydrocephalus'. On the other hand, in some hydrocephalics where there is little obvious intellectual impairment detected by methods at our disposal nor any motor disability, the effect of hydrocephalus nervertheless may show itself as an emotional liability and lack of self-reliance which lead eventually to performing in life below, and sometimes considerably below, what would be expected by their test results.

Summary

Hydrocephalus may be due to oversecretion or underabsorption of cerebrospinal fluid, or to obstruction of the cerebrospinal fluid pathways, the last accounting for nearly all the cases seen clinically. The malformations are described, such as aqueduct forking, and the Arnold-Chiari anomaly with spina bifida and the inflammatory lesions secondary to both trauma or meningitis, that may cause this obstruction. It is pointed out that in hydrocephalus associated with spina bifida, inflammatory lesions are frequently superimposed upon malformations that are already present. The sequence of anatomical changes which occur as the ventricular system dilates, such as progressive white matter reduction, are described.

The incidence of hydrocephalus is about 3 per 1000 births, in most cases it is associated with spina bifida, while a few are due to birth trauma or meningitis. With modern treatment more than 60% of those will survive to school age.

With increasing hydrocephalus there appears to be decreasing performance in intelligence tests, whether the hydrocephalus is acquired or is associated with spina bifida cystica. However, these patients do not only suffer from the effects of a ventricular dilatation, but also from parenchymal brain damage as a result of the condition which leads to the hydrocephalus. Consequently, very grossly retarded children with focal lesions are found, especially in those with acquired hydrocephalus. The specific neurological and psychological features, including the 'cocktail party syndrome' peculiar to patients with hydrocephalus, are described.

REFERENCES

Granholm, L. and Radberg, C. (1965). *Acta Radiol.* **3,** 156.
Granholm, L. and Siesjo, B. K. (1970). *Develop. Med. Child Neurol. Suppl.* **22,** 73.
Grotte, G. and Lundberg, N. G. (1961). *Acta paediat. (Uppsala)* **50,** 617.
Hadenius, A. M., Hagberg, B., Hyttuas-Bensch, K. and Sjögren, I. (1962). *Acta Paediat. (Uppsala)* **51,** 117.
Hagberg, B. and Sjögren, I. (1966). *Amer. J. Dis. Child.* **112,** 1152.
Hassler, O. (1964). *Acta Neuropath.* **4,** 65.
Ingram, T. T. S. and Naunton, J. A. (1962). *Develop. Med. Child. Neurol.* **4,** 287.
Laurence, K. M. (1959). *Ann. Roy. Coll. Surg. Engl.* **24,** 388.
Laurence, K. M. (1964). *Arch. Dis. Childh.* **39,** 41.
Laurence, K. M. (1969). *Arch. Neurol.* **20,** 73.
Laurence, K. M. (1972). 'Handbook of Neurology' (P. J. Vinken and G. W. Bruyn, eds). Amsterdam: North Holland Publ. (in press).
Laurence, K. M., Carter, C. O. and David, P. A. (1968). *Brit. J. prev. soc. Med.* **22,** 146.
Laurence, K. M. and Coates, S. (1962). *Arch. Dis. Childh.* **37,** 345.
Laurence, K. M. and Tew, B. J. (1971). *Arch. Dis. Childh.* **46,** 127.
Lorber, J. and Grainger, R. G. (1963). *Clin. Radiol.* **14,** 98.
McKeown, T. and Record, R. G. (1960). In 'Ciba Symposium on Congenital Malformations' (G. E. W. Wolstenholme and C. M. O'Connor, eds), p. 2. London: Churchill.
Russell, D. S. (1949). *MRC. Spec. Rep. Ser.* No. 265. London: H.M.S.O.

DISCUSSION

Kirman: I discerned, probably wrongly, that the cases of hydrocephalus that come up at three months, and perhaps even later, without spina bifida might be due to a congenital malformation showing the effect later. Would these all be acquired?

Laurence: I think so. Practically all cases of truly congenital hydrocephalus are recognised very soon after birth, and it is very dangerous to assign hydrocephalus of late onset to a congenital origin, except when it is associated with spina bifida.

Crome: I would agree with Dr. Laurence. I think that quite a number of cases of hydrocephalus arise *in utero.*

Laurence: By congenital hydrocephalus I mean a lesion which is present at the time of birth, but I do not necessarily mean a malformation.

Kirman: But some of the cases that manifested themselves some time after birth, nonetheless were due to a malformation.

Laurence: I think you would be on slippery ground in believing this.

Jellinger: I would not agree. We have looked at the incidence of hydrocephalus due to overproduction of CSF, obstruction etc. More than 27% of all malformations were accompanied by hydrocephalus, most of them progressive, but sometimes non-progressive ones occurred. By contrast one-third of the post-infective defects was associated with hydrocephalus. Cases of aqueduct stenosis, which are of course congenital and developmental in origin, arise some weeks after birth. Among 24 cases of spina bifida and Arnold-Chiari malformation we only found this twice, whereas in five cases of severe hyperplasia of the cerebellum only one was accompanied by forking of the aqueduct. In most of the other cases we found a peculiar brain stem-cerebellar syndrome which may be in part an abortive form of Arnold-Chiari malformation. This was associated with a peculiar embracement of the ventral medulla by the hypertrophic cerebellum. We believe that the ventral displacement may be one of the causes of hydrocephalus in these cases. This deformity is not typical Type II Arnold-Chiari formation.

Laurence: I think this is a matter of semantics. I would regard this as part of the Arnold-Chiari type of deformity. I have found the Arnold-Chiari malformation absent in only three or four times out of 200 or 300 p.m.'s of cases of myelocoele.

Crome: I would agree with that. If hydrocephalus occurs without Arnold-Chiari malformation the meningocoele is very small and insignificant.

Laurence: What do you mean by meningocoele? I think you have to distinguish the meningocoele which does not involve the cord and the myelocoele which does. The myelocoele is almost always associated with some form of hind brain malformation complex.

Crome: Dr. Wigglesworth should know about this.

Wigglesworth: Most of our cases do not die in the neonatal period. I wondered whether hydrocephalus occurred with anterior spina bifida?

Laurence: I have seen two cases of anterior spina bifida both of whom had hydrocephalus.

Giroud: I wanted to add something about experimental conditions. Hydrocephaly can be induced in the embryonic stage, and perhaps also at the onset of the foetal stage. Many factors can induce this. The best known are folic acid deficiency and excess vitamin B_{12}. Some people think that the CSF is increased due to failure of growth of the nervous system, because it is very early in development, when the choroid plexus is more or less inactive. The increase of CSF appears to correlate with absence of growth of the brain, and accumulation of CSF may occur for this reason.

Dobbing: Has anyone any idea whether CSF production ceases entirely when the choroid plexus becomes sclerosed? Dr. Davson considers its function of regulating the *milieu* of the brain as a lymphatic system, to be a very important one.

Laurence: The CSF remains more or less normal in such cases, so that it must also be formed and absorbed elsewhere.

Dobbing: Davson attaches a lot of importance to reabsorption of substances by the choroid plexus as well as secretion of fluid.

Laurence: You can still get progressive hydrocephalus after all the choroid plexus has been ablated.

Cavanagh: Only a proportion, surely, of the CSF comes from the choroid plexus, a certain amount comes from the brain itself.

Dobbing: There is a lot of exchange, but it is difficult to conceive of a flow in this way.

Kleihues: You mentioned that there was a considerable reduction of the capillary bed as the result of progressive hydrocephalus. Does the vascular bed disappear faster than the cortex itself?

Laurence: No, it is probably a concomitant change, and as a result some neuronal anoxia must occur.

Hanefeld: We have found that the protein content of the CSF is always rather high if there is no secretion of CSF.

Laurence: Protein in CSF is high in post-inflammatory hydrocephalus, but in spina bifida without any ventriculitis the protein content remains more or less normal. However, a high percentage develop ventriculitis, and so many have a high CSF protein.

Dobbing: CSF physiologists are agreed that it is in equilibrium with brain extracellular fluid, and that this is the environment of our nerve cells, but not, of course, the astrocytic space.

Harris: At what stage was the I.Q. analysed in your cases? In the early years this is not a static state, of course.

Laurence: They were all cases of arrested hydrocephalus and the average age was about 12. Their hydrocephalus in all but one had been arrested for a number of years. The assessment of the degree of hydrocephalus was done during the acute phase, when they were first investigated in the neurosurgical department.

Stern: In making these series comparable, do psychologists correct their tests for physical disabilities?

Laurence: The psychologists, of course, correct for the neurological problems and physical disabilities so far as this is possible.

Jellinger: In Vienna at the Department of Child Neurology a study of 28 cases was made after surgical treatment and no correlation was found between the degree of hydrocephalus in the acute stage at the operation and the subsequent intelligence level. Almost none of these cases had neurological deficits, and they argued that there was almost complete recovery of function.

Laurence: I would agree with this. The cerebral mantle seems to return towards normality again provided the hydrocephalus has not become severe. I cannot conceive that when it is reduced to 3 mm it will ever return to anything like normality. Presumably in the Vienna series those children were operated upon early.

Jellinger: Yes, it was early, but the hydrocephalus was very severe in many cases.

Cavanagh: It is well known, of course, that white matter can withstand a good deal of stretching provided this is slow, with good restoration of function when the reason for the stretching is removed.

Sylvester: May I ask about Dr. Laurence's views on early detecting and possibly prevention, because I can foresee that the spina bifida child is likely to replace the mongol population in the long-stay hospital.

Laurence: At the moment early detection of spina bifida by X-rays and ultrasound is not really reliable. In any case, these methods cannot be used early enough in the pregnancy to enable termination to be carried out easily, should an abnormality be found. However, a new technique is being developed at the moment where spina bifida and anencephaly (a closely related condition) can be detected by 'foetoscopy' or direct inspection of the foetus at about the 16th-18th week. The instrument, a modified baby cystoscope, needs further development before it can be used, other than experimentally on pregnancies which are going to be terminated anyway for one reason or another. All these methods are in any case only applicable to high-risk pregnancies–usually where the mother has previously had a pregnancy with a major dysraphic neural tube malformation.

Non-specific Developmental Abnormalities and Unclassified Mental Retardation

L. CROME

Introduction

Possibly the first thing to be said about the neuromorphology of undifferentiated mental deficiency is the absence of any watertight partition between the changes in this group of cases and in those with recognised syndromes. For example, many of the classified metabolic diseases, such as phenylketonuria, are associated with smallness of the brain, but such smallness is also the most common single finding in the unclassified cases. Prosencephaly may occur in unclassified cases, being also a very common malformation in cases of D trisomy. Extensive demyelination with gliosis may place a case into the category of the leucodystrophies, but lesser changes of a similar kind will often be encountered in unclassified or in doubtful cases. This principle applies to almost all the changes enumerated below as well as to brains without ascertainable lesions.

Although a very wide, almost kaleidoscopic, variety of changes may be present in undifferentiated cases, a certain, possibly limited, number of identifiable *patterns* of malformation can nevertheless be discerned amongst them. In severity each of these ranges from the extremely severe which are incompatible with long survival, to those discovered accidentally in otherwise normal individuals. It is as if motor cars coming off an assembly line had a fault in wheel size ranging from a scarcely ascertainable smallness to unmistakable mini-wheeliness and then down to total wheel-lessness and immobility. In mental retardation we are dealing with a limited span in the possible range of severity of a given pattern of changes. The lower limit is set by viability and the upper by normal mentality. However, the upper limit is never clear-cut; there is inevitably an overlap with the normal. It is these factors that complicate numerical analysis of malformations, and one must admire the expertise and courage of workers like Prof. Jellinger who have grappled with this problem despite all difficulties.

It is also noteworthy that, on the whole, lesions associated with undifferentiated mental retardation are burnt-out, non-progressive, although certain secondary complications and crises may well occur. For example, the ventricles in cases of congenital or acquired hydrocephalus may go on enlarging although the initial cause of the obstruction has long since ceased to operate. Epileptic fits may cause further damage to an already abnormal brain.

Morphological changes fall into two main not mutually exclusive groups: malformations and reactive encephalopathies. The main patterns of both groups are considered below.

Malformations

As already indicated, the most frequent change is some reduction in the size and weight of the brain–*micrencephaly*. The smallest brains are also the rarest in the mentally retarded. The smaller the brain the less intelligent the patient and the shorter his expectation of life.

The micrencephalic brain may be equally small in all its parts but, more commonly perhaps, some parts are more affected than others. Thus the cerebellum may be relatively smaller or larger than the cerebrum. Micrencephaly is often associated with other anomalies, some of which are described below, and with reactive changes–particularly gliotic encephalopathy.

It has been suggested that microcephaly or micrencephaly may either be 'true' or 'secondary', the brains of the 'true' micrencephalics showing only smallness, and those of the others being associated with other anomalies. It is however difficult to see any advantage in this distinction. Thus Penrose (1963) considered that 'true' microcephaly is a recessively inherited defect and described their clinical state as being characteristic. Norman (1963) defined what he regarded as a characteristic anatomical picture in such 'recessive familial' microcephaly. These observations are, however, not entirely convincing, and we have presented elsewhere critical observations on this subject (Crome and Stern, 1967). Nevertheless, there is no doubt that familial and genetically determined syndromes associated with microcephaly do exist, but they are by no means homogeneous either clinically or morphologically (McKusick *et al.*, 1966; Hooft *et al.*, 1968).

Microcephaly is not always ascertainable at birth. The head

circumference and the brain may at first be well within the normal range and then begin to fall behind in their rate of growth.

Associated hypoplasia or atrophy may be present in areas connected with each other by fibre tracts. For instance, the ventrolateral thalamic nuclei may be small when lesions are present in the parietal lobe. Contralateral cerebellar atrophy or hypoplasia may be associated with lobar or hemispheral cerebral smallness. The pattern of convolutions is often 'simplified', the shorter tertiary gyri and sulci being absent. On the cut surface, the cerebral white matter is usually too thin in relation to the cortex.

It would seem reasonable to accept as a working hypothesis that the total number of nerve cells in the cerebral cortex, parts of it, or the subcortical formations is reduced in cases of undifferentiated mental retardation. All attempts, however, to demonstrate this by counting have so far come up against redoubtable practical difficulties, particularly in regard to controls.

Hydrocephalus is dealt with in this symposium by Dr. Laurence, but passive ventricular dilation ('ex vacuo') due to atrophy or underdevelopment of the overlying tissue, particularly in association with micrencephaly, is a very common finding and should, perhaps, be mentioned here.

The cerebral hemispheres are normally formed by the transformation of the single prosencephalic vesicle into two telencephalic ones. Arrest of this process results in some degree of persistence of abnormal union betwen the hemispheres–*prosencephaly*. This anomaly may be extreme, as in cyclopia, or, at the other end of the range, quite mild and insignificant, taking the form of an abnormally stout connexus thalamicus. Somewhere in the middle of the spectrum is fusion of the two cingulate gyri. In severe prosencephaly there is always absence of the corpus callosum and of the olfactory nerves or more proximal parts of the rhinencephalon. For this reason there is often a tendency among workers to identify the three conditions, viz. prosencephaly with *absence of the corpus callosum* and *arhinencephaly*. This, however, is wrong, since these malformations occur often independently of each other.

Since the corpus callosum is the main commissural connection between the two cerebral hemispheres, and these, as mentioned, are so frequently abnormal, it is not surprising that the corpus callosum is also often abnormal in retarded individuals. One of these anomalies is agenesis or hypoplasia. The corpus callosum develops by growing dorsally from the embryonic commissural plate. Only the posterior part of the definitive formation will be absent if the development is arrested at some stage *after* the start of the development (Loeser and Alvord,

1968). If completely absent, the structure is usually represented by a thin membrane. In some cases a lipoma, cyst or meningioma occupies the site of the absent corpus callosum. It should be noted that some cases with absent corpus callosum are of normal intelligence.

The normal outward migration of primitive neuroblasts from the periventricular areas may be interrupted or arrested. The resulting patterns of malformation are *microgyria* (also known as micro-polygyria), *pachygyria* and *ectopia.*

Microgyria is much more common than pachygyria. In the affected areas gyri are replaced by numerous closely-set small convolutions, the appearance after the meninges are stripped being like cobblestones or morocco-leather. Although usually symmetrical and bilateral, the condition may be unilateral or, apparently, restricted to an area supplied by one or other of the cerebral arteries (Morsier, 1952). The abnormal pallium so formed is characterised by a four-layer lamination. The first, marginal, layer contains, as in the normal cortex, few neurones. The second layer is densely cellular and is separated from the fourth, similarly cellular, layer by a thin sparsely cellular zone containing axis cylinders, some of which become in due course myelinated.

In cases of pachygyria, the gyri are few and broad while the sulci are short, shallow and straight. The extreme degree of this pattern is *agyria.* The histological picture is again four-layered and, in principle, of the same character as in microgyria. Large neurones are often present in layer 2.

The morphogenesis of these malformations is similar. Owing to interference with migration the outward movement of neuroblasts is interrupted at a time when a certain number of them, represented by abnormal layer 2, have reached the cortex. The axis cylinders of these cells course in the abnormal layer 3 and, when migration is resumed, prevent the remainder of nerve cells from reaching those in layer 2. Recent experimental work has brought to light some details of the migration process (Hanaway *et al.*, 1968). It appears that cells, reaching the cortex relatively late, move to more superficial positions by 'leap-frogging' past earlier immigrants. It is in this way that large neurones, originally destined to lodge in the normal layer 5, remain in pachygyria in the superficial layers.

Interference with the migration process may result in other anomalies. In nodular *ectopia* nerve cells remain at their original site where they form tumour-like nodules which may project into the ventricles or be implanted anywhere in the white matter of the cerebrum or cerebellum. They show varying degrees of differentiation and, sometimes, even indications of definitive cortical lamination.

Similar anomalies may occur in the vicinity of the basal ganglia and the brainstem. A form of nodular ectopia has been observed in Down's syndrome, viz. tuber of the cerebellar floccular peduncle. This is, however, also common in other cases of mental retardation and even in normal individuals.

Porencephaly is a rather ambiguous term. Solitary or multiple cavities are a very common finding in all kinds of encephalopathies, especially in association with reactive gliotic encephalopathy. It seems worth while to reserve the term porencephaly for brains presenting only a single or double cavity, *porus*, which communicates with the ventricle and is lined by ependyma. In some cases pori are roundish holes covered externally by a thin membrane formed by fused leptomeninges and ependyma. The extreme degree of this malformation, when both hemispheres are almost wholly replaced by such a membrane, is *hydrencephaly*.

Reactive Changes (Gliotic Encephalopathy)

It is thought that disease or injury in the early stages of morphogenesis causes simple liquefaction of tissue which results, if the embryo survives, in some malformation such as one of those described in the preceding section. Later, the brain, like other tissues, acquires the ability to limit and repair the damage by proliferative and reparative processes, chiefly on the part of glial cells and their fibres. Such scarring (gliosis) is one of the commonest findings in the brains of mental defectives. The extent of the gliosis and its intensity vary enormously. The whole brain may be affected or only one of the hemispheres, a lobe, a group of gyri (ulegyria), or parts of gyri (granular atrophy). Such scarring is associated with partial or complete disappearance of neurones and their processes. In the cerebral cortex neuronal loss may be focal, diffuse or laminar. The surviving neurones are often distorted in shape and orientation by the scar tissue. Some may be enlarged. Decaying neurones and their processes may show a variety of changes, such as calcification or ferrugination, i.e. incrustation with granules giving a positive reaction for calcium, iron or both of these elements (Taslor *et al.*, 1971). Another change occasionally seen in degenerating axis cylinders is *neuroaxonal dystrophy* (Kamoshita *et al.*, 1968).

Gliosis of the cerebral cortex is often associated with that of the white matter, but the degree of involvement can be very different in the two formations. Scarring of the white matter can take many different forms. It can extend, for example, like the veins of a leaf from the centrum semiovale into the digital white matter of the gyri (Crome and Foley, 1959).

Scarring at any level may not be sufficient to close over the destroyed part and gliosis is therefore frequently associated with *cavitation, cystencephaly* or *encephalomalacia.* In the early stages of brain destruction there may be considerable cellular proliferation with phagocytic activity of the microglia. The cells contain at that time sudanophilic cholesterol ester and triglycerides. Later they tend to disappear and be replaced by astrocytes, but many persist for a long time, especially if encysted in the cavities.

A change that is not fully understood is *'marbling'.* It occurs in the cortex and/or the basal ganglia. In the basal ganglia the picture is that of irregular thin white streaks (like the veins of marble) upon the background of gliotic tissue. Microscopically, there is always intense fibrous gliosis and, seemingly, an excess of myelinated fibres, which can be particularly dense around blood vessels. Whether or not this represents true hypermyelination is perhaps still questionable, although there is some recent electron microscopical work supporting this theory (Borit and Herndon, 1970). Marbling is very often associated with a history of birth injury, particularly anoxia.

Another relatively frequent change which may occur in the grey or white matter is rarefaction of the tissue, which may assume the form of so-called *spongiform encephalopathy.* It is worth mentioning that some workers have referred to this change as being characteristic of inborn errors of metabolism, but this is by no means so.

A relatively frequent finding is fibrous gliosis of the white matter without ascertainable demyelination. This may occur at all levels of the CNS.

Brains with no Ascertainable Lesions

Some of the brains in cases of classifiable *and* unclassifiable mental retardation show no ascertainable change. The proportion of such cases will no doubt vary with the type of population studied. At our hospital, which deals with a large number of severely subnormal children, the figure for such lesion-free brains has been running at about 8%. It may well be higher in higher-grade individuals, but most of our lesion-free brains have come from very severely retarded individuals, some of whom were also epileptic.

In order to explain this phenomenon some workers have tended to attach significance to minor or marginal morphological changes. This tendency should be resisted: some such anomalies may be found, if looked for hard enough, in almost all people.

One factor accounting for the lesion-free brains is undoubtedly the relative crudity of the available methods of anatomical study. Future refinement of techniques will certainly permit recognition of still unknown changes, especially on the ultrastructural level. Indeed, claims to have observed significant ultrastructural lesions in otherwise normal brains have already been made (Gonatas and Goldensohn, 1965; Gonatas, 1967; Gonatas *et al.*, 1967). In a few other lesion-free brains the changes may be entirely molecular, as they are perhaps in some of the reversible instances of adult psychosis. The proportion of such cases cannot be large. Some cases diagnosed as childhood autism have shown obvious brain lesions at autopsy.

REFERENCES

Borit, A. and Herndon, R. M. (1970). *Acta neuropath. (Berl.)* **14,** 304.
Crome, L. and Foley, J. (1959). *J. ment. Defic. Res.* **3,** 63.
Crome, L. and Stern, J. (1967). 'The Pathology of Mental Retardation', p. 100. London: Churchill.
Gonatas, N. K. (1967). *Nature* **214,** 352.
Gonatas, N. K., Evangelista, I. and Walsh, G. O. (1967). *J. Neuropath. exp. Neurol.* **26,** 179.
Gonatas, N. K. and Goldensohn, E. S. (1965). *J. Neuropath. exp. Neurol.* **24,** 539.
Hanaway, J., Lee, S. I. and Netsky, M. G. (1968). *Neurology (Minneap.)* **18,** 791.
Hooft, C., Hanwere, R. de and Acker, J. K. van (1968). *Helv. paediat. Acta* **23,** 1.
Kamoshita, S., Neustein, H. B. and Landing, B. H. (1968). *J. Neuropath. exp. Neurol.* **27,** 300.
Loeser, J. D. and Alvord, E. C. (1968). *Neurology (Minneap.)* **18,** 745.
McKusick, V. A., Stauffer, M., Knox, D. L. and Clark, D. B. (1966). *Arch. Ophthalm.* **75,** 597.
Morsier, G. (1952). Proceedings of the First International Congress of Neuropathology, Rome, Vol. II, p. 212. Torino: Rosenberg and Sellier.
Norman, R. M. (1963). In 'Greenfield's Neuropathology', p. 348. London: Arnold.
Penrose, L. S. (1963). 'The Biology of Mental Defect', p. 172. London: Sidgwick and Jackson.
Taylor, D. C., Falconer, M. A., Bruton, C. J. and Corsellis, J. A. N. (1971). In press.

DISCUSSION

Laurence: One thing we must get quite clear is that birth is only an incident in brain development and there is no real distinction between maldevelopment and acquired lesions. Many malformations happen to be acquired lesions early in intrauterine life.

Kirman: From what Dr. Crome was saying he looks upon these cases as part of a continuum. Hydrocephalus, however, we put among the classified disorders, but have we any evidence about the epidemiology of any factors linking the malformations with any of the other abnormalities that give rise to mental retardation?

Laurence: I think we have to treat hydrocephalus separately from the dysraphic lesions. This is clear from family studies. Most of the cases of hydrocephalus are difficult to sort out. Some are undoubtedly genetic, but the majority are acquired lesions. Hydranencephaly is a good example. Most are burnt out by the time of birth, while occasionally the cataclysmic process occurs near delivery and the haemorrhagic lesions can be seen in the brain.

Balázs: Dr. Crome has shown that most of the mentally retarded children had smaller brains. It was surprising to me that Dr. Laurence's enormous hydrocephalic brains appear to function normally. It seemed to me in this instance that the amount of functioning brain tissue can be greatly reduced, but the distribution of the I.Q. is very similar to that of the normal population. What is the real situation?

Laurence: Firstly, the spina bifida hydrocephalic at birth has a normal amount of brain for its length or age. This becomes less with time. I am afraid my message could not have been quite clear on this point. In the hydrocephalic, however large the brain is, there is considerable intellectual deficit. The distribution is normal, but there is a considerable 'shift to the left'. There is a diffuse neuronal loss in severe hydrocephalus.

Jellinger: I got the impression that reduction in brain weight is always called 'micrencephaly'. In a large series of cases, including reactive encephalopathies, many are by definition not micrencephaly, they are atrophic brains due to loss of substance. True micrencephaly means a developmental disorder leading to reduction of brain volume with or without associated cerebral malformation. Quantitative studies on hemi-megalencephaly on the other hand have been made by Bignami and collaborators (Bignami, A., Palladini, G. and Zappella, M. (1968) *Brain Res.* **9**, 103) in which they found more DNA in the larger half of the brain. In the future we will get new tools for quantitating brain features, and I would not want to see any mixing of a small brain due to loss of brain substance with a primarily maldeveloped brain that failed to develop. This separation is important.

Dobbing: Dr. Crome said the smaller the brain the greater the defect, but I am sure he means to exclude from this generalisation the great variation in brain size in normal people. It must be remembered that there was a considerable range in Coppelletta and Wolbach's figures, and that a lot of Dr. Crome's upper figures would fall within that range. If one expressed brain size in terms of body weight, on which it is very dependent, one might be much more precise.

Crome: Certainly there is a great variation and the correlation of expectation of life with degree of micrencephaly is also an over-simplification.

Kleihues: From recent experimental studies, especially with drugs, etc., we generally find that the dose required to cause considerable reduction in cell number is usually less than that to cause disturbances of cell migration. In those cases where there is a severe migration disorder, are their brains lower in weight, or can this happen with a normal brain weight?

Crome: You find both. In microgyria there is also a reduction in brain weight, in general, but ectopic nodules occur in brains of fairly normal weight and often in hydrocephalic brains. But I have not made a special study of this point. With regard to Prof. Jellinger's cases of hemi-megalencephaly, in my experience of this condition they show a tremendous admixture of astrocytes as well as neurones. I think that there is loss of nerve cells and a large increase of astrocytes.

Cavanagh: Of course, ectopias do occur in otherwise apparently normal brains. Perhaps in Dr. Crome's cases the brain may tend to be small by virtue of the material he gets. You can get this focal migration defect in apparently normal persons.

Giroud: If the number of cells is important, I believe that differentiation is much more important, particularly arborisation and the completeness of the synaptic system. Do you suppose, Dr. Crome, that there is one period at which mental retardation is produced, or does this occur at many different times? I suppose that it may be produced at both the foetal and the post-foetal stages. It is difficult to envisage a late action here, because these mentally retarded children have anatomical malformations which are produced very early. These are usually small malformations such as can be easily found in prosencephaly. The evolution of the nervous system is a sequence of events which are linked with each other. If there is an early disturbance, perhaps the later ones are dependent upon these. What do you think about that?

Crome: I do not know, but I would say that there is a continuous and sometimes a cumulative process which can originate at various stages of ontogenesis.

Holt: Could I ask a bit about the clinical features of some of the children without histological lesions? In Dr. Kirman's account 50% of cases were referred to as unclassified, whereas you found pathological lesions in the majority. One in five, therefore, of the unclassified clinical cases must fall into the category of having no pathological lesions at p.m. Is it possible to distinguish these clinically? Do they have, for instance, a normal head circumference, normal growth, etc. absence of congenital stigmata, etc., or are they completely indistinguishable from all the others?

Crome: They have a normal head circumference that may serve to distinguish them, and they have a normal brain weight, but they may have any of the other features of mental retardation. Thus they may be idiots, or imbeciles, they may have epilepsy or not, they may be hyperkinetic and so forth. They may have EEG changes as the only abnormality.

Laurence: Is there growth retardation amongst those with apparently normal brains?

Crome: I haven't looked into that.

Jellinger: These cases are of all ages. They have no variation in somatic growth. They may be adults with or without seizures, with or without neurological disturbances. From the histories there is no detectable difference from the cases of so-called classified mental retardation.

Cavanagh: This is clearly the hard core cases of mental retardation where we have absolutely no idea as to what is going on.

Kirman: If we look at phenylketonuria, for example, it is of course possible to find anatomical changes, but in some it is minimal or absent. Function may be at a grossly retarded level but there is nothing demonstrable in the brain. One can well imagine that something of the same kind may be present in those other cases.

Laurence: A note of caution should be sounded, for sometimes quite gross abnormalities may be found in cases with no apparent brain disturbance.

Neuropathological Features of Unclassified Mental Retardation

K. JELLINGER

Introduction

The progress of modern efforts to prevent and to treat mental retardation greatly depends on the nature of the underlying pathological conditions. Considering the aetiology of mental deficiency, two main factors can be recognised—genetic and environmental (exogenous). What information there is relates predominantly to severe grades of retardation which require admission to hospital or an institution, and which are either associated with inborn errors of metabolism or, more often, with recognisable structural brain damage (Crome and Stern, 1967). Not infrequently, however, the brains of mental defectives fail to reveal any clear-cut pathological changes when examined by light microscopy. Recent EM biopsy studies suggest that abnormal synapses and mitochondria (Gonatas *et al.*, 1967; Suzuki and Rapin, 1969) or abnormal astrocytes (Miyakawa *et al.*, 1970) may be the sole significant abnormality and possibly causal in some cases of mental retardation and seizure disorders. Although classical neuropathology cannot be expected to elucidate the causes of mental deficiency, much can be derived from evaluating a large series of pertinent specimens. It is, however, difficult to compare the results of the various post-mortem studies (Meyer, 1949; Benda, 1952; Malamud, 1952; Gross and Kaltenbäck, 1962; Christensen *et al.*, 1965; Freytag and Lindenberg, 1967) because of differences in the interpretation and because of the nature and source of the material examined (Table 1). The present observations are based on a series of randomly collected post-mortem material from 1130 cases of mental deficiency *clinically manifest within the first three years of life.* Although, for reasons of selection, this series does not reflect the actual incidence of the different disease entities in a population of mentally retarded persons,

TABLE 1

Number of Cases According to Nosological Entities in Various Post-mortem Series

Nosological condition	*Meyer 1949*		*Benda 1952*		*Malamud 1952*		*Freytag-Lindenberg 1967*		*Present series*	
	No	*%*	*No*	*%*	*No*	*%*	*No*	*%*	*No*	*%*
Mongolism	*		55	19	97	19	31	8.7	97	8.7
CNS malformations. Phacomatoses (Hydrocephalus included)		19	48	17	117	23	97	27.0	265	23.5
Cerebral tumours	*		–	–	*		6	1.7	30	2.7
Metabolic disorders	*		6	2	10	2	13	3.6	92	8.1
Thyreogenous encephalopathy (cretinism)	*		*		?		5	1.5	12	1.0
Anoxic-vascular lesions		40	61	21	86	17	90	25.0	290	25.7
Post-infectious lesions and meningoencephalitis		3	37	13	27	5	29	8.1	75	6.6
Post-traumatic defects	*		*		*		3	0.8	3	0.3
'Cryptogenic' epilepsies	*		*		*		*		75	6.6
Idiocies without findings		31	40	14	175	34	55	15.3	76	6.7
Others and unclassified		10	29	10	–		30	8.4	115	10.2
Total	385	100	287	100	512	100	359	100.0	1130	100.0

*Not mentioned.

TABLE 2

Age at Death in Whole Series of 1120 Cases

Years	*No.*	*Percent*
Under 1	197	17.4
1-2	184	16.2
2-5	300	26.7
5-10	207	18.3
10-15	144	12.7
15-20	74	6.6
Over 20	24	2.1
Total	1130	100.0
Males	642	56.8
Females	488	43.2

it is hoped that the data presented puts the broad morphological field of unclassified mental deficiency into perspective, and for the purposes of this meeting the various already classified disorders will not be subjects for discussion.

Materials and Methods

The material, collected during a 30-year period (1940-1970) in the files of the Neurological Institute of Vienna University and the Boltzmann-Institute for Research of Cerebral Malformations (formerly the Neurohistological Laboratory of the Vienna Psychiatric Hospital) was received from different hospitals and institutions in Austria. Only patients surviving birth for at least two months and showing clinical signs of mental retardation under the age of three years were included. Hence, severe CNS malformations not compatible with long survival were excluded. There was also a certain selection from the pathological point of view, as the brains were often examined where positive results were anticipated from clinical and laboratory findings. Other disorders in which no CNS abnormalities could be expected, e.g. mongolism, were less often received. On the other hand, our sample also includes several cases of metabolic disorders clinically suspected or proved in the laboratory.

The cerebral findings were classified by nosology (Table 3) and by pathology, regardless of their aetiology (Table 4). Seventy questionable or not yet completely examined cases were excluded, thus reducing the number evaluated to 1060.

TABLE 3

Frequency of Seizures and Neurological Disorders in the Various Nosological Groups

Nosological condition	*Seizures* %*	*Neurol. symptoms* %
Mongolism	15.3	–
Craniostenosis	33.3	25.0
CNS malformations	41.8	47.6
Tumours	50.0	56.7
Metabolic disorders	45.0	71.4
Thyrogenous encephalopathy	41.7	41.7
Anoxic-vascular lesions	71.4	63.4
Postinfectious lesions	76.0	47.3
Posttraumatic lesions	–	
'Cryptogenic' epilepsy	100.0	
Idiocy without changes	53.8	28.4
Others and unclassified	15.5	
Total	47.5 (52.2*)	47.6

* Of 1035 cases with sufficient histories.

TABLE 4

Main Types of Morphological CNS Lesions

Type of lesion		*No. of cases*	*%*
'Normal brain'		202	19.2
Idiocy without findings	61		
Mongolism	97		
Craniostenoses	10		
Cranio-facial dysplasia	11		
'Cryptogenic epilepsy'	23		
Negative findings except for mongolism		105	10.0
Developmental disorders (see Table 7)		275	24.0
Tumours and hamartomas		30	2.9
Metabolic disorders (see Table 11)		92	8.7
Cicatricial defects and cerebral atrophies (anoxic-vascular; post-infectious)		351	33.1
Cerebral atrophies (thyreogenous; unclassified)		47	4.5
Progressive hydrocephalus		39	3.6
Other inflammatory defects		9	0.9
Meningo-encephalitis		10	1.0
Degenerative and atrophying processes		12	1.1
Total material analysed		1060	100.0
Unclassified cases (excluded)		70	

Results

Table 2 shows the sex incidence and the ages at death of the whole series, the majority (61.2%) dying between 1 and 10 years. Fits were reported in 47.5%. Since adequate histories were present in only 1035 cases (Table 3), the frequency of fits increased to 52.2%. In about 60% of them the onset of seizures was before the age of six months and in 90% convulsions began within the first year of life (Jellinger, 1970). 47.6% of the patients showed spastic syndromes or other neurological defects (Table 3).

Classification Remarks

Without reference to the case history, the clinical picture of the condition alone would have enabled a correct diagnosis in 15% of all cases, and by addition of laboratory and biochemical tests (excluding organ biopsy) recognition was possible in 28.9% of the sample (Table 5). In 18.5% of all patients, obscure clinical syndromes could be clarified by the case or by the family history. If exact medical records had been available in each patient, a clarification of the diagnosis would have been possible in about 30%. However, this information was of little value in almost 60% and even misleading in 13%, especially with paranatal accidents. Those were recorded in 49.6% of the cases with sufficient clinical data, but only in 14.1% of these was the morphological brain damage reasonably referable to birth injury or other paranatal distress (Table 6). Under optimal circumstances the clinician would not have been able to reach a correct diagnosis in more than half the cases (Gross *et al.*, 1968). Since this material originates from the period 1940 to 1970 the percentage of correct clinical diagnoses was much lower because of lack of adequate clinical diagnostic facilities. Hence, a considerable part was clinically considered as 'unclassified' mental and neurological disease.

TABLE 5

Proportion of cases in which clinical diagnosis was obvious, independent of the medical history

Condition	*No.*	*Percentage*
Developmental disorders	238	65.5
Tumours	20	66.6
Thyreogenous encephalopathies	12	100.0
Metabolic disorders	57	61.9
Total	327	28.9

TABLE 6

Proportion of cases, with histories available, showing paranatal distress (i.e. birth injury, abnormal delivery, birth asphyxia, etc.)

Nosological entity	*Number with birth history available*	*Percentage with paranatal distress*
Mongolism	78	38.4
Developmental disorders	229	36.1
Tumours	26	11.5
Metabolic disease	82	5.0
Thyreogenous encephalopathies	11	27.3
Anoxic-vascular lesions	210	81.3
Postinfectious lesions	58	16.7
'Cryptogenic' epilepsies	67	14.9
Idiocy without changes	56	44.6
Others and unclassified	96	35.4
Total	913	40.6
Paranatal lesion (clinically excluded)	81	
Paranatal lesion (clinically suggested)	290	31.8
Paranatal CNS lesion (morphologically confirmed)	160	14.1

On the basis of the morphological findings in the CNS, a satisfactory diagnosis was possible in almost 80% of the material, while combined clinical and pathological evaluation enabled a clarification of the morbid entity in about 90%. Genetic and developmental abnormalities, including mongolism (8.7%), ranked highest in frequency (32%), followed by anoxic-vascular defects predominantly of paranatal origin (25.7%), metabolic disorders (8.1%), post-infectious lesions, 'cryptogenic' epilepsies and idiocy without changes (6.6% each), while 10% of the material presented rare entities or remained unclassified (Table 1).

Most of the problematical cases fell into the categories of probable 'idiopathic' epilepsy, mental defects 'without substrate' and unclarified cases. These three groups represented 23.5% of the total and might be regarded as 'unclassified' mental retardation *sensu strictiori.* The group of 'cryptogenic' epilepsies includes all those cases of generalised fits of undetermined origin which showed no neuropathological changes or which only showed non-specific scars, considered to be the result of seizures rather than causative. Almost 70% of the adequately examined brains of such patients showed symmetrical Ammon's Horn sclerosis. Idiocy 'without substrate' comprises all forms of retardation without significant morphological or biochemical lesions, probably a major part being unrecognised genetic or metabolic disorders. This group includes inherited forms of retardation, cranio-facial dysplasias without cerebral changes, and cases with non-specific minor developmental abnormalities. The remainder without neuropathological findings or with questionable and still unclarified lesions was 135, i.e. 12.1% of the total. Exclusion of 70 insufficiently examined brains reduces this number to 65 or 5.8% of the total material.

Neuropathological Findings

Among the adequately examined cases, 80.8% showed organic brain damage as a cause of the clinical deficit. If Down's syndrome was excluded from the 'negative' cases, the frequency of genetically and organically determined retardations increased to 90. More specific data on the relevant categories listed in Table 4 are given below.

Developmental Disorders

Table 7 shows the main types and frequency of malformations encountered in 275 cases. Malformations of the forebrain system were found in 43.6%, and developmental arrest and other dysmorphies in 55%. Combined developmental abnormalities were prssent in almost one-third of the cases. Twenty-seven per cent of the developmental anomalies were associated with hydrocephalus, mostly of severe and progressive forms. In a further 14 cases hypertensive hydrocephalus without malformations was present, the origin of which remained undetermined.

The cerebral malformations easy to classify clinically include dysgenesias and dysraphias of the forebrain system (almost half of the cases) due to frequently associated craniofacial dysplasias and the AEG demonstration of malformations of the telencephalic ventricles, and closure defects of the caudal neural tube (20%), while for rhombocerebellar dysraphias, representing about one-third of this group (Table 8), clinical diagnosis is rather difficult (Table 5). Half of our 12 cases of *holoprosencephaly* were associated with median facial clefts. Two occurred in trisomy 13-15, while in a two-year-old boy with semilobar holoprosencephaly, a missed abortion with quinine was reported between the 50th and 60th day after the first day of the last menstruation. *Agenesis of the corpus callosum,* present in 28 cases, was often associated with facial and other malformations (median clefts–2; acrocephalosyndactylia–2; hyperteleorism–one-third; microcrania–4; microphthalmia–2; spina bifida–2; cardiac and renal malformations–4 each). In two cases it was accompanied by familial hypersecretory hydrocephalus; in nine instances other CNS malformations were noted which might have played a role in producing clinical symptoms. In one

TABLE 7

Dysplasias and Dysmorphias of the CNS

		Subtotal	*Total*
1. Migration disorders			93
Agyria, Pachygyria		2	
Microgyria, Ectopias		62	
Agyria of Dentate and Olivary nuclei		1	
Agenesia of Septum pellucidum (without other malformation)		11	
Cortical Microdysgenesias		17	
2. Migration disorders with defects			28
True Porencephaly			
Cerebrum		26	
Cerebellum		2	
3. Disproportionate brain growth			81
Micrencephaly		59	
Megalencephaly		19	
Megacerebellum		1	
Hemimegalencephaly		2	
	Subtotal		202
4. Phacomatoses			38
Tuberous sclerosis		26	
Localised cortical dysplasia		2	
Sturge-Weber disease		2	
Angiodysgenesia, Angiomas		8	
	Total		240

case the absence of corpus callosum was associated with mid-line fusion of the frontal lobes, and twice with uni- or bilateral agenesis of the olfactory bulbs or tracts, thus demonstrating their relationship to other telencephalic dysgenesias (Loeser and Alvord, 1968). Abnormal chromosome findings were reported in one single case showing a 47-XXY pattern, characteristic for Klinefelter's syndrome. *Rhombo-cerebellar and caudal dysraphias* are often associated with progressive internal hydrocephalus, the pathogenesis of which may not be completely understood. While Arnold-Chiari's deformity is considered as an almost constant accompaniment of lumbar meningomyelocoele, in our material of 25 necropsies, it was only present four times. Five cases showed cerebellar hypoplasia, while the others revealed a peculiar cerebellar-brain stem syndrome characterised by funnel-shaped deformity of the posterior fossa, hypoplasia of the vermis, and crestlike

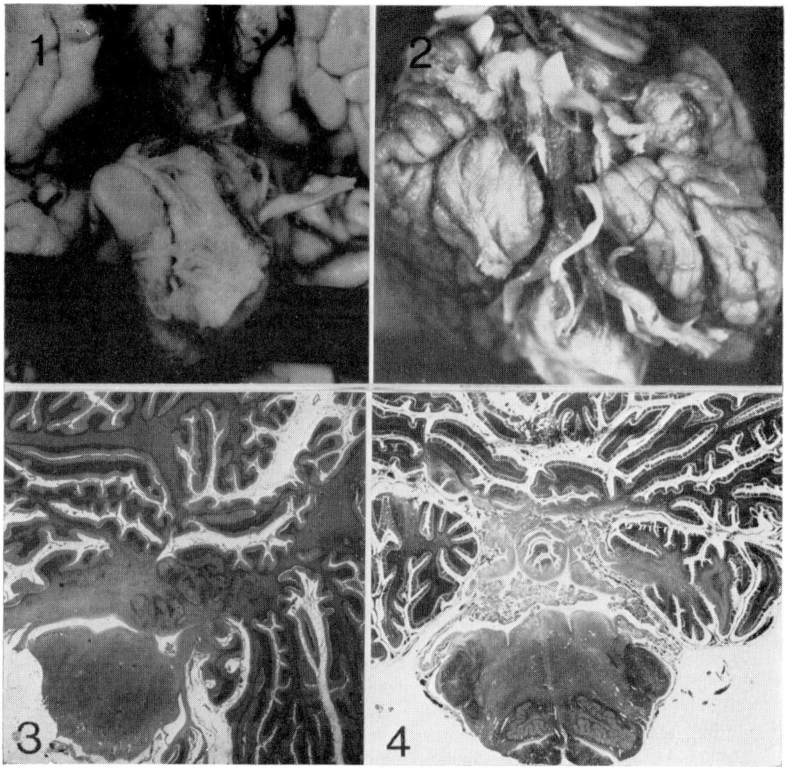

Fig. 1. Cerebellar hypoplasia in hydrocephalic infant with lumbar myelomeningocoele.

Fig. 2. Embracing of brain stem by ventrally displaced parts of cerebellum in hydrocephalus associated with spina bifida.

Fig. 3. Cortical dysplasia in inferior cerebellar vermis in hydrocephalic infant with lumbar meningocoele.

Fig. 4. Scarring and membranous adhesion of atrophic inferior vermis to the medulla oblongata in hydrocephalic child with caudal myelomeningocoele.

[To face p. 300

Fig. 5. Microcephalia vera in 24-year-old female idiot.

Fig. 6. Coronal section of microcephalic brain with agenesis of corpus callosum, multiple nodular heterotopias, pachygyria of the temporal lobes and dystopic Ammon's horn.

Fig. 7. "Blastomatous" hemimegalencephaly with unilateral fibrillary gliosis in 13-year-old epileptic girl with hemiplegia. Kanzler-Arendt stain.

Fig. 8. Large abnormal glial cells in the cortex of hemimegalencephalic brain. H. & E. × 400.

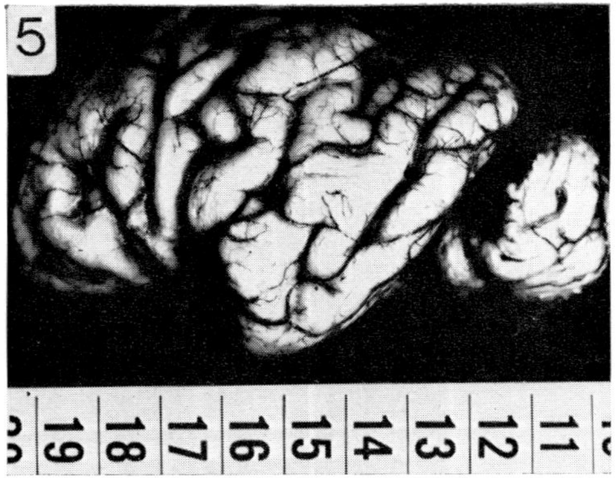

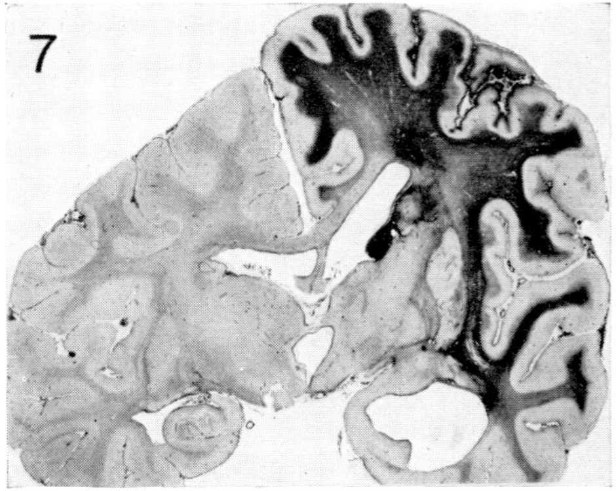

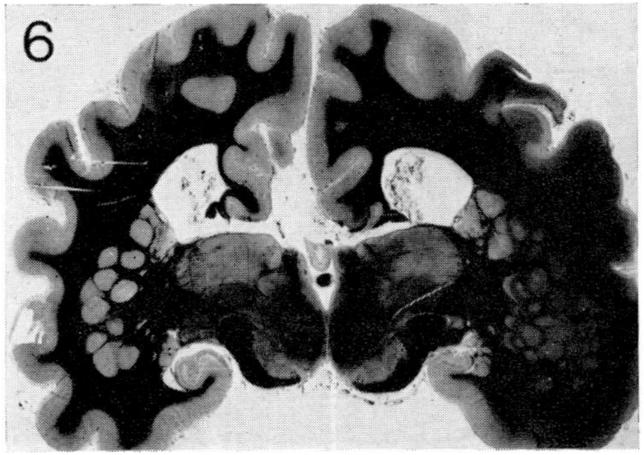

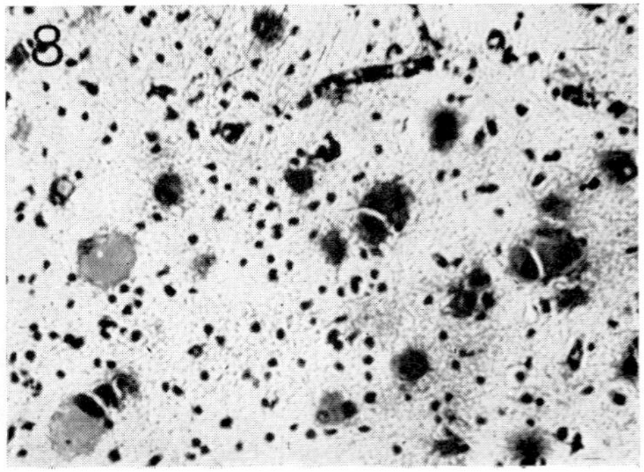

TABLE 8

Cerebrospinal Dysgenesias and Dysraphias

	Subtotal	Total
1. Meningoencephalocoele (parietal, occipital)		3
2. Holoprosencephaly (Arhinencephaly)		12
3. Prosencephalic Dysraphic disorders		44
Agenesia of Corpus Callosum	29	
Agenesia of Anterior Commissure	1	
Absence of Rhinencephalon	1	
Pseudomonoventriculia	2	
Dysraphic equivalents (Cavum septi pellucidi, etc.)	11	
4. Rhombo-cerebellar Dysraphias		35
Cerebellar Hypoplasia	4	
Aplasia (Hypoplasia) of Vermis	16	
Dandy-Walker syndrome	1	
Rhombencephalosynapsis	2	
Arnold-Chiari malformation	2	
Aqueductal malformation	5	
Others	5	
5. Caudal Dysraphias (Meningomyelocoele sacralis)		25
With hydromyelia	2	
syringomyelia	3	
diplomyelia	1	
Total		119

encircling of the brain stem by ventrally displaced parts of the cerebellum causing closure of the lateral foramina (Gross and Jellinger, 1969) (Figs 1-4).

Among the other developmental anomalies, dysmorphism and disorders of the relationship in cerebral masses showed about equal frequency (Table 7). Microgyria is much more common than pachygyria. Unusual agyria of the dentate and olivary nuclei associated with disorders of the cerebral cortical cyto-architecture was noted in a one-year-old retarded and tetraplegic boy. About one-third of the migrational disorders (micropolygyria), particularly in the claustrum and Reil's insula were associated with porencephalic defects apparently resulting from secondary vascular defects superimposed on primary developmental anomalies (Gross and Kaltenbäck, 1960). These are the only cases of dysmorphism which are clinically recognisable (Table 5).

Apart from gross developmental anomalies, a large variety of *minor malformations* were observed, and occasionally represented the sole findings in the brains of idiots and epileptics (Benda, 1952; Peiffer, 1970). Veith and Wicke (1968) commented upon cortical microdysgenesias which include an increase in the number of Cajal-Retzius cells, subpial multipolar cells, persistent superficial granular layer, small rims and nodules of superficial neurones, marginal gliosis of the cortex, small heterotopic islands of CNS tissue in the subarachnoid space, etc. Such insignificant anomalies were the only findings in the brains of 14 patients aged from 7 months to 24 years, half of whom had early manifestation of epilepsy. One of them suffered from inherited oligophrenia, another was a 'cri-du-chat' syndrome, another was a Pierre-Robin syndrome, and a further two were associated with small cicatricial defects. Since these microdysgenesias are also found in the brains of non-epileptic infants without mental retardation, often associated with cardiac malformations, the significance of these findings needs further statistical evaluation. Bérard-Badier *et al.* (1965) drew attention to groups of indifferent cells, referred to as spindle and round cell dysgenesias in the dentate nuclei of young infants. We noted such anomalies in several premature and term infants up to the age of 46 days (not included in this series), usually associated with extracerebral malformations and in trisomy D, while Terplan *et al.* (1970) and Sumi (1970) reported them in trisomy 18. These and other findings are important in so far as they indicate the developmental, and probably genetically determined origin of such minor abnormalities. Up to the present, however, it is not possible to state how much these are variations of the normal or whether they are truly pathological and responsible for the mental state.

Anoxic-Vascular Defects

This group, 33% of the total, comprises all cases in which the clinical defects were caused by circulatory disorders of various nature during different periods. The lesions ranged from large cystic and cicatricial defects–hydranencephaly, lobular sclerosis, ulegyrias and hemispheral cavities–to multiple sclerotic foci. To this group, 45% of 'simple' cerebral atrophies were added, since they showed minor forms of anoxic defects, i.e. loss of nerve cells with glial scarring. This raises the incidence of cicatricial defects to 32.8% of the total. In more than half of the cases, the lesions probably originated at birth, because there was a history of difficult birth, forceps delivery, birth asphyxia or other paranatal distress, while in 22 kernicterus was reported. Prenatal lesions were mentioned in 11 cases including five cases of hydranencephaly, while in 22 cases post-natal origin of vascular defects was anticipated by the history of early infantile cardiac arrest, cranio-cerebral injuries or embolic softenings in congenital heart failure. In the remainder (27%) it could not be decided whether the lesion was para- or post-natal in origin.

Post-Infectious Lesions

This group, 6.7% of the total, included 26 cases with vascular damage following meningo-cerebral inflammatory disease, 24 cases of post-infectious hydrocephalus and 10 cases with active meningo-encephalitides or their sequelae. These were mostly post-natal infections except for foetal toxoplasmosis (six cases), cytomegalia (one), foetal rubella syndrome (two) and one case of chronic necrotising panencephalitis of probable intrauterine origin.

Metabolic Disorders

This group, amounting for 8.7% of this material, is listed in Table 9 according to the biochemical or morphological entities.

'Degenerative' Processes

Among the unclassified cases a small group (1%) was characterised by peculiar system-bound degenerative lesions. They include an infantile case of ponto-cerebellar atrophy with associated degeneration of cortico-spinal and dentato-rubral systems (Gross and Kaltenbäck, 1959), one case of Werdnig-Hoffmann disease with idiocy associated with gliosis of the cerebellar white matter, dentate nuclei and brain stem with defective myelination of the corticospinal tracts (cf. Norman and Kay, 1965), and six cases of oligophrenia with or without neurological signs or seizures in which pronounced fibrillary gliosis of the cerebellum and brain stem were the sole findings. These changes resemble those in certain amino acidurias (Martin *et al.*, 1968) suggesting some unrecognised metabolic origin, but should be distinguished from fibre gliosis limited to ventral parts of the brain stem in young infants who died from acute disease (Martin *et al.*, 1969). In two male sibs with retardation and choreiform-cerebellar symptoms, symmetrical atrophy of the inferior olives and vestibular nuclei were present, while a 12-year-old idiot with petit mal seizures and torsion dystonia only showed symmetrical degeneration of the dentate nuclei. The nosology of system degenerations in young age needs further elucidation.

Conclusions

The fact that 90% of this series of cases of mental retardation—including mongolism—showed organic brain damage is noteworthy. This incidence is higher than that of others, despite similar frequencies in disease entities (Table 1) perhaps due to selection of the more severe cases.

TABLE 9

Metabolic Disorders

Leukodystrophies		27
Orthochromatic Ld	4	
Pelizaeus-Merzbacher type	4	
Metachromatic Ld	12	
Spongy Ld (Canavan)	4	
Globoid type (Krabbe)	3	
Lipidoses		20
GM_2 gangliosid. (Tay-Sachs)	10	
Late infantile (Batten)	3	
Infantile Gaucher's disease	5	
Niemann-Pick disease	1	
Wolman's disease	1	
Mucopolysaccharidoses		13
Gargoylism	13	
Amino acid disorders		13
PKU	5	
Phenylalaninuria	1	
Hyperammonaemia	6	
Maple syrup urine disease	1	
Neuroaxonal dystrophies		7
Infantile NAD	5	
Hallervorden-Spatz disease	2	
Others		13
Leigh's disease	5	
Alper's disease	4	
Galactosaemia	1	
Glycogenosis	1	
Glial poliodystrophy	1	
Total		92

Genetic and developmental disorders (32%) ranked highest in frequency, in conformity with other authors and most were well-known anomalies. However, in some cases, ranging as 'idiots without substrate' or 'cryptogenic epilepsies', minor malformations were the sole findings. Since similar insignificant abnormalities were seen in normal controls and in the brains of infants with extracerebral malformations, more information is needed of a statistical nature before their significance to this problem can be evaluated.

The second largest group in the whole series (close to 30%) had brain damage from circulatory disorders of various aetiology, the greater part probably of paranatal origin.

In 45% of the brains showing 'simple atrophy' minor anoxic lesions were present, putting the group of circulatory disorders to 33% of the total series and thus almost reached the frequency of developmental abnormalities. Hippocampal sclerosis must be added to this group since 70% of idiopathic epileptics showed this change.

Proved metabolic disorders represented 8.7% of the morphologically evaluated cases, which was higher than in other post-mortem series.

Other groups of minor importance were progressive hydrocephalus of post-infectious or undetermined origin (3.6%) and other inflammatory diseases and their residuals (1.8%). Of particular interest is a small group of infantile system degenerations associated with mental and neurological defects which are probably related to still unknown metabolic disorders. The number of cases without significant anatomical findings amounted to 10% of all sufficiently examined specimens. Inclusion of questionable and unclarified cases raises their proportion to 12% which is slightly less than in other post-mortem series (Benda, 1952; Freytag and Lindenberg, 1967).

What was once an almost uniform entity, 'mental retardation', has been fragmented under the incessant scrutiny of biological science into a veritable mosaic of aetiologically distinct conditions. The broad spectrum of these disorders ranging from gross malformations and circulatory damage to specific enzymatic and genetic defects, is generally known, but more information is desirable on the frequency distribution of these causes. In a considerable proportion of these disorders the neuropathological features are non-specific or still undetermined, and the aetiology is obscure. The search of biological factors in this wide range of conditions by multidisciplinary efforts including molecular neuropathology, biochemistry and genetics, will be one of the most rewarding areas of investigation in the field of unclassified mental deficiency.

REFERENCES

Benda, C. E. (1952). 'Developmental Disorders of Mentation and Cerebral Palsies'. New York: Grune & Stratton.

Bérard-Badier, M., Colmant, H.-J., Jacob, H. and Solcher, H. (1965). *Acta neuropath.* **5**, 243.

Christensen, E., Melchior, J. C. and Bredmose, G. V. (1965). 'Proc. Internat. Congr. Scientific Study of Mental Retardation' (J. Øster, ed.), Vol. 1, p. 427.

Crome, L. and Stern, J. (1967). 'Pathology of Mental Retardation'. London: Churchill.

Freytag, E. and Lindenberg, R. (1967). *Johns Hopkins Med. J.* **121**, 379.

Gonatas, N. K., Evangelista, L. and Walsh, G. O. (1967). *J. Neuropath. exp. Neurol.* **26**, 179.

Gross, H. and Jellinger, K. (1969). *Wien. Z. Nervenheilk.* **27**, 9.

Gross, H., Jellinger, K., Kaltenbäck, E. and Rett, A. (1968). *J. neurol. Sci.* **7**, 551.

Gross, H. and Kaltenbäck, E. (1959). *Dtsch. Z. Nervenheilk.* **179**, 388.

Gross, H. and Kaltenbäck, E. (1960). *Morph. Jahrb.* **100,** 517.
Gross, H. and Kaltenbäck, E. (1962). In 'Proc. IVth Internat. Congr. Neuropath',' (H. Jacobs, ed.), Vol. 1, p. 24. Stuttgart: G. Thieme.
Jellinger, K. (1970). 'Second Internat. Congr. Assoc. for the Scientific Study of Mental Retardation', Warsaw.
Loeser, J. D. and Alvord, E. C. Jr. (1968). *Brain* **91,** 553.
Malamud, N. (1952). 'Proc. 1st Internat. Congr. of Neuropath., Rome', Vol. II, p. 261. Torino: Rosenberg & Sellier.
Martin, J. J., van Bogaert, L. and Guazzi, G. C. (1968). *Conf. Neurol.* **30,** 97.
Martin, J. J., Guazzi, G. C. and de Barsy, Th. (1969). *J. Hirnforsch.* **11,** 7.
Meyer, J. E. (1949). *Z. Kinderheilk.* **67,** 123.
Miyakawa, T., Sumiyoshi, S., Deshimaru, M. and Tatetsu, S. (1970). *Acta neuropath.* **16,** 25.
Peiffer, J. (1970). In 'Epilepsy, Mod. Probl. Pharmacopsychiat.' (E. Niedermeyer, ed.) Vol. 4, p. 42. Basel-New York: Karger.
Sumi, S. M. (1970). *Brain* **93,** 821.
Suzuki, K. and Rapin, I. (1969). *Arch. Neurol. (Chicago)* **20,** 62.
Terplan, K. L., Lopet, E. C. and Robinson, H. B. (1970). *Amer. J. Dis. Child.* **119,** 228.
Veith, G. and Wicke, R. (1968). 'Cerebrale Differenzierungsstörungen bei Epilepsie, Jahrbuch, Landesamt für Forschung, Nordrhein-Westfalen', pp. 515-534. Köln-Opladen: West-deutscher Verlag.

DISCUSSION

Cavanagh (Chairman): Perhaps the discussion might be opened by Dr. Hanefeld who has made a clinical study of this problem in Berlin and may have some important points to add.

Hanefeld: After hearing about so many pathological aspects of unclassified mental retardation, it might be valuable to look at the problem from a clinician's standpoint. Going through the clinical notes of all children going through the University Hospital for Children in Berlin from 1965-1970, I have chosen from them those cases who were more than six months old when admitted for investigation of delayed mental development. Most were not more than three years old. In six years there was a total of 17,723 cases (Table 1) admitted of whom 359 (2%) presented as cases of mental retardation. In 196 (55%) the history and investigations gave us some insight into the aetiology of these. I found those with perinatal distress (91 cases) formed 25%, but this included every child with a history of hyperbilirubinaemia, or any respiratory or other problems. This was done since it is well known that the development of kernicterus is often multifactorial, and there is a higher risk of this in premature infants with acidosis and respiratory infections and so forth, even when the level is well within the normal range. Those who were retarded following infections formed 9%, while 5.3% had genetic disorders, amongst which are all the various

Table 1

	1965	1966	1967	1968	1969	1970	Total	%
Number of admissions	2964	2990	3090	2990	2675	3014	17,723	100
Referred with mental retardation	58	49	55	63	52	82	359	2.0
Perinatal distress	16	14	15	12	9	25	91	25.3
Infections of the CNS	10	2	5	5	5	6	33	9.2
General diseases (not chromosome anomalies)	2	3	2	5	4	3	19	5.3
Malformations	6	2	5	2	6	3	24	6.7
Trauma	0	0	0	2	1	2	5	1.4
Metabolic disorders	1	1	2	6	5	9	24	6.7
Unknown	23	27	26	31	22	34	163	45.4

syndromes, such as Laurence-Biedl-Moon syndrome. Moreover, not included in this group studied are Down's syndrome. Moreover, not chromosomal disorders. Malformations were a surprisingly small group forming only 6.6%. This is almost certainly due to the fact that many children with spina bifida were directly transferred to the neurosurgical department, not part of the hospital. Trauma formed only 1.4%, while metabolic disorders formed about 6.6%.

In the remaining 45% (163) cases we were not able to find a cause, or to name a syndrome or a disease.

Looking more closely at the clinical picture (Table 2), we found that 56 (34%) had normal muscle tone, 36 (22%) were hypertonic (spastic) and 71 (43%) were hypotonic or athetoid. Of those 163 cases with unclassified mental retardation, 39 of them had epilepsy and 12 of these had had infantile spasms. Seventeen cases (10%) were microcephalic and six of these also showed hydrocephalus which was proved by air encephalogram. Fourteen cases (8.5%) had hydrocephalus, short stature, obesity, cataracts and optic atrophy were also found in those patients.

Wigglesworth: We have had some mention of kernicterus with normal bilirubin levels, but in my experience I have only seen this in babies dying in extreme hypoxic circumstances, where I assumed that the staining was merely the manifestation of the hypoxia preceding death. In very premature babies we have never seen one develop signs of

Table 2

Clinical Findings in 163 Children with Unclassified Mental Retardation

Muscle tone		No.	%
Normal		56	34.4
Hypertonic-spastic		36	22.1
Hypotonic or athetoid		71	43.5
	Total	163	100
Epilepsy		39	24
Microcephaly		17	10.4
Hydrocephaly		14	8.5
Short stature		5	3.1
Obesity		5	3.1
Cataract		4	2.4
Optic atrophy		3	1.8
No abnormalities		70	42.9

kernicterus during life with bilirubin below 20. We have not, in fact, been impressed with the occurrence of low bilirubin kernicterus, except as a terminal event.

Hanefeld: This is a matter of definition. It would be better termed 'bilirubin encephalopathy' which is not only a pathological diagnosis. Premature children in several studies have certainly been shown to have clinical symptoms, such as vertigo, deafness, athetosis, etc., with a history of relatively low bilirubin levels, respiratory distress and acidosis.

Crome: By and large I think I agree with Dr. Wigglesworth. One sees an occasional case of kernicterus with septicaemia.

Kirman: As regards the neurological studies, I agree that the correspondence with the clinical aspect of these cases is quite limited, and usually we are in ignorance of the precise anatomical findings until they are revealed.

Laurence: With arhinencephaly you said you get this median cleft syndrome. I have seen a number of such conditions, even the extreme holoprosencephaly variety, without any median facial or palatal cleft at all. Although there is a tendency for some sort of a cleft to be present, all variations seem to occur, and I cannot see any reason for an invariable association between arhinencephaly, clefts and trisomy 13/15. Perhaps someone can enlighten me?

Jellinger: You know the papers of De Meyer (De Meyer, W. and Zeman, W. (1963) *Confin. Neurol.* **23**, 1; De Meyer, W., Zeman, W. and Palmer, C. G. (1964) *Pediatrics* **34**, 256) where holoprosencephalies were found to be associated with median or bilateral cleft syndromes. In half our cases of holoprosencephaly there were associated various types of median clefts. They are or may not be associated with a corpus callosum defect. They may predict the state of the brain or they may not. I do not know what the correlation is between these lesions and either genetic or exogenic processes. That is dependent probably on the time when the lesions are acting. I do not think anyone knows the association between trisomy 13/15 and the cleft syndromes. We know that some of these cases can be diagnosed by air encephalography and also recently by angiography.

Laurence: We have published results with both angiography and air encephalography, but we were unable to confirm De Meyer's dictum (Bligh, A. S. and Laurence, K. M. (1967) *Clin. Radiol.* **18**, 383) about the face predicting the brain lesion or vice versa.

Balázs: In some of these brains there were ectopias. Someone early on mentioned that one cause of cell death is if a neurone cannot make contacts with an end organ. What happens with these ectopias? Do they innervate anything?

Jellinger: A recent paper of De Meyer (De Meyer, W. (1967) *Arch. Neurol.* **16**, 203) some experiments were done in the foetal rat showing that a sufficiently early lesion could stop neuroblast migration. Ectopic nodules of undifferentiated nerve cells developed near the ventricular wall. This may be one possible cause of such lesions, but we do not know if they are functioning cells. No electrophysiology has been done on them.

Balázs: What do they do, then?

Jellinger: I do not know, but one indication that they may function is found in telencephalic haematoma associated with pubertas praecox which are localised nerve cell nests in the base of the third ventricle, which probably act in the same way as the cells of the infundibular nuclei to produce gonadotropin-releasing hormones. Some are and some are not associated with pubertas praecox, so we can suggest that they may become functionally intact.

Kirman: Taking Dr. Laurence's point about malformation that some were genetically determined and some not, perhaps, like laboratory animals, we may have evolved rather differently in some areas of the world. Thus, it is suggested that Chinese are more resistant to factors inducing mental retardation, while Sikhs, like the Irish, are more sensitive. Moroever, it seems that West Indian women keep up a better level of B_{12} during malnourishment. In Social Class V, if this capacity to nourish the infant is stressed, then any defect would be more readily displayed in some people than in others. The notion of genetic predisposition could be combined, therefore, with an environmental factor.

Laurence: There was an interesting report (Naggan, L. and MacMahon, B. (1967) *New Engl. J. Med.* **277**, 1199) on the CNS malformations in the various ethnic groups in Boston where it was found that the Irish, particularly the poor Irish, have the highest and the Negroes the lowest incidence. The Chinese are also low wherever they live, so there is clearly a strong genetic factor operating (Searle, A. G. (1959) *Ann. Human Genet.* **23**, 279; Stevenson, A. C. *et al.* (1966) *Bull. Wld. Hlth. Org.* **33**, Suppl. (Congenital Malformations).

On the subject of environmental trigger mechanisms, we are currently looking at the folic acid and B_{12} state during the first month of pregnancy when it matters most, but it is too early yet to say anything about this. I suspect that there are too many factors to enable us to get the answer from this kind of investigation, except on a much larger scale.

Crome: It seemed to me that Dr. Hanefeld's figures were rather low for mental deficiency in a general population. Were they low?

Hanefeld: I cannot say whether this is so, the population is selected in that we mainly see young children. If chromosomal anomalies were also included the figure would be about 3%, which probably reflects the incidence in the country.

Clayton: In Great Ormond Street it is about 400 for 12,000 admissions per year, but this also is too low a figure.

Holt: I took this low incidence to be due to a high admission rate of acute infections which might mirror the population of a general children's hospital rather than a specialist hospital like Great Ormond Street.

Crome: There is another point. Anencephaly is said to be very rare in Central Europe, and more frequent in the Western Seaboard. Is this Dr. Jellinger's experience?

Jellinger: In Hungary it is about 1 per 1000 live births (Czeikel, A. and Revesz, C. (1970) *Brit. J. Prev. Med.* **24**, 205) and about 1.5 per 1000 in W. Germany (Tunte, W. (1968) *Humangenetik* **6**, 225).

Laurence: That is about half the incidence in the U.K.

Giroud: It seems there is less in some regions, and we have thought recently about the water being responsible. But in some parts of Europe there is some connection with rickettsial infection. In those with anencephaly, infection is four times more common than in controls. But there must be many more causes responsible, including genetic factors, since there are population differences.

Prestige: I wanted to ask about microgyria, because here is a defect in organogenesis in which the structure has compensated for the defect in a beautiful way. Are there other studies of this condition?

Crome: There are a number of studies on the morphology of

microgyria, and on the experimental aspects. Helena Riggs in Philadelphia (Riggs, H. E., McGrath, J. J. and Schwartz, H. P. (1956) *J. Neuropath. Exp. Neurol.* **15**, 432) has produced something like this by irradiation on the 11th day in rat brains. This produced a migration defect of the same general sort as in humans. I think that microgyria can also be produced by cytomegalic inclusion virus at a much later stage, for migration of cells occurs almost up till birth and you can interrupt this at any stage.

Jellinger: We saw one case of CO intoxication at the 24th week of gestation, the baby being born spontaneously 6-8 weeks later and living for 3½ hours. Almost the whole brain was destroyed, except for the hippocampus and medial temporal lobe. Between the destroyed and the intact cortex there were symmetrical microgyric areas. This appears to be the latest date for an exogenous lesion producing microgyria.

Cavanagh: In the ectopias, the collection of cells fails to migrate at all from the subependymal plate region, while in microgyria the cells seem to come too late when a fibre barrier has already been formed. There seems therefore to be two sorts of defect here, at different stages of migration.

Balázs: Does the EEG show any differences in such circumstances, where there is almost two layers of cortex in the same place?

Harris: We might relook at this in the course of time.

Jellinger: These cases are associated with focal seizures.

Cavanagh: I do not think that this change was found in any of the temporal lobe series of the Maudsley Hospital.

Jellinger: We never saw them in the temporal lobe either, and none had temporal lobe epilepsy. These were local Jacksonian fits. Pachygyria, on the other hand, is rather frequently reported in infantile spasms.

Harris: The EEG does not, in fact, help here, for the abnormality is so severe and global. I have seen cases, when the infantile spasms have disppeared, and in whom the gross EEG abnormality has disappeared and then focal features can be seen.

General Discussion

OPENED BY P. E. SYLVESTER

Mr. Chairman, it was suggested that I should be complementary to Dr. Crome. You may think that perhaps the last word has been spoken by the morphologists, but I shall try and destroy that impression. Starting with Dr. Jellinger's observation that not infrequently the brains of mental defectives show no clear-cut pathological changes, both he and Crome agreed to a conservative figure of 10-12% for their incidence. They, of course, deal with children, and I would like to shift the emphasis to the older subject. The graph (Fig. 1) shows wet brain weights from Roessle and Roulet (Roessle, R. and Roulet, F. (1932) Mass und Zahl in der Pathologie, in 'Pathologie und Klinik in Einzelldarstellungen' (L. Aschoff, ed.), Vol. 5. Vienna and Berlin: Springer) in adult males and upon this has been drawn a curve from a sample of 188 adult mentally handicapped males and you can see that those two lines are quite closely related. If one takes a standard of 1300 gm as being a normal brain weight, then 50-60% of this population compare closely with the normal population.

Two-hundred-and-seventy brains examined over the last 10 years from St. Lawrence's Hospital have shown obstructive hydrocephalus in only 3%, usually the result of infection or malformations. Many (17%), on the other hand, have ventricular dilatation judged to be compensatory, but this may be begging the question somewhat when, perhaps, it should be related in some way to cell nutrition. Cortical atrophy which was a common feature of both Crome's and Jellinger's material was found only in 8%. In the cerebellum, however, quite a lot of abnormality turns up, and roughly speaking about 20% of the brains show this. Amongst these, hypoplasia, i.e. merely reduction in weight and little else, occurred in 11%, while sclerosis accounted for 9%. This seemed rather out of proportion by comparison with the findings of Crome and Jellinger, neither of whom have commented on the significance of cerebellar disease.

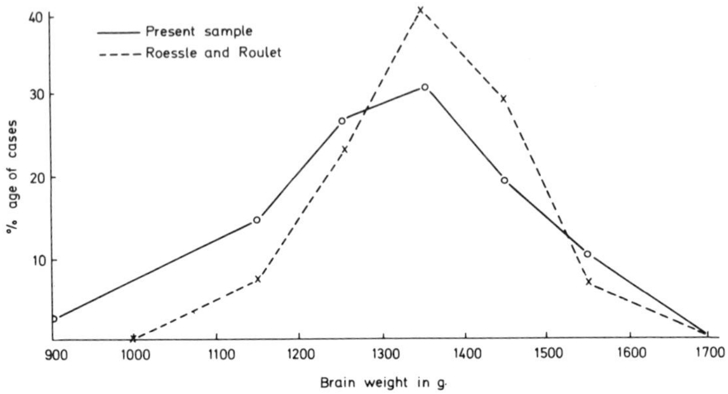

Fig. 1. Curve of distribution of 157 male patients aged 15-59 years (continuous line) compared with Roessle and Roulet's curve for 893 normal males from 16-60 years (interrupted line). The mean weight of the defectives was 1263.04 g and for the normals was 1374.55 g.

By comparison with children, in adults peri- and post-natal problems seem a long way off. While Crome may have a glut of information about early history, with a population of adult mental defectives such information is scanty or absent. This defect may, however, prompt one into looking elsewhere for answers. Older children and adults may suffer from acquired brain disease, so that the virus infections discussed by Dr. Zlotnik may bear no relation to their mental handicap. In a community of long living mentally handicapped persons consideration of the causes of their problem is not very realistic, but what is important is an understanding of the mechanisms behind their disability. I have tried to approach this problem by measuring and weighing, particularly the parietal lobe, and I find that in 9.5% of my population this region of the brain seems to be quite small, while the rest of the brain seems normal. Moreover the body of the corpus callosum through which the transhemispherical fibres pass is also small and thinned. I related this back to the clinical story. Several had been epileptic, two of whom were seriously handicapped in performance tests, such as picture-completion, block designs and mazes. It was next tried to extrapolate this information to the living subject, and with the help of Mrs. Blundell, the psychologist, we set up samples of epileptic and non-epileptic subjects, where the epilepsy dated from early childhood. Mrs. Blundell demonstrated that the epileptics had serious difficulty with space concept (*J. ment. def. Res.* (1966) **10**, 141). One would not dare to conclude too much from these findings, because it has yet to be shown that the living subjects have the anatomical defect defined.

Concerning the counting of neurones I think one should continue to make the effort to count them, despite what people say. I have done this in part of the temporal lobe, involving lamina V of the fusiform gyrus. There seems to be, in a control group, a strong correlation between cell density and the patient's age, and up to a certain age this is related to increasing synaptic and dendritic development. In a population of mentally handicapped people, no such correlation was found. So far as this goes, it means that we certainly should continue with this approach. Our concept of what is happening in unclassified mental retardation is going to hinge upon what information we are going to get from the neurones, both about numbers and enzyme activity.

Returning to the question of brain weights, it seems that our material, in the last few years, may be approaching the material of Dr. Crome in that our brains certainly seem to be getting much smaller. This may be a sign of a change in a population of a large hospital for the subnormal.

Balázs: Up to what age is the graph you showed linear in the control population?

Sylvester: It started at 18 and went to 60 years. In small children the cell density gets less rather quickly and then it tapers off. We have found that it continues to increase until about the age of 20.

Balázs: I was trying to compare it with the rat where a similar situation seems to exist. Here the increase is simply a reflection of the increase in cell size and also in myelination. Due to this there are fewer cells per unit volume. A 35-day-old rat would in fact probably compare with a 20-year-old man, so that this would correspond to a general phenomenon of cell differentiation.

Jellinger: What were these cerebellar hypoplasia and sclerosis cases? So many conditions can produce these changes, of course. Thus, about one-third of our cases of vascular encephalopathy had cerebellar atrophy. Hypoplasia occurred in about 2% of our total series.

Sylvester: Hypoplasia I take to be merely reduction in size, as in mongolism. Sclerosis is different in that the anatomical pattern is disturbed. Such sclerosis may be linked with cortical atrophy, and all cases were epileptic. I do not know what it means, but there may be a possible role in epilepsy here.

Balázs: To return to your graph, to go one step further, when looking at your mentally handicapped population, your finding that the neuronal density does not change indicates that the cell differentiation is arrested.

Sylvester: There are discrepancies, however, in our results, which make us distrustful of our technique, but we must look into this further.

Balázs: Until we know this basic information we are more or less in doubt. If a cell count is done in conjunction with a DNA estimate in a given area, we would get also an idea of the total cell number. The two methods should be complementary. If this were done one might get information that could suggest that neuronal differentiation was at fault in some way. Perhaps the dendritic arborisation was much less, as in the thyroid-deficient animal.

Jellinger: This approach could well lower the percentage of 'negative' cases. Similar studies are being done on schizophrenics' brains using automatic counting machines and computers. In untreated schizophrenics a reduced number of cells was found in some regions (Colon, E. J. (1971) *Acta Neuropath.* (in press)) and it was considered that this was not due to loss of neurones, but to a reduction of the arborisation.

O'Connor: I would like to ask Dr. Sylvester whether, in this particular instance, where the parietal lobes were affected, one would expect this only on the right side? If the corpus callosum is restricted, perhaps the left is affected too. In that case, why does one get the pattern of the high verbal defective? This is a problem that has always troubled me. If there is going to be any cell counting, perhaps it could be done in the two parietal lobes to see how differentiation occurs.

Sylvester: The question is which part to start counting on. I began on the temporal lobe simply because S. T. Bok (Bok, S. T. (1959) 'Histonomy of the Cerebral Cortex', Amsterdam: Elsevier Publ. Co.) in his book discussed the temporal lobe, and I could localise the fusiform gyrus accurately.

Cremer: How do those cells stay alive when they are undifferentiated and so small? Are their oxygen requirements low?

Sylvester: They appear to be similar to the normal cells, but I cannot say whether something has happened previously to take some of the cells out. There are, of course, severely subnormal patients with I.Q.'s of 50.

Balázs: May I put in a plea to measure the cerebellum, too, as this is a relatively late developing region? It may be possible simply by weighing and getting the ratio to pin-point times when possible insult may have been inflicted. Moreover, some parts of this organ that can be easily dissected out may be developing much earlier than other parts. This could possibly show whether the insult was late or early in development. It might then be determined what proportion of cases are inflicted after birth, a rather neglected time about which something can be done.

Cavanagh: I think the time has come now to ask Dr. Kirman, as Chairman of this Symposium, if he could summarise some of the many ideas for future work that have been thrown up over the last three days.

Chairman's Summary

B. H. KIRMAN

This Study Group has been very valuable. It has brought together a number of specialists in different fields each one of whom has a useful contribution to make to the study of the brain in unclassified mental retardation. The discussion has been intense, informed and lively. It is clear that considerable cross-fertilisation has taken place and that this will be a further stimulus to those already engaged in the field and may attract others to it.

The definition of the group of cases under consideration gives rise to some difficulty though it is agreed that it is very large. Both Dr. Crome and Prof. Jellinger find that the majority of children with severer degrees of mental handicap show structural lesions of the brain, and Dr. Crome stresses that in most of these it is not possible to recognise a process with a specific aetiology. On a clinical basis a majority, even of the more severely retarded with an I.Q. below 50 on standard tests, cannot be assigned to a diagnostic category with known aetiology and in this sense are unclassified. With the more numerous mildly retarded the proportion unclassified is even greater. The work reported by Dr. Drillien and others emphasises, however, that adverse experience in early life may also be an important factor in determining the intellectual status of this group, although multifactorial aetiology must be particularly common in this degree of retardation. Consideration of the adequacy of the educational and cultural environment must be included in any attempt to understand the origin of mild mental handicap.

In considering the nature of damage to the brain in unclassified mental retardation Dr. Crome stressed the relative non-specificity of the structural changes in response to a whole range of possible noxious factors, so that, although neuropathology permits timing of the insult in some cases, it is often unable to determine its precise nature. There is also in unclassified cases a tendency to widespread damage to the CNS which equates with the difficulty expressed by Dr. O'Connor of determining in the majority of such cases any specificity of psychological defect. Rather there is a tendency to diffuseness of dysfunction, a global defect, which may be expressed as a deficit of attention or arousal.

The same type of difficulty is no doubt responsible for the limitation, indicated by Dr. Ruth Harris, to the contribution which electrophysiology can make at the present to clarification of the difficult problem of the as yet unclassified cases. Electrophysiology is useful in that, where it shows marked asymmetry, convulsive features or other clear-cut anomalies, it can establish the existence of an organic basis for dysfunction, thus clarifying one aspect of the vexed problem of childhood psychosis and autism.

It seems likely, as suggested by Prof. Clayton, that further fragments will be won away from the total of unclassified cases of mental handicap by recognition of new factors in aetiology. Dr. Zlotnik made a particularly valuable contribution in this connection by pointing out that, on an experimental basis, viruses, which have not been recognised to have this effect, can have devastating consequences when acting before birth or in early life. It seems possible that there are as yet unrecognised viral effects of this kind in humans. There is also a warning to public health authorities to pay particular attention to the risk which would possibly result from the use of a live attenuated vaccine during pregnancy.

A vivid illustration of another type of man-made hazard which constitutes a potential threat to the development of the brain was illustrated by the work of Dr. Wechsler and Dr. Kleihues on the role of alkylating agents which may act either by provoking tumours or by producing destruction, much depending in this case as with other noxious factors on the time of the insult to the brain. As explained by Prof. Magee this action is a real threat since substances with this type of effect are known to be produced by interaction in the stomach between nitrites, or nitrates and food amines. Nitrites are used in food preservation, and nitrates are now a very general contaminant. Several speakers, particularly Drs Crome and Zlotnik, emphasised that gross structural lesions may exist in the brain without obvious neurological symptoms. The deficit may need sophisticated behavioural tests to be made manifest, comparable to the rigorous psychometry required in mildly retarded human children, to demonstrate the handicap. Dr. Zlotnik's work, like that of a number of other members of the Study Group, shows that existing techniques are only now being brought to bear on the problem of damage to the brain which may result in mental handicap.

Several speakers emphasised that in considering abnormalities of the brain attention can also usefully be paid to co-existing or resultant somatic anomalies. Dr. Rundle's long-term study of growth in unclassified mental handicap adds point to this observation, and again emphasises the severity of the growth deficit in a high proportion of cases. This type of patient study may provide further clues to classification, if only by focusing attention on that minority of cases who are well grown.

There are different levels of classification in mental handicap and the use of descriptive terms, such as hypertensive hydrocephalus or obstructive hydrocephalus, already implies the existence of a classifiable group, but in one sense this merely displaces the question of aetiology one stage further. So that Dr. Laurence's summary of the problem of mental handicap and hydrocephalus is very pertinent, and it is useful to have this model of multifactorial aetiology. One of the baffling clues, mentioned in this connection by Prof. Giroud, was the link between malformation of the nervous system and soft water, and even if such connections are only secondary they are valuable pointers.

The sensitivity of the developing nervous system which Prof. Giroud took as his theme was emphasised throughout the sessions by all speakers, and it is evident that the professions concerned, and the public, are not sufficiently informed as to the fact that agents, which may be quite innocent to the formed brain, are injuriious during the formative period which, in the case of man, extends long after birth. Professor Giroud stressed the role of nutritive balance and adequacy, pointing to the irreversible effects on the nervous system which can result from excess or inadequacy of a particular constituent of the diet. Dr. Woollam, who is also well known for his work in this field, elaborated in particular the part played in brain development by the vascular supply, and suggested that in much of brain development it is this which mediates the final structure of the brain. Dr. Prestige's contribution on numbers of brain cells gave insight into the dynamic nature of cerebral cell growth and some assessment of the role of controlling factors which may give a clue to the reasons for sub-optimal development. The hormonal regulation of cerebral development was outlined by Dr. Balázs, whose contribution again made clear the need for further work in this important field.

The reasons for the apparent inhibition of brain growth in human infants prior to birth are not always clear, but Dr. Wigglesworth, whilst giving an account of some experimental growth factors again emphasised the role of nutrition which is gradually receiving attention both at the pre-natal and neonatal levels. This point was further stressed by Dr. Drillien who attributes improvement in results with newborn low-weight babies, at least, in part, to an appreciation of the need for early feeding.

Attention was paid during the sessions of the Study Group to the importance of critical periods in brain development coinciding with growth spurts in neurones and glia in different areas of the brain. It became clear that many aspects of knowledge relevant to an understanding of the development of the human brain are also undergoing 'growth spurts' and are desperately in need of appropriate nutrition. If one of these aspects can be singled out without detriment to the others, it is perhaps that of enzymology, which should, if pursued to its logical conclusion, permit a more general evaluation of the structural basis of normal and abnormal variation in human intelligence. Dr. Cremer reminds us that almost nothing is known about the mechanisms controlling the rates of synthesis and removal of enzymes in brain cells. This is true of the rat, but it is even more true of ourselves, since we have more information in this respect about the rat brain than the human.

The contributions bristle with important questions and the discussion poses many of these. It is to be hoped that the necessary resources will be found and organised to implement at least some of the suggestions for further enquiry into this important field of human inadequacy, and that the publication of the proceedings will attract the attention of those who can carry the work a stage further.

List of Participants

R. Balázs, MD, PhD	Neuropsychiatric Research Unit, Medical Research Council Laboratories, Carshalton, Surrey
J. B. Cavanagh, MD, MRCP	(Adviser) Professor and Director, MRC Research Group in Applied Neurobiology, London
B. E. Clayton, PhD, MD, MRCP, MRCPath	Professor and Cons. Chemical Pathologist, The Hospital for Sick Children, London, and the Institute of Child Health (University of London)
J. E. Cremer, PhD	Biochemical Mechanisms Section, MRC Toxicology Research Unit, Medical Research Council Laboratories, Carshalton, Surrey
L. Crome, MC, MRCP, FRCPath	Cons. Neuropathologist, Queen Mary's Hospital for Children, Carshalton, Surrey
A. N. Davison, BPharm, PhD	Professor and Head of the Department of Biochemistry and Organic Chemistry, Charing Cross Hospital Medical School (University of London)
J. Dobbing, BSc, MB, MRCPath	Department of Child Health, University of Manchester
Cecile M. Drillien, MD, MRCP(Edin)	Department of Child Life and Health, University of Edinburgh
A. Giroud, MD	Professor at Laboratoire d'Histologie, Faculte de Medecine de Paris, Universite de Paris a la Sorbonne
F. A. Hanefeld, MD	Children Hospital of the Free University, Berlin, W. Germany

Ruth Harris, MD, DCH	Cons. Electrophysiologist, Bethlem Royal and Maudsley Hospitals and Queen Mary's Hospital for Children, Carshalton, Surrey
K. S. Holt, MD, FRCP, DCH	The Director, Wolfson Centre and Department of Developmental Paediatrics, Institute of Child Health (University of London)
K. Jellinger, MD	Professor at Neurologisches Institut der Universität, Wien, Austria
B. H. Kirman, MD, DPM	(Chairman) Cons. Psychiatrist, Fountain and Carshalton Group; Hon. Associate Physician, St. George's and Maudsley Hospitals, London
P. Kleihues, MD	Max-Planck-Institut für Hirnforschung, Abteilung für Allgemeine Neurologie, West Germany
K. M. Laurence, MA, MB, ChB, MRCPath	Senior Lecturer (Paediatric Pathology) Department of Child Health, Paediatric Pathology Laboratory, Llandough Hospital, Penarth
P. N. Magee, BA, MB, BChir	Phillip Hill Professor of Biochemistry, Courtauld Institute of Biochemistry, Middlesex Hospital Medical School (University of London)
N. O'Connor, MA, PhD	The Director, MRC Developmental Psychology Research Unit, London
Ruth Porter, MTCP, DCH	Deputy Director, Ciba Foundation for the Promotion of International Co-operation in Medical and Chemical Research, London

M. C. Prestige, MA, PhD	Department of Physiology, University of Edinburgh
D. Richter, PhD, MRCP	Director, MRC Neuropsychiatric Research Unit, Medical Research Council Laboratories, Carshalton, Surrey
A. T. Rundle, BSc, MIBiol	Principal Biochemist, Pathology Department, St. Lawrence's Hospital, Caterham, Surrey
J. Stern, BSc, PhD	Principal Biochemist, Pathology Department, Queen Mary's Hospital for Children, Carshalton, Surrey
P. E. Sylvester, MRCS, LRCP, DCH, MRCPath	Cons. Psychiatrist and Director of Neuropathology Department, St. Lawrence's Hospital, Caterham, Surrey
W. Wechsler, MD	Max-Planck-Institut für Hirnforschung, Abteilung für Allgemeine Neurologie, West Germany
J. S. Wigglesworth, MD, MRCPath	Neonatal Department, Institute of Child Health (University of London)
D. H. M. Woollam, MA, MD, ScD, MRCP	Department of Anatomy, and Fellow and Tutor of Emmanuel College, University of Cambridge
Dr. I. Zlotnik, PhD, BVSc, MRCVS	Pathologist, Microbiological Research Establishment, Ministry of Defence.

Index

Abortion, small for dates babies and, 160, 163
Abstraction, behaviour and, 250, 253
Acrocephalosyndactyly, 266
Actinomycin D, 27
Adenoviruses, 114
Aetiology of mental retardation, 188, 192, 205, 261, 294, 295, 317
Aflatoxin, 148
Alertness, 255
Alkylating agents,
  effects, 117-132, 318. *See also under specific agents*
    acute, 123
    carcinogenic, 133
    comparative studies, 122
    on amino acids, 141, 142
    on nucleic acids, 125, 126
    on protein synthesis, 128
    on RNA synthesis, 139
  metabolism and distribution, 123
  tumour induction by, 122
  types of, 118
Alzheimer disease, 263
Amino acids,
  alkylation of, 141, 142
  cerebral transport, 265
  conversion from glucose carbon, 63, 64
  disorders of metabolism, 304
  importance in brain development, 32
Aminoaciduria, 213, 218, 261
δ-Aminolaevulinic acid dehydratase, 219
Ammonia in blood, 263
Androgens, effects of, 69, 70
Anencephaly, 105, 310
  soft water and, 45
Anoxia,
  effects of, 201
  importance in cerebral vascularisation, 4, 10
Anoxic-vascular defects, 302
Antibiotics, teratogenic effects, 24
Antibodies,
  and the developing brain, 30, 37, 44
  sympathetic nervous system and, 45
  transmission, 114
Anticonvulsants, effect on enzymes, 90
Antimyelin antibodies, 38
Anti-tumour agents, teratogenic effects, 24
Apert's syndrome, 88
Aphasia, 245, 253
Arhinencephaly, 308
Arnold-Chiari malformation, 10, 271, 280, 300
Arousal, subnormal, 244
Arteriosclerosis, cerebral, 250
Astrocytes,
  abnormal, 293
  effect of infection, 115
'At risk' registers, 206
Autism, 197-198, 201
  digit-span, 257
  EEG changes, 242, 254, 256
Azoethane, 120

Babbling in mongols, 256
Barbiturates, effect on enzyme activity, 90
Basal ganglia, marbling, 288
Behaviour, 251
  abstraction and, 250, 253
  effect of corticosteroids, 66
  effect of hormones on development, 65-70
  effect of thyroid hormone, 64
  hippocampus and, 150
  imposed patterns, 196-197
  modification of, 191
  unacceptable, 197

Bilirubin,
causing neurological damage, 30, 307
levels, 261, 307
Biochemistry, mental retardation and, 213
Biochemistry of brain, correlation with structure, 93
Birth injury, 298
Birthweight, low. *See Low Birthweight*
1,3-Bis(2-chloroethyl)-1-nitrosourea, 137
Block design imitation, 246
Blood sugar in mental retardation, 214
Blood vessels,
in cretinism, 73
Blood vessels of brain, 319
development, 3-12
importance of anoxia, 4
foetal, anatomical and physiological significance of, 6-7
functional aspects, 3, 10
mental defect and, 8-9
relation to neurones, 6
Blue tongue disease, 31
Body weight, relation to brain weight, 14, 15, 16
Brain. *See also under other headings Embryonic brain, Foetal brain, Blood vessels, etc.*
abnormalities of, 208, 209
amino acid transport, 265
arteriosclerosis, 250
association with behaviour, 245
atrophy, 285, 304
disorders, tryptophan metabolism in, 216
dysfunction, 257, 258
ectopias, 286, 291, 309
growth, 319
hypoplasia, 285
injury,
defined by psychology, 244, 252
intelligence and, 252
mental subnormality and,. 243-259
review of studies, 246-251
in schizophrenia, 316
malformations,
mental retardation and, 285
motor disturbances in, 246
maturation, effect of lead, 223
Brain—*cont.*
size, 290, 314
structural lesions, 317
weight of, 315
Breast milk, composition, 85

Camberwell Survey, 207, 241, 242
Capillaries,
definitions, 5
in cretinism, 8
intra-cerebral, 5, 11
relation to metabolic requirements, 6
Carbon monoxide intoxication, 311
Carcinogenesis,
by alkylating agents, 117, 133
by nitrosamines, 145
Caudal dysraphias, 300
Cells. *See also Neurones*
effect of alkylating agents on, 124
numbers, malformations and, 50
organ population, biochemical approach, 50-52
sizes, malformations and, 50
weight of, 57
Cell contact, 21
Cell death, 4, 11, 43
control of, 18
radiation, 24
Cell division, control of, 17
Cerebellar ataxia in hydrocephalus, 277
Cerebellum,
abnormalities, 313
cell growth in, 77
chemical factors affecting, 30
DNA content, 78
development of, 41
effect of hormones on, 67, 73
effect of irradiation, 30
effect of thyroid gland, 62, 67
hypoplasia, 315
measurement of, 316
sclerosis, 315
Cerebral cortex,
gliosis, 287
marbling, 288
Cerebral hemispheres, malformation, 285
Cerebral palsy, 171
Cerebrospinal dysgenesias and dysraphies, 301

Cerebrospinal fluid,
changes in, from inflammatory causes, 272
maldevelopment causing obstruction, 271
overproduction, 270
pathway defects, 269-282
pathway obstruction, 270-271, 280, 313
protein content, 281
role of, 10, 13
underabsorption, 270
Cerebrum, DNA content, 78
Chemotherapeutic agents, 137
Chicken-pox, 105
1-(2-Chloroethyl)3-cyclohexyl-1-nitrosourea, 137
Chorionic gonadotrophin, 183
Chorioretinitis, 104
Choroid plexus, 271, 281
papillomata, 270
Chromosomes,
alterations, 27
analysis, 96
Citrullinuria, 95
Classification of mental retardation, 190, 205, 297, 319
Community services for mentally handicapped, 194
Comprehension, speed of, 247
Congenital anomalies,
low birthweight and, 161, 162
transient dystonia associated with low birthweight and, 167
Congenital disabilities, infertility associated with, 159
Congenital heart disease, mental retardation and, 182
Congenital malformations, brain weight and, 142
Contraceptive pill, 73, 99
Copper deficiency, 34
Corpus callosum,
abnormality of, 285
absence of, 300
agenesis of, 299
Corticosteroids,
effects
on developing brain, 64-65
on development of behaviour, 66
on hypothalamus, 69
on neurones, 74
Corticosteriods–*cont.*
effects–*cont.*
on pituitary, 69
in infantile spasms, 74
Coxsackie B virus infection, 105, 106
Cretinism, 91
capillary bed in, 8
cerebral blood supply in, 73
'Cri-du-chat' syndrome, 302
Cycasin, 30, 147
Cyclamates, 143
Cycloheximide as growth inhibitor, 54
Cystencephaly, 288
Cytochrome oxidase activity, 94
Cytomegalic inclusion disease, 104, 113, 311

Dandy-Walker syndrome, 273
Deafness, 104
Degenerative processes, 303
Delinquency, mental retardation and, 196
Demyelination, 283
Deoxyribonucleic acid,
amounts in developing brain, 77-78, 81
effect of alkylating agents on, 125
synthesis, 17
effect of alkylating agents, 128
effect of corticosteroids, 64, 74
effect of thyroid hormone, 62, 63
Developmental abnormalities, mental retardation and, 283-292, 298, 299
Diabetic mothers, overweight babies of, 171
Diet,
growth and, 184
maternal, effect on CNS, 217
Diethylhydrazine, effects, 120
Differentiation of brain, 28, 29, 43
Digit-span in autism, 257
Dimethylnitrosamine,
carcinogenesis by, 145
effects on nucleic acids, 125
Dimethylnitrosourea, effects, 119
Dimethyl sulfonate, effects, 120
Disaccharidase activity, 214, 221, 222
Down's syndrome, 9, 10, 75, 252, 299, 307
among small for dates babies, 161
babbling in, 256
cost of, 97

Down's syndrome–*cont.*
ectopia in, 287
EEG patterns, 238
epilepsy in, 257
testicular function in, 185

Eastern equine encephalitis, 106
Economic factors in growth, 177
Electroencephalography,
abnormal, 227
abnormal response in photic stimulation, 235, 238
changes, 292
in autism, 242, 254, 256
in epilepsy, 227, 229, 233, 237
in hydrocephalus, 241
in hypocalcaemia, 242
in infantile spasms, 232, 233, 238
in spina bifida, 241
during sleep, 235, 238, 239
effect of hypothyroidism, 73
in mental retardation, 225-242
alpha rhythm, 234
lambda waves, 235
serial recordings, 236
normal patterns in mental retardation, 241
serial records, 239
techniques, 226, 263
Embryonic brain, sensitivity of, 24-27
Emotions, effect of corticosteroids, 68
Encephalitis,
aetiology, 115
eastern equine, 106
von Economo's, 106
Japanese B, 106
measles, 106
St. Louis, 106
western equine, 105, 106
Encephalomalacia, 288
Encephalomyelitis, experimental, 38
Encephalopathy,
bilirubin, 308
of unclassified mental retardation, 113
spongiform, 288
Endocrine disorders, 61
Environmental factors in mental retardation, 193, 309
Enzymes, polymorphism, 210
Enzyme activity, 266
effect of drugs on, 90
in developing brain, 77-90
in rat, 78-80
in relation to metabolic rate, 81-86
patterns, 78
foetal and adult, 88
measurement in post-mortem material, 89
Enzyme systems, effect of corticosteroids, 68
Ependymomas, 123, 136
Epidemic hepatitis, 105
Epilepsy, 225
cryptogenic, 304
diagnosis, 237
EEG changes, 227, 229-233, 237
serial recordings, 236, 239
idiopathic, 298
in Down's syndrome, 257
minor malformation and, 301
postmortem, 235
Ethylmethanesulphonate, 146
Ethylnitrosourea,
effects, 120, 128, 136
oncogenic, 133, 135
teratogenic, 133, 135, 142
toxicity, 134
metabolism, 124
Ethylurea, reaction with sodium nitrite, 148, 149
Exencephaly, 27
Exercise, growth hormone secretion and, 185
Eye opening, 44

Flicker-fusion tests, 255
in schizophrenia, 247
Foetal brain
protein metabolism in, 29
sensitivity of, 28-34
Foetus,
cerebral blood supply,
anatomical and physiological significance of, 6-7
growth retardation, 49, 148
protection against viral infection, 103
Folic acid antagonists, 27
Forebrain, malformations of, 299
Fructosaemia, 264
Fructose excretion, 214

Galactosaemia, 94, 264
Galactose altering brain cell division, 217
Genetic aspects of mental retardation, 195, 202, 293, 298
Genetic counselling, 203
Glial cells, effect of infection on, 110
Gliomas, induction, 122, 136
Gliotic encephalopathy, 287
Glucose carbon, conversion to amino acids, 63, 64
Glucose excretion, 214, 216
Grey matter,
  blood supply, 5
  in hydrocephalus, 273
Growth,
  anomalies,
    frequency, 174
    intelligence and, 181-182
    mental retardation and, 218
    sexual development and, 179-180
  autism and, 202
  causation of defects, 177
  dietary factors, 184
  excess, 180
  foetal retardation in rat, 53
  head circumference and, 59
  inhibition, 52, 49-59
  in severe mental retardation, 173-186
  institutional factors, 184, 185, 186
  intrauterine, 175
  phases of, 50
  social and economic factors, 177
  thyroid dysfunction and, 178
  velocity of, 184
Growth hormone,
  production, 183, 185, 223
    exercise and, 185
Growth of brain, 28, 34, 41
  effect of corticosteroids, 66
  effect of uterine vessel ligation, 53
  post-natal, 51
Gyri, atrophy, 287

Haemoglobin, 222
Halstead tests battery, 249-250
Halstead impairment index, 246
Head circumference, 291
  brain cell population and, 52
  relation to growth, 59
Height, mental retardation and, 180
Hemi-megalencephaly, 291
Hepatitis, epidemic, 105
Herpes simplex infection, 106
Hippocampus,
  destruction of, behaviour and, 150
  microneurone formation in, 68
  results of infection, 110
Histidinaemia, 98
Holoprosencephalies, 299, 309
Homocysteinuria, 95, 223
Hormonal aspects of brain development, 61-76
Hormones in psychiatric disorders, 262
Hydrocephalus, 9, 285
  aetiology, 269, 280
    inflammatory changes, 272-273
    malformations, 271
  anatomical effects, 273-274, 281
  associated with other anomalies, 290-291, 299
  associated with spina bifida, 271, 272, 274, 279, 280, 290
  chronic brain syndrome of, 278
  congenital, 279
  degree of and performance, 275-278
  development, 279
  EEG changes, 241
  enlarged ventricles in, 284
  incidence, 274
  infective factors, 25
  intelligence in, 276, 278, 281
  obstructive, 313, 319
  progressive, 305
  virus infection and, 104, 105
Hydroxybutyrate dehydrogenase activity, 82, 87
5-Hydroxytryptamine, 70, 91
Hydroxyurea as growth inhibitor, 54, 58
Hyperammonaemia, 263
Hyperbilirubinaemia, 307
Hypercholesterolaemic drugs, 25
Hypernatraemia, 261
Hyperprolinaemia, 238
Hypocalcaemia, EEG changes in, 242
Hypoglycaemia, 216
Hypothalamus, effect of thyroid hormones on, 68
Hypothyroidism,
  EEG patterns in, 238
  in children, 73
Hypoxia, low birthweight and, 162

Imbeciles, trainable, 189
Infantile spasms, 307, 311
ACTH and, 74
EEG changes, 226, 232, 233, 238
pathological changes, 241
Infection causing hydrocephalus, 272
Infertility,
associated with low birthweight infants, 160, 161, 162
congenital anomalies and, 159
Influenzal virus infection, 105, 113
Institutional neurosis, 196
Intelligence,
brain damage and, 252
brain weight and, 13, 14
growth defects and, 181-182
in hydrocephalus, 276, 278, 281
Iodine deficiency, 32, 34
Iproniazid, effect on enzyme activity, 90
Isle of Wight study, 198
Isocitrate dehydrogenase, 214
activity in brain development, 79, 82
Isoleucine, 213
Isoniazid, effect on developing brain, 30

Jacob-Monod hypothesis, 94
Japanese B encephalitis, 106
Jejunal biopsy, 214, 215

Kernicterus, 307, 308
Ketone bodies, 81, 90
Ketotic hypoglycaemia, 88
Kidney, tumours in, 146
Klinefelter's syndrome, 300

Lactose excretion, 214
Langate TP 21 virus, infection with, 107
during pregnancy, 108
neonatal, 110
transplacental, 111
de Lange syndrome, 88
Laurence-Biedl-Moon syndrome, 307
Lead intoxication, 219, 221, 223, 262
Learning, 14, 151
comparative aspects, 15
deficits, 75
Leigh's encephalomyelopathy, 11, 96
Lesch-Nyhan syndrome, 94
Leucine, 213
Leukodystrophies, 304
Leuco-encephalitis, subacute sclerosing, 229
Lipidosis, 241, 304
Liver disease, maternal, effect on child, 264
Louping-ill, 38, 115
Low birthweight,
transient dystonia associated with, 156, 165, 171
congenital anomalies and, 167
incidence, 165
intrauterine growth and, 167
later status, 166
post-natal complications and, 168
Low birthweight infants. *See also Small for dates infants*
aetiology, 157
brain damage in, 217
characteristics, 161
congenital anomalies in, 161, 162
height and social class of mother, 157, 161, 169
maternal characteristics, 157, 160, 169
mental development of, 155
post-natal nutrition of, 163, 170
post-natal weight loss in, 161
teeth of, 207

Malformations, mental retardation and, 285
Malformations of nervous system, mechanisms of, 27
Malnutrition, 265
brain damage and, 217
brain development and, 32, 85, 86
causing mental retardation, 163
effects of, 46
effect on growth, 50
enzyme activity in, 89
Maple sugar urine disease, 95
Massa intermedia in mental retardation, 8, 10
Measles, 105
Median cleft syndrome, 308
Meningitis,
anatomical lesions following, 273
mental retardation following, 248
vascular damage following, 303
Meningocoele, definition, 280
Meningo-encephalitis, 110

Meningomyelocoele, 203
Mental excellence, 208
Mental Health Act 1959, 196
Mentally handicapped, parental attitudes, 203
  potential of, 189
Metabolic disorders, causing retardation, 303, 304
Metabolic rate, enzyme activity in relation to, 81
Metabolism,
  of brain,
    foetal, 29
    inborn errors of, 94
    relation to capillaries, 6
Metachromatic leucodystrophy, 94, 266
Methionine, 261, 264
Methioninaemia, 217
Methylazoxymethanol, effects, 30, 117, 120
Methylmethanesulphonate, effects, 120, 146
    acute, 123
    carcinogenic, 118
    on nucleic acids, 125
Methyl nitrosobiuret, effects of, 119
Methylnitrosourea,
  effects, 117, 119, 128, 136
    acute, 123
    liver, 140
    on nucleic acids, 125
    protein synthesis, 128
  metabolism, 124, 146
  toxicity, 124, 125
  tumour induction by, 122
Microcephaly, 59
  from alkylating agents, 142
  virus infection and, 104
Microencephaly, 285, 290
Microgyria, 104, 286, 291, 301, 310
Microneurones,
  effect of hormones on, 67
  post-natal proliferation, 64
Microphthalmia, 104
Micropolygyria, 301
Mitochondria, abnormal, 293
Multiple sclerosis, 250
Mumps, 105
Myelination, 44, 93
  defective, 52, 303
Myelocoeles, 271, 276
Myoclonus, 241
Neonatal brain,
  development, 28
  ketone-body utilization by, 83, 87
Nerve conduction velocity, 258
Nervous system,
  carcinogenic effects of alkylating agents, 117
  development of sensitivity, 23-39
  dystrophies and dysmorphias of, 300
  effect of maternal diet, 49, 217
  effect of sex hormones on, 69
  effect of thyroid hormones on, 64
  malformations, 295
    in different ethnic groups, 310
    mechanism, 27
    types, 296
  sensitivity, time factors, 37, 38
Neurinomas, malignant, 123
Neuroaxonal dystrophies, 291, 304
Neurolipidosis, 232
Neurones, 13-22. *See also Microneurones*
  cerebral blood supply and, 6
  contact between, 21, 22
  control of division of, 16
  death of, 4, 11, 43
    control of, 18
    radiation causing, 24
  disordered integration, 22
  disturbances of, causing malformation, 27
  effect of androgens on, 69
  effect of thyroid hormone on, 61, 66, 67
  growth spurt, 320
  in tissue culture, 44
  many cells–one function, 16
  migration, 17
  numbers of, 21, 44, 285, 315
    congenital malformations and, 50
    control of, 16
    deficiency in, 256
    effect of corticosteroids, 64, 74
    effect of malnutrition, 51
    effect of protein metabolism, 33
    head circumference and, 52
    importance of, 291
    in developing brain, 77
    in mental retardation, 22
    in schizophrenia, 316
    phylogenic factors, 14

Neurones–*cont.*
numbers of–*cont.*
total, 13
variation in, 51
within groups, 16
oestrogen receptors in, 74
over-production of, 19
post-natal formation, effect of hormones on, 64, 66, 67
protein synthesis in, 141
selective differentiation, 18
size, congenital malformation and, 50
types of, 21
Neuropathological features of mental retardation, 293
Nitrosamides, effects, 117
Nitrosomethylurea, carcinogenesis by, 145
Normality, 208
Nucleic acids, alkylation of, 125, 126
Nutrition, 319
effect on brain development, 32, 42-43
maternal, impairment of, 49
post-natal in low birthweight babies, 163, 170
sensitivity of embryonic brain to, 25
thyroid function and, 185

Oedema of brain, 57
Oestrogens, effects, 73
Oligodendrogliomas, 123
Orotic aciduria, 94

Pachygyria, 286, 301, 311
Panleukaemia, 142
Parents,
attitudes towards patients, 194-196, 203
counselling, 193, 203
rejection by, 194, 204
Parietal lobe, size of, 314
Parkinsonism, post-encephalitic, 113
Perception, 248
Perinatal damage, 201
Phenylalanine, 34, 222
Phenyl dimethyltriazene, 119
Phenylketonuria, 42, 95, 98, 201, 209, 217, 222, 262, 263, 283
anatomical changes, 292
incidence, 223
Photic stimulation, EEG changes in, 235, 238
Pica, 219, 221
Pierre-Robin syndrome, 302
Pituitary function, nutrition and, 185
Pituitary gland, effect of corticosteroids, 69
Placenta, infection crossing, 111
Poliomyelitis,
intrauterine infection, 105, 114
post-natal infection, 106
Polysomes, 140
Ponto-cerebellar atrophy, 303
Porencephaly, 287
Pregnancy,
complications associated with low birthweight infants, 162
oestrogen levels in, 261
smoking during, 148, 149
Propansulfone, effects, 120
Prosencephaly, 283, 285
Protein,
amounts in developing brain, 77-78, 81
cellular, 50
cerebral activity, 141
content of CSF, 281
restriction, effect on brain cell division, 217
role in developing brain, 32-34
synthesis,
effect of alkylating agents, 128
in foetal brain, 29
inhibition of, 54
in neurones, 141
Protein factors, 74
Psychiatric aspects of mental retardation, 187-204
Psychology, definition of brain injury by, 244
Psychosis, 197-198
Psychotherapy of mentally handicapped, 191, 193
Puberty, growth abnormalities and, 175, 179-180
Pyramidal tract, blood supply, 5
Pyridoxine, 30, 32, 216

Reactive changes in brain, 287
'Reeler' syndrome, 266
Rejection by parents, 194, 204
Retrolental fibroplasia, 11
Rhombocerebellar dysraphies, 300

Ribonucleic acid, effect of alkylating agents on, 125, 128, 139
Rickettsia burneti, 31
Rubella, 103, 104, 209

Sarcoma, induction by alkylating agents, 122
Schizophrenia, 95, 247
Schwann cells, neoplastic, 123
Screening of children, 46
Seizures, frequency of, 296
Serotonin, 70, 91
Sex hormones, effect on CNS, 69
Sexual behaviour, 69
Sexual development,
growth anomalies and, 179-180
mental retardation and, 174
Shape perception, 248
Sleep, EEG records in, 235, 238, 239
Small-for-dates infants, 51, 58, 157, 161, 170
infertility associated with, 160, 161, 162
threatened abortion and, 160, 163
Social aspects of mental retardation, 204
Social factors in growth, 177
Sodium nitrite, reaction with ethylurea, 148, 149, 318
Spasticity in hydrocephalus, 277
Speech in autism, 202
Spina bifida, 104, 202, 204, 271, 299, 307
associated with hydrocephalus, 271, 272, 274, 279, 280, 290
detection of, 282
EEG changes, 241
massa intermedia in, 10
soft water and, 45
St. Louis encephalitis, 106
Stimuli, speed of reaction to, 151
Streptocytosin, 147
Structural changes and mental retardation, 91
Structure,
correlation with biochemistry, 93
versus function, 95
Subacute sclerosing panencephalitis, 106
Subnormality compared with normal, 98
Succinic dehydrogenase activity, 93
Sucrosuria, 262-263
Swayback, 46
Sylvius, aqueduct of, 271, 280
Sympathetic nervous system, antibodies and, 45
Synapses,
abnormal, 293
cerebral blood supply and, 5, 10
connections in mental retardation, 22

Tay-Sachs disease, 232, 238
Teeth of low birthweight children, 207
Telencephalic haematoma, 309
Temporal lobe epilepsy, 113
Testicular function in Down's syndrome, 185
Thiouracil, effect on developing brain, 30
Thyroid gland,
dysfunction, growth retardation and, 178
effect on brain development, 61
function, nutrition and, 185
Thyroid hormones,
effects,
cerebellum, 62, 67
cortex, 255
developing brain, 30, 66
hypothalamus, 68
neurones, 62
Tic de salaam. *See Infantile spasms*
Toxoplasmosis, 31
Trace elements in water, 45
Transient dystonia associated with low birthweight, 156, 165, 171
congenital anomalies and, 167
incidence, 165
intrauterine growth and, 167
later status, 166
post-natal complications, 168
Triiodothyronine,
effect on developing brain, 73
effect on neurones, 63
Trimethylnitrosourea, effects, 119
Trisomy D, 302
Tryptophan metabolism in mental retardation, 216
Tuberous sclerosis, 88, 98
Tumour induction,
by alkylating agents, 117
classification of, 122
by nitrosamines, 145
renal, 146
Tyrosinaemia, 217

Ulegyria, 287
Uterine growth, 175
Uterus, vessel ligation, effects on brain weight, 53

Valine, 213
Ventricles, dilation, 284, 285
Ventriculo-atrial shunts,269, 275
Vigilance, measurement, 252, 255
Viral infections, 209, 314
  brain development and, 25, 32, 103-115
  during pregnancy, 108
  experimental, 107
  post-natal, 105
  pre-natal, 104
Vitamin B_{12}, effect on brain, 217
Vitamin deficiencies, 25, 27, 32, 34, 37

Water, softness of, 45
Weight of brain,
  alteration in age, 11
Weight of brain–*cont.*
  congenital malformations and, 142
  mental subnormality and, 22
  relation to bodyweight, 14, 15, 16
Werdnig-Hoffman disease, 303
Western equine encephalitis, 105, 106, 107
  infection with,
    during pregnancy, 108
    neonatal, 109
West Nile fever, 106
White matter,
  blood supply, 5
  gliosis, 287, 288
  in cerebral atrophy, 285
  in hydrocephalus, 273, 282
  shrinking of, 11

X-rays, effect on developing brain, 24, 26, 30, 39

Zinc deficiency, 25
Zona vasculosa, 271